Changing Body Composition through Diet and Exercise

Michael J. Ormsbee, Ph.D.

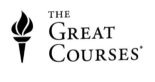

THE
GREAT
COURSES

PUBLISHED BY:

THE GREAT COURSES
Corporate Headquarters
4840 Westfields Boulevard, Suite 500
Chantilly, Virginia 20151-2299
Phone: 1-800-832-2412
Fax: 703-378-3819
www.thegreatcourses.com

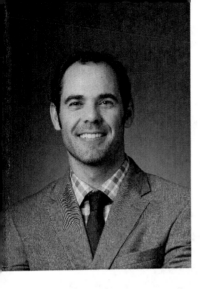

Michael J. Ormsbee, Ph.D.
Assistant Professor in Nutrition, Food, and Exercise Sciences
Florida State University

D r. Michael J. Ormsbee is an Assistant Professor in the Department of Nutrition, Food, and Exercise Sciences and the Interim Director for the Institute of Sports Sciences and Medicine at Florida State University (FSU). He is a faculty affiliate of the Center for Advancing Exercise and Nutrition Research on Aging and the Institute for Successful Longevity at FSU. Dr. Ormsbee is also an Honorary Research Fellow at the University of KwaZulu-Natal in Durban, South Africa. He earned his B.S. in Exercise Science and Business from Skidmore College, his M.S. in Exercise Physiology and Sports Nutrition from South Dakota State University, and his Ph.D. in Bioenergetics from East Carolina University. Dr. Ormsbee's research and expertise involve the interaction of exercise, nutrition, and supplementation to achieve optimal body composition, human performance, and health in both athletes and clinical populations.

Prior to arriving at FSU, Dr. Ormsbee taught and conducted research at Skidmore College. His major research contributions have included investigation into meal composition and frequency, exercise type and duration, nighttime feeding, and the use of supplements to alter body composition and performance. Dr. Ormsbee started Ormsbee Fitness Consulting in 2006 and has worked with everyone from Olympic athletes to everyday people. He is a sought-after speaker both nationally and internationally on issues related to exercise, diet, and performance nutrition.

While at FSU, Dr. Ormsbee won the 2013–2014 University Teaching Award, the Excellence in Online Course Design Award, the Excellence in Online Teaching Award, and the 2013 Transformation through Teaching Award. He was also selected for the Guardian of the Flame Faculty Award by the Burning Spear leadership honor society in 2015. In 2012, Dr. Ormsbee was elected as a Fellow of the International Society of Sports Nutrition, and in 2014, he was elected as a Fellow of the American College of Sports Medicine.

Dr. Ormsbee regularly publishes his research in the top scientific journals in his field and presents at national and international conferences. He is active in education and outreach, giving seminars to academics, athletes, and the public. Dr. Ormsbee and his work have been featured in many popular magazine, radio, podcast, and television outlets, including *The Washington Post, Men's Health, Shape, Philly.com,* and *O, The Oprah Magazine.* ∎

Table of Contents

Disclaimer

This series of lectures is intended to convey general health, fitness, and nutritional information and is for educational purposes only. It is not a substitute for, nor does it replace, professional medical advice, diagnosis, or treatment of health conditions. Please consult your physician or other health-care professional before beginning or changing any fitness or nutrition program to make sure that it is appropriate for your needs. If you have any concerns or questions about your health, you should always consult a physician or other health-care professional. Do not disregard, avoid, or delay obtaining medical or health-related advice from your health-care professional because of something you may have seen or heard in these lectures. Current health and fitness research may exist that could affect the educational information provided in these lectures, and advice found herein may not be based on the most recent findings or developments. Therefore, the use of any information provided in these lectures is solely at your own risk. By continuing with the programs, exercises, advice, information, or diets discussed in these lectures, you recognize that there are risks of injury or illness that can occur because of your use of the aforementioned information, and you expressly assume such risks and waive, relinquish, and release any claim that you may have against The Teaching Company as a result of any future physical injury or illness incurred in connection with, or as a result of, use or misuse of the programs, exercises, advice, diets, and/or information discussed in these lectures. The opinions and positions provided in these lectures reflect the opinions and positions of the relevant lecturer and do not necessarily reflect the opinions or positions of The Teaching Company or its affiliates.

The Teaching Company expressly DISCLAIMS LIABILITY for any DIRECT, INDIRECT, INCIDENTAL, SPECIAL, OR CONSEQUENTIAL DAMAGES OR LOST PROFITS that result directly or indirectly from the use of these lectures. In states that do not allow some or all of the above limitations of liability, liability shall be limited to the greatest extent allowed by law.

Acknowledgments

Sam Kramer

Brittan Allman

Katie Gorman

Stacy Cappadona

Amber Kinsey

Palmer Johnson

Chris Bach

Morgan Clift

Beth Miller

Changing Body Composition through Diet and Exercise

Scope

Improving body composition by losing body fat and optimizing lean muscle mass is not about vanity—it's about health. It's not about how quickly you can lose weight or how small you can become. It's about how to become stronger and healthier while decreasing your body fat and increasing your muscle mass. It's about changing your body composition through diet and exercise in a safe way that supports you holistically and helps you achieve optimal health and performance. This course is about the science of nutrition and exercise that can lead to lasting changes in body composition.

In the first section of the course, you will learn why body weight is not the best way to determine your health status and why understanding more about exactly how much body fat you have and how much muscle mass you have is the key to improved health and performance. You will discover what happens to food from the moment it enters your mouth—where it goes and how it supports your cellular functions. You will learn about what carbohydrates, fats, and proteins are and how they are broken down in your body to provide energy for everything you do. You will also discover that as you age, your nutrition needs change.

The next part of the course explores how to evaluate a nutrition label, and you'll discover that the calories from a bag of chips are entirely different from the same number of calories from a piece of fruit or lean meat. You'll consider how not only your food choices, but also when you eat and how frequently you eat might influence how you feel, look, and perform day to day in your normal life and also while you exercise. You'll also uncover myths and facts about dietary supplements that are designed to help you lose body fat or gain muscle mass all within the context of energy balance and weight control.

The third segment of the course examines the caloric cost of exercise, and you'll learn some simple strategies that help increase your activity level. You will discover why certain types of exercise might be most beneficial for losing body fat or gaining muscle mass. This section allows you to draw conclusions for the most optimal way for you to incorporate various types of exercise into your life to meet your goals. You'll also discover why weight training is good for everyone and won't just make you big and bulky. You will also explore certain hormones and the influence they have on your body composition.

The final lectures will use science to dispel myths about unrealistic methods that are marketed to improve body composition and provide evidence for what really works. You'll also discover the best practices for handling travel, boredom, and a busy schedule while keeping your nutrition and workout plan consistent. You will learn why improvements in body composition tend to plateau and how the set point influences your outcomes. You'll discover the science behind popular diets and how to build sustainable habits for successful loss of body fat and gain in muscle mass.

By the end of this course, you will learn to avoid the quick-fix mentality and find simple strategies to keep discipline, hard work, and fun in your plan to improve body composition. You will appreciate the complexity of the human body and understand why smart nutrition and purposeful exercise are both critical for improving body composition, health, and performance.

Body Composition: Managing Our Expectations

This course is about the science of nutrition and exercise that can lead to changes in body composition. The goal of the course is to provide you with the tools to make the decisions that you want to make, when you want to make them, to produce lasting results, not necessarily fast results. This course will provide you with all of the information you need to make big or small changes to live a fit life. The field of nutrient metabolism, exercise physiology, body composition, and performance—also known as performance nutrition—involves studying how energy is derived from foods and how this energy fuels exercise and human movement.

Body Composition

What is body composition, and why should it be used as your indicator of health instead of body weight? We all get crazy about body weight when what we should be talking about instead is how much muscle and how much fat we have. A two-pound fat loss and a two-pound gain in muscle would improve your body composition, health, and functionality, but it would not change your body weight.

Body mass index (BMI), which is your weight in kilograms divided by your height in meters squared, is useful in some situations but not others. The way you hold your weight—how much fat and how much muscle you have—contributes a lot to how you look, feel, and perform (in the context of the real world—in your job, with your family, and with your general energy and enthusiasm for life—not simply on an athletic field).

The nutrition that feeds your body and fuels the physical activity that can change your body composition is also a major component of the

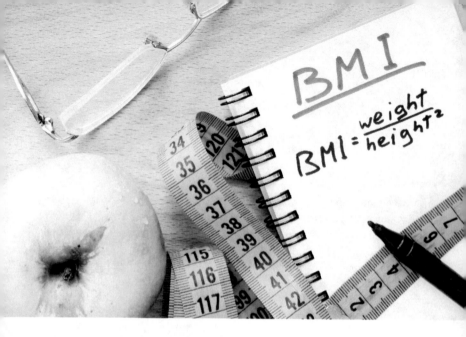

science of body composition. Nutrition is directly linked to your health and well-being. It influences your body composition and your energy levels for work, play, and exercise.

Energy Balance

A lot of controversy surrounds the topic of energy balance. Energy balance is the balance of the calories you take in from foods and beverages (energy intake) with the calories that you expend (energy output) for all of your biological processes necessary to live, such as breathing and thinking, plus the calories you expend from walking around and from exercise.

To alter body composition, to lose fat (for example), you want an energy deficit. Just burn more than you take in. But if it were that easy, maybe we wouldn't have the obesity epidemic that we have today.

The quality of our calories has as much of an impact on our body composition and overall health as the total number of calories that we eat daily. Your body needs certain foods. In fact, you should probably eat more protein in your diet. Your body works harder to digest and absorb protein than it does carbohydrates and fats. This is probably why eating protein gives you the largest increase in metabolism when you eat it.

A number of research studies have been designed to measure metabolism after a meal containing protein versus fat versus carbohydrates, and the majority of these indicate that the greatest impact on increasing metabolism comes after eating protein. Some foods come with a little bit of a metabolic advantage, and this can have an impact on goals you're setting for changing body composition.

Twenty years ago, we were served smaller portion sizes. The National Institutes of Health tells us that a bagel 20 years ago was typically around 3 inches in diameter and 140 calories. Today, a bagel is typically 6 inches in diameter and contains nearly 350 calories—more than twice as many calories as just 20 years ago.

You don't have to begin counting calories, because that takes a lot of time and is not fun. Getting bogged down with the numbers complicates it all and can get you fixated on the wrong kinds of details. Instead, try using your hands as a way to gauge how much you should eat.

For example, most women can go with one palm-sized portion of lean protein to meet their needs at a particular meal. Men, who typically have bigger and thicker hands, can go with two palm-sized portions of lean protein. You simply adjust this based on your goals and the food you are eating. Carbohydrates, for example, could be a fist-sized portion of vegetables or rice.

Learning to pay attention to what you eat and how you feel will help you achieve your optimal body composition and lead to improved health and performance. When you eat, just eat. If you're distracted while you eat—rushed, or stressed, or not paying attention—you are more likely to eat more than your body really wants or needs. Most of the time, the simple practice of eating just enough becomes overcomplicated by massive amounts of media propaganda, misinformation, or family habits.

Exercise

How much exercise do you need to do, and how often do you need to do it? What exercise or activity works best if you want to gain muscle mass, and what works best if you want to lose fat?

Data shows that we lose about 5 percent of our muscle mass per decade. Over the span of 50 years, you could lose as much as 25 percent of your muscle mass. That's not something we want. It can make you weak and frail and lower your metabolism a lot, too.

But the fact is that the overall decrease in your metabolism is only one to three percent during the aging process, which really doesn't amount to much—and you can easily offset this with the nutrition and exercise strategies that you'll learn throughout this course.

Many people think that being sedentary is easier than being active. Screen time—the time that people watch television, use the Internet, play video games, or look at their phones—is increasing every year. This is likely a big problem because during these activities, we're usually not moving.

In a national sample of girls and boys, it was found that those who watched less than two hours of television per day had about a 10 percent chance of becoming obese, but those who watched more than five hours per day had close to a 30 percent chance of becoming obese.

For adults, this is also an issue—typically from too much sitting and sedentary time during the day. In fact, a number of research studies link daily sitting time to a number of health concerns, including risk of obesity, cardiovascular disease, and cancer.

The obvious answer is to exercise. Unfortunately, planned exercise and unplanned activity typically slow down as we age and make it likely for us to gain weight and fat. You need to make a real effort to stop this reduction in metabolism and work for your optimal body composition.

Having the body composition of your dreams is certainly a great goal, but keep in mind that just being active is extremely helpful for improving your health. The good news is that following even the most basic of recommendations brings many benefits.

In fact, just a 5 to 10 percent loss in total body weight will improve your blood pressure, cholesterol, and sugar levels. And even if you're still in the "overweight" or "obese" range, this modest weight loss can decrease your risk factors for chronic diseases related to obesity.

A major point of information about body composition that most people don't know is that if you are trying to lose weight, you should be lifting weights. This might go against what you've always been told, but long and slow aerobic exercise is no longer the recommended way to lose fat. While it is part of the plan, many other types of exercise are needed if you really want a fighting chance to lose fat but keep or add muscle mass.

Particularly when trying to lose weight, it's important to lift weights so that your muscle mass has the best chance of staying around and your metabolism stays as high as possible.

Quick changes in body composition should not be expected. Instead, look for changes to come over a period of time, after you've dialed in a nourishing eating plan based on quality foods and a consistent and effective exercise regimen.

Nutrition

Overall, the health benefits of exercise and eating right are clear. If a pill existed with even half of the same benefits, there's no doubt that it would be the best seller.

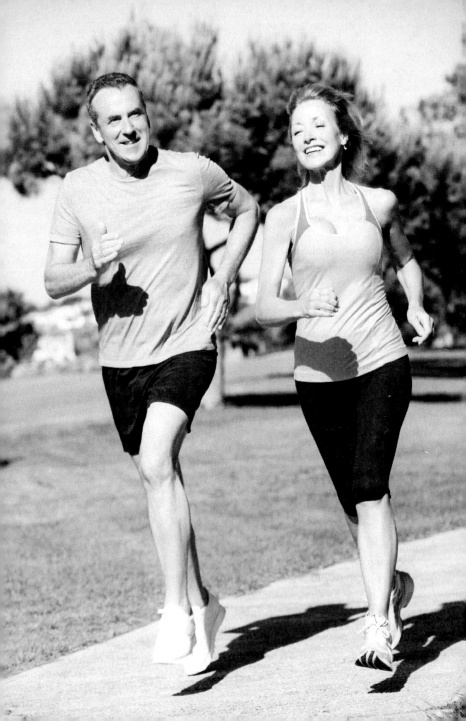

Even if you are overweight or obese, simply being physically active can ward off metabolic disease and keep you healthy. Health is not always about weight. Of course, they are related, but the key for your health is that you exercise and work on ways to improve how you eat.

However, simply exercising more and eating less is not the key for improving body composition. We've been preaching this for a long time, but it doesn't work very well. The science of healthy body composition is not weight loss science; it's the science of a healthy balance of fat and muscle mass and how we can achieve that.

Choosing both quality exercise and quality foods is the way to make lasting improvements. And weight loss might be a consequence of changing eating and exercise habits, but it is not the goal.

It's also important to keep in mind that things like your genetics, your environment, and even chemical pollutants are factors that might contribute to gaining fat. But even though our ability to alter our body composition depends on many things, the take-home message is that exercise and quality nutrition do a body good.

In fact, exercise and nutrition must be combined for a healthy body composition. You can make it pretty far with one or the other, but healthy does not just mean "not overweight."

Your journey to better health is not about a quick fix; it's about a lifestyle change that works for you. It's not about how quickly you can lose weight or how small you can become. It's about how to become stronger and healthier while lowering your body fat and increasing your muscle mass. It's about changing your body composition through diet and exercise in a safe way that supports you holistically and helps you achieve more day to day.

Try This

Write down the biggest hurdle you see as standing in the way of achieving your optimal body composition and health.

Questions to Consider

1. What is the easiest and most sustainable change that you think you can make for big improvements in your body composition, health, and performance?

2. What exercise or nutrition myth was busted by this lecture?

Body Composition: Managing Our Expectations

This course is about the science of nutrition and exercise that can lead to changes in body composition. That's the key—this is science. And it's my aim to provide you with the tools to make the decisions that you want to make, when you want to make them, to produce lasting results, not necessarily fast results.

Maybe you just never think about body composition because your weight has been stable for years and you've just never considered what adding a little bit of muscle or losing a little bit of fat may do to make you feel different and perform better in your daily life. I'll provide you with all of the information you would ever want and more, so that you can make big or small changes when you're ready to achieve more and live life fit. And I'll share all of this excellent information with the scientific research to back up all of the concepts that I will tell you about.

In my field of nutrient metabolism, exercise physiology, body composition and performance—also known as performance nutrition—we study how energy is derived from foods and how this energy fuels exercise and human movement. You see, our energy comes from breaking down the food we eat, and we'll talk about that. We also need to talk about dietary supplements and when it's appropriate to incorporate them into your nutrition plan. And once we understand energy intake from foods and drinks—that is, how they are metabolized and used for energy—then we'll talk about energy expenditure, or the energy you use to keep alive and allow you to move and exercise.

In the course, we'll study all types of exercise, and how intensity and duration influence your body fat and muscle mass. We'll talk about what the caloric cost of exercise really is and what types of exercises are best to burn fat or gain muscle. We'll also look at hormones and how they influence your hunger, exercise, health, and body composition. All of these topics align to let us understand how to change body composition if you choose to, and how to best apply all of the information that we learn from the science of performance nutrition.

You know, one interesting thing about exercise and nutrition is that a lot of people believe they are experts on these topics even if they have little to no formal education or experience. And a quick comparison to other jobs makes this almost funny. Let's say that you're cooking a meal for your family one night. Something distracts you and the dish catches on fire. Luckily, you react quickly and put the fire out. So, are you now a trained firefighter? Of course not, but in the fitness and nutrition fields, I often find that if someone reads a book or watches an infomercial all of a sudden they feel like an expert. This is taken advantage of way too often, and what's left is an overload of misinformation, half-truths, and lots of myths. We'll discuss these myths in many of the lectures.

Recently, a new client of mine told me that he had great nutrition and exercised daily, but that he couldn't lose any weight and he had no energy. After months and months of trying all the popular diets, he'd had zero success. In fact, despite his perfect efforts, he'd actually gained weight over the past year. And what's worse, after a recent checkup, he was told by his doctor that he needed to be placed on blood pressure medication. Unfortunately, this is an extremely common scenario in health, nutrition, and fitness. But how is it even possible to have great nutrition and consistent physical activity patterns and not change weight? Well, for an overweight person it would be unlikely, but maybe you feel the same way as my client did—no matter what you do, nothing seems to work.

By now we know that nutrition and fitness are two keys to living well. And whether we're talking about lowering your risk for disease, keeping your brain fit, changing your body composition, or just feeling your best, eating well and exercising have to be included. But do you find yourself wondering what nutrition and exercise advice you should listen to? I mean, you've seen the diet and exercise section at the bookstore that's stocked with thousands of guides and self-help DVDs. Every magazine on the rack has a headline offering you weight loss advice. And you've probably noticed advertisements on TV, and they're trying to sell you a new device, pill, or potion to help you lose fat. You're probably asking, "Why are there so many choices? Do any of them work?"

Well, now imagine that you could easily sift through the mountains of media headlines and infomercials to find the real solution to your weight loss goals. Well, that's my goal for this course. We'll sift through all of the science and bring clear messages about how to change your body composition and what you can really expect.

At a corporate seminar I gave recently, a woman stood up and said, "I heard that our metabolism slows as we age, so does it really matter what we do if we're all destined to gain fat and lose muscle?" She believed that her weight gain over the past 15 years was unstoppable simply due to the consequences of aging. But is it really inevitable? Well, the short answer is no, and in this course you'll learn why, and what you can do about it.

The focus of my research over the past 14 years has been to study how nutrition, supplementation, and exercise influence optimal body composition, performance, and health. We'll talk about the evidence for what works and what doesn't from my research and from research that has been published in this field. I need to say here that many of the research studies that we'll discuss have been completed using male subjects. This happens often because the female menstrual cycle induces hormone changes that researchers must control for—so, by default, men are typically used as subjects in studies. This is changing though, and when it's possible, I'll discuss sex-specific differences that occur with nutrition and exercise training.

But, sometimes, we just have to use the information we get from men— or from women—to make the best lifestyle choices we can for ourselves. Many times, data from animals like mice or rats is used initially to later set up human research trials. Animal research has a critical role in the development of the science, but you'll also learn that animals and humans don't always respond identically. The absolute generalizability of some data can only be to a very specific group of people or animals, but, again, we have to use the information provided in an attempt to make the most optimal choices we can to provide performance benefits for health and body composition.

Luckily, in this field, many common threads have emerged, and I'm going to share those with you throughout the course. I'll cover evidence-based steps to help you increase your metabolism, improve your health, and create the best possible conditions for achieving your optimal body composition. I'll go into detail about ways to change your body fat and muscle mass to meet the goals that you have. It's important for me to say again that this is a no gimmicks type of course. What you'll get are just the facts based on cutting-edge research from my lab and from many other colleagues around the globe.

Let's begin by going into what body composition is and why it should be used as your indicator of health instead of body weight. We all get crazy about body weight, when the thing we should be talking about is how much muscle and how much fat we have instead. Even on popular weight loss shows, what you don't learn is how much fat versus how much muscle was lost in the process. Any day of the week, I'd take a 2-pound fat loss and a 2-pound gain in muscle. This would improve my body composition, health, and functionality, but it wouldn't change my body weight.

We'll also talk about BMI, or body mass index, which is simply your weight in kilograms divided by your height in meters squared and how it is useful for some situations but not others. For example, if you are 5'2" and weigh 180 pounds, you're classified as obese according to the body mass index. But this identical BMI can also describe a professional athlete who's 6'2" and 255 pounds. See, the way you hold your weight—that means how much fat and how much muscle you have—contributes a lot to how you look, how you feel, and how you perform. And by perform, I mean this in the context of the real world, not simply performance on an athletic field. To me, improving your performance can happen in your job, with your family, or with the general energy and enthusiasm for life that is true to performance.

The nutrition that feeds your body and fuels the physical activity that can change your body composition is also a major component of the science of body composition. We'll discuss everything from how your food is digested, to where it goes in your body, to your cellular function, because, believe it or not, this matters in a big way. It is directly linked to your health and well-being; it influences your body composition and your energy levels for work, play, and exercise. If you've ever thought about cutting out fat or carbohydrates from your diet, we'll go into that, too. I'll detail what carbohydrates, fats, and proteins are and why you should care about them. We'll even cover when a low-carb diet might be best for you, and when a high-carb diet might be better, and answer questions like, "Should I eat fat or not?" and "Is gluten-free the healthiest choice for me?"

What about calories? Do they matter? You may know a lot about the controversy that surrounds the topic of energy balance. Energy balance is quite simple really—it's the balance of the calories you take in from foods and beverages, or energy intake, with the calories that you expend, or energy output, for all of your biological processes necessary to live, things like breathing and thinking, plus those calories you expend from walking around and from exercise. For the most part, we understand that in order to alter body composition, to lose fat for example, you would want an energy deficit—just burn more than you take in. But, if it were that easy, maybe we wouldn't have the obesity epidemic that we do today.

The question becomes: "Are all calories created equal?" For example, if you drink 800 calories from soft drinks, does this do the same thing to your metabolism and body composition as eating 800 calories from broccoli? Well, that's a topic for a bit later when we go into more detail, but we need to understand that the quality of our calories will have as much of an impact on our body composition and overall health as the total number of calories that we eat daily.

Other important topics in this field include the best foods to eat before a workout, or to recover after a workout; what to do at night before bed; and whether you should eat breakfast or skip it. I'll also talk about some major hormones that influence how we look and feel. I'll also break a few myths along the way. I'll talk about your needs for certain foods, and specifically why you probably should eat more protein in your diet. Your body works

15

harder to digest and absorb protein than it does carbohydrates or fats. This is probably why eating protein gives you the largest increase in metabolism when you eat it. A number of research studies have been designed to specifically measure metabolism after a meal containing protein versus fat versus carbohydrate, and the majority of these indicate that the greatest impact on increasing metabolism comes after eating protein. So, some foods come with a little bit of a metabolic advantage, and this can have an impact on the goals you're setting for changing body composition.

Many of the questions I get are about nutrition and supplements, so we'll talk about which ones might work for your goals, and which ones you should just leave on the shelf. For example, did you know that creatine, a popular sports performance supplement, is now being used for neurological disorders, brain protection as we age, improving muscle mass, hydration, and sports performance? Well it is, and the effectiveness, or not, of some other supplements I discuss may surprise you. We'll discuss food portion sizes too, and some simple ways to manage how much you eat.

Did you know that 20 years ago we were served smaller portion sizes? It's true. The National Institutes of Health tells us that a bagel 20 years ago was typically about 3 inches in diameter and 140 calories. Now compare that to today: a bagel is typically 6 inches in diameter and now contains nearly 350 calories, more than twice as many calories than just 20 years ago. Or what about a fast food cheeseburger? Twenty years ago, it had about 330 calories, nearly 1/2 when compared to the almost 600 calories today, and sometimes more than 600 calories in a cheeseburger. And french fries 20 years ago were typically a 2.4-ounce serving containing 210 calories. But today, your standard serving of fries weighs in at 6.9 ounces and will set you back around 610 calories.

Now, you don't have to begin counting calories, because that takes a lot of time and, let's face it, it's no fun. Getting bogged down with the numbers complicates it all and can get you fixated on the wrong sorts of details. So, what's the solution? Try using your hands as way to gauge how much you should eat. For example, most women can go with one palm-sized portion of lean protein to meet their needs at a particular meal. Men typically have bigger and thicker hands, and they can go with two palm-sized portions of lean protein—you simply adjust this based on your goals and the food you're eating. Carbohydrates, for example, could be a fist-sized portion of vegetables or rice. Much easier, isn't it?

I'll go over all of the recommendations for these major nutrients, and micronutrients too, things like vitamins and minerals that you should pay attention to. It is important to be aware of the fact that food is big business, so there are all sorts of economic pressures involved with labeling and marketing. For example, you should remember that the most common recommendations we have for food to eat, and how much to eat, are influenced by companies that have a big stake in selling food products. So it is important to have the most education you can about the science behind what foods you choose to eat.

Here's a secret: Learning to pay attention to what you eat and how you feel will help you to achieve your optimal body composition, and lead to improved health and performance. When you eat, just eat. If you're distracted while you eat, rushed, or stressed, or not paying attention, you are more likely to eat more than your body really wants or needs. Most times it is the simple practice of just getting enough becomes overcomplicated by massive amounts of media propaganda, misinformation, or family habits.

Over and over, I'll discuss how exercise fits into the equation, too. How much do you need to do and how often do you need to do it? We'll talk about questions like, "What exercise or activities work best if you want to gain muscle?" or "What works best if you want to lose fat?" We'll talk about lifting weights, implementing high-intensity interval training, and finding activities that you love to do.

Remember the woman I mentioned who was asking whether metabolism tends to slow as we age? With data that shows that we lose about 5% of our muscle mass per decade, it's a bit sad. And over the span of 50 years, you could lose as much as 25% of your muscle mass. And that's not something we want—it can make you weak and frail, and lower your metabolism a lot, too. But the fact is, the overall decrease in your metabolism is only about

1%–3% during the aging process, which really doesn't amount to much, and you can easily offset this with nutrition and exercise strategies that we'll discuss throughout the course.

Now, I know that many people think that being sedentary is easier than being active. Consider this: screen-time, or the time that people watch TV, use the Internet, play video games, or look at their phones is increasing every year. This is likely a big problem because, during these activities, we're usually not moving. In a national sample of girls and boys, it was found that those who watched less than 2 hours of TV per day had about a 10% chance of becoming obese. But, those who watched more than 5 hours per day had close to a 30% chance of becoming obese.

For adults, this is also an issue, typically from too much sitting time and sedentary time during the day. In fact, a number of research studies link daily sitting time to a number of health concerns including obesity, cardiovascular disease, and cancer. Sitting all day sometimes is called the sitting disease, so the obvious answer is to exercise. Unfortunately, planned exercise and unplanned activity typically slow down as we age and make it likely for us to gain weight and fat. You need to make a real effort to stop this reduction in metabolism and work for your optimal body composition. You see, it's often said—and for good reason—that we don't stop being active because we get old, we get old because we stop being active. I'll show you evidence for this, too.

I'll also ask you to do some thinking and really identify what your strong and weak points are in this transformation process. Are you great at exercising but lousy at making healthy meals? Do you eat veggies all day but have no idea if you're getting enough protein? Do you like to exercise but just don't know what to do? Here's a great starting point: Can you name one thing you could change today, the easiest possible thing you can think of, that would help you improve your body composition, health, and performance?

Well, here are some suggestions. Could you take the stairs more often? That's a pretty easy change. Could you eat more fruit? That's really easy. What about working out a little more effectively? Sure, with some coaching.

If you know what your easiest obstacle is to overcome, that is the perfect place to start. I'll work to have you understand not only how to identify your weak points but to come up with a strategy for how to work with them, and not just temporarily, but to change for good, to truly implement a new strategy as part of your lifestyle.

Having the body composition of your dreams is certainly a great goal, but keep in mind that just being active is extremely helpful for improving your health. The really good news is that following even the most basic of recommendations brings many benefits. In fact, just a 5%–10% loss in total body weight will improve your blood pressure, cholesterol, and even your sugar levels. And even if you're still in the overweight or obese range, this modest weight loss can decrease your risk for chronic diseases related to obesity.

A major point of information about body composition that most people don't know about is that if you're trying to lose weight, you should be lifting weights. I know this may go against what you've always been told, but no longer is long and slow aerobic exercise the recommended way to lose fat. Sure, it's part of the plan, but many other types of exercise are needed if you really want a fighting chance to lose fat and keep or add muscle. Particularly when trying to lose weight, it's important to lift weights so your muscle mass has the best chance of staying around, and your metabolism stays as high as possible.

I was part of a research team that looked at medical weight loss programs for massively obese individuals. Part of the study was to add weight lifting to one of the groups on a very low calorie diet as directed by their physician. We compared the weight lifting group to another group that was also on a low calorie diet but did not lift weights, and we found that the resistance exercise— that is, weight lifting—was critical for helping to maintain their muscle mass while they were losing large amounts of weight. In fact, the group that did not lift weights lost far more muscle mass than the group that did.

It's been estimated that energy expenditure required for about 2 pounds of muscle is 13 calories per day, but only 4 1/2 calories per day for fat tissue of the same weight. So, a higher amount of muscle will help keep you lean and fit. But keep in mind that only 13 calories per day is quite low, even when you multiply this by our total amount of muscle mass. So, quick changes in body composition should not be expected. Instead, look for changes to come over a period of time, after you've dialed in a nourishing eating plan based on quality foods and consistent and effective exercise strategies.

Overall, the health benefits of exercise and eating right are clear. If a pill existed with even half of the same benefits, there's no doubt that it would be a best seller. Even if you are overweight or obese, simply being physically active can ward off metabolic disease and keep you healthy. Health is not always about weight. Sure, they are related, but the key for your health is that you exercise and work on ways to improve how you eat.

But simply exercising more and eating less is not the key for improving body composition. We've been preaching this for a long time but it doesn't work all that well. The science of healthy body composition is not weight loss science, it's the science of a healthy balance of fat and muscle, and how we can achieve that. Choosing both quality exercise and quality food is the way to make lasting improvements. And weight loss may be a consequence of changing eating and exercise habits, but it is not the goal.

It's also important to keep in mind that things like your genetics, your environment, and even chemical pollutants are factors that contribute to you gaining fat. But, even though our ability to alter our body composition depends on many things, the take home message is that exercise and quality nutrition do a body good. In fact, exercise and nutrition must be combined for a healthy body composition. You can make it pretty far with one or the other, but healthy does not just mean not overweight. For example, I know many skinny but unhealthy people.

I want you to have the science-based knowledge so that you can make informed decisions about your health and body composition whatever your age, sex, or physical condition. Sometimes the hardest part is not in understanding but in applying what you learn. With that said, it's been my experience that the hardest part about having a client or research participant begin a transformation is not in deciding to change—because, let's face it, making the decision is the easy part. The trick comes in actually doing the work to change.

Let's take a commonly used example from motivational speakers around the world. Three frogs are sitting on the edge of a pond. Two decide to jump in. How many frogs are now left on the side of the pond? Well, most people think the answer is one—one frog left on the side of the pond—but the real answer is three frogs are left on the side. Why? Because deciding to do something doesn't mean that you actually do it; it only happens when you leap.

But let's not leap blindly, let's have a plan, because this journey is not about a quick fix; it's about a lifestyle change that works for you. It's not about how quickly you can lose weight or how small you can become, it's about how to become stronger and healthier while lowering your body fat and increasing your muscle mass. It's about changing your body composition through diet and exercise in a safe way that supports you holistically and helps you achieve more day to day. Try this: write down the biggest hurdle you see as standing in the way of achieving your optimal body composition and health.

A Healthier Way to Measure Body Composition

B
ody weight offers no indication of how much fat versus muscle a person carries on his or her frame. This relative proportion is critical, because it is related to what the status of our overall health is, how our body moves and behaves, and how we look and feel aesthetically. How can we better quantify success with weight management? After this lecture, you will have a better, healthier idea of what's happening to your body during weight loss, which benchmarks are typically used to indicate success, and why success goes far beyond simply what the scale tells you.

Body Mass Index and Fat-Free Mass Index

- Body mass index (BMI) compares your body weight (in kilograms) to your height (in meters squared). A note of caution: Measures like BMI or body weight may be relevant only in certain situations. The usefulness of BMI is not great when considered on an individual-to-individual basis. In practice, BMI is most appropriate for large sample populations or in a clinical situation to quantify risk for a patient who is clearly overweight and overfat at the same time.

- There are four main categories of BMI.
  - Underweight: a BMI of less than 18.5.
  - Normal weight: 18.5 to 24.9.
  - Overweight: 25 to 29.
  - Obese: more than 30.

- Research has consistently shown a positive association between a high BMI and greater risk of cardiovascular, pulmonary, and metabolic disease. If you are curious about your own body mass index, calculate it or look online for a free website that can give you the information.

The problem is that BMI only considers your body weight and body height and does not account for the proportion of muscle mass or fat mass—which is the composition of your body weight.

For example, a typical NFL running back is very strong, has lots of lean muscle mass, and has very little body fat. Assuming that this running back is about 6 feet tall and a little more than 230 pounds (due to all of the muscle mass), his BMI would be more than 31 kg/m^2. According to BMI standards, this professional, healthy, lean athlete would be considered obese, even though common sense tells us otherwise.

Body composition is different from body weight and body mass index. Body composition is the relationship between the different types of tissue that comprise your body—in other words, how much muscle and how much fat make up your body weight.

To account for fat-free mass and not just total body weight, the fat-free mass index (FFMI) was developed. It is similar to the BMI, but it takes your fat-free mass, or muscle mass (again, in kilograms), divided by your height (in meters squared).

This index can quantify your body composition more accurately when you know that you have extra weight that is mostly muscle. It is not always a better index, but it is a different index, and like any index will be more or less useful depending on the specific need for the information.

While the FFMI is not used nearly as much as the BMI, a few research papers have attempted to come up with normal FFMI values for men and women. A paper from 2002 in the *International Journal of Obesity and Related Metabolic Disorders* found that the average FFMI for young women is about 15 kg/m^2 and for young men is 19 kg/m^2. These values change slightly after age 35, showing that fat mass is gained as we age, most likely due to a more sedentary lifestyle.

These indices are important to consider because they can be helpful for knowing your health status and risk for certain kinds of disease, such as cardiovascular disease, pulmonary disease, and metabolic disease. It is well established that if you have a lot of fat deposition, particularly around your waist and belly (near your major organs), your chance of developing these types of diseases increases dramatically.

In addition, knowing your current body composition gives you greater clarity about your starting point for an upcoming weight loss intervention. You will better be able to track your body's changes over time and have a bigger picture of "success."

MYTH
Muscle Weighs More Than Fat

This myth is just like saying that one pound of bricks weighs more than one pound of feathers. Of course, if you have one pound of each, then they both weigh one pound.

But here is the difference: Muscle has more density than fat. This is a key to understanding why two people can weigh exactly the same at the same height but look entirely different.

If you look at five pounds of fat and five pounds of muscle, they weigh exactly the same, but the amount of muscle is smaller than the same amount of fat. The muscle is about a third to a half smaller than the fat because of its increased density.

When you add muscle, you might weigh the same, but you could be an entirely different shape.

Body Fat and Muscle Mass

In terms of body composition, your total body fat includes both essential body fat and storage body fat. Essential fat includes fat in your organs, such as the heart, liver, kidneys, intestines, muscles, and bone marrow. This type of fat is required for normal physiological functioning and differs greatly between men and women. In fact, it accounts for most of the major body fat differences between genders. Women have about 12 percent essential fat, while men have about 3 percent essential fat.

Women have more essential fat mostly because of its biological function for reproduction. Women need extra fat stores during pregnancy. Regardless of whether a woman ever has children or not, she will most often have slightly more fat than a man.

There is another type of fat that is also required for normal body function. It is called storage fat, which is fat stored until it can be used for energy when needed. It includes the visceral fat, or deep fat, around your organs and the fat just underneath your skin, which is called subcutaneous fat.

Storage fat can insulate your body, helps to maintain your body temperature, and provides vital protection for your organs. The amount of storage fat is more similar between men and women—usually just 2 to 3 percent higher in women.

Health issues arise when storage fat becomes excessive. Body fat is important for supporting daily function and health, but excess amounts will contribute to overweight and overfat conditions.

The other component of body mass that is not comprised of fat is called fat-free mass or lean body mass. These terms are often used interchangeably; however, they are technically different. Fat-free mass is only the muscle mass that you have, while lean body mass also includes your muscle mass, bone mass, connective tissue (such as ligaments and tendons), internal organs, and any essential fat stored in these tissues.

In practice, body composition is often described as a two-compartment model: fat mass and fat-free mass (or lean body mass). And if you know these values, it can help you avoid getting stuck in the rut of only measuring and talking about body weight. It will also give you much more information about your overall health.

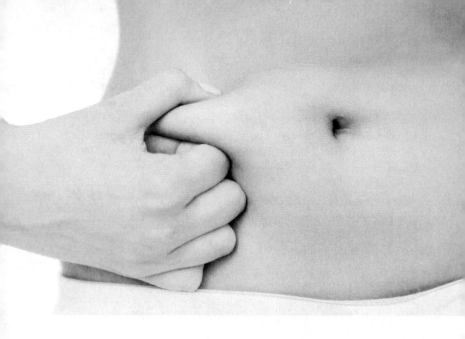

Typically, body fat levels are broken into "optimal health" and "optimal fitness." These terms are very similar, but in general, "health" refers to the optimal level for reduced risk of disease, and "fitness" takes a step further to the optimal level for physical fitness. We should all strive for at least optimal health, and then optimal fitness.

For women, optimal health is a body fat range of 18 to 30 percent and optimal fitness is 16 to 25 percent. For men, optimal health is 10 to 25 percent and optimal fitness is 12 to 18 percent. Consider your own goals to determine which range you should fall into. Then, the next step is to determine your current body composition.

Measuring Body Composition

Many methods of assessing body composition exist, including direct and indirect measurements. Direct measurements include dissolution of the body and physical dissection. This means that to truly know your body composition, you will have to wait until after you have passed away and donate your body to science. This is obviously not a viable option.

Luckily for us, multiple indirect methods are available to assess body composition and are fairly easy to get access to. But because each method is indirect, each will have its own inherent error threshold based on the accuracy compared to the direct method. That error threshold is usually somewhere between one and four percent.

Depending on the modality, if you are measured at 30 percent body fat with a method that has an error threshold of plus or minus 4 percent, your "true body fat" could really be anywhere between 26 and 34 percent body fat.

While this is somewhat disappointing, these assessment tools are great for tracking changes over time, as long as the same machine and same technician is doing the measuring. The skill of the technician can also make big differences in the measurement that is made in some instances.

Some of the more expensive and laboratory-based methods include the following.
- Dual-energy X-ray absorptiometry (DEXA)
- Hydrostatic, or underwater, weighing
- Air-displacement plethysmography, or what is commonly known as the "bod pod"
- Skinfold measurements using skinfold pinches
- Bioelectrical impedance analysis using an electrical current
- Advanced clinical methods, such as computerized tomography (CT) or magnetic resonance imaging (MRI)

With each technique, we are able to assess body density through your body volume in water (such as with underwater weighing) or in air (such as with the bod pod), or via some sort of imaging technique, such as DEXA, CT, or MRI.

For most of these tests, you can either ask your local gym personnel to administer them or search for a human performance or exercise science laboratory at a local college or university.

Body Shape

All of these methods can only estimate your relative fat and lean components. But just how much body fat you have is not the whole picture. It turns out that where you store that fat may be more important than how much fat you have.

Typically, fat is stored either around your abdomen in the typical "apple shape," called android fat, or around your hips and buttocks in the typical "pear shape," called gynoid fat. Depending on where you store your fat, you can often predict your risk of future health complications.

The android pattern of body fat indicates a lot of fat stored around your organs, which is called visceral fat, in addition to fat also underneath your skin, which is called subcutaneous fat. This fat distribution is much

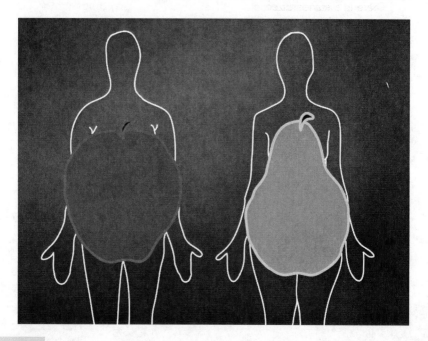

more common in men and is associated with more disease risk than the gynoid fat distributions.

The gynoid fat deposition is typically thought of as the female pattern of weight gain. This might actually be protective against disease for women. However, after menopause, when estrogen production tapers off, women tend to shift more toward the android obesity that is associated with men.

A measurement called waist-to-hip ratio, or waist and hip circumference, was developed to quickly and easily allow physicians to crudely estimate body composition as well as determine risk based on where fat is located. The size of your waist (smallest part of your abdomen) in relation to your hips (greatest protrusion of the buttocks) can quickly paint the picture of your fat distribution.

There is a standardized set of values that can identify your risk based on both measurements. For example, your disease risk increases with a total waist circumference measurement of more than 35 inches (88.9 cm) for women and more than 40 inches (101.6 cm) for men. And this is for just for your waist, regardless of hip circumference.

Similarly, a waist-to-hip ratio of greater than 0.86 for women or greater than 0.95 for men indicates an increased risk for disease. The closer to 1 or above, meaning a bigger belly than buttocks, gives you the apple shape. In both cases, improvements in body composition are recommended to avoid these associated health problems.

Another way that body shape is often described is according to somatotype, or physique shape. The three clearly defined shapes include ectomorphs, who are naturally thin with longer limbs and small joints; mesomorphs, who are naturally muscular with broad shoulders and narrow waists; and endomorphs, who are more round and soft with thicker joints.

Most people can identify with one of the categories even if they are a hybrid of two groups. Just keep in mind that the type of body shape you might naturally be might be hidden or morphed by years of beating up your body with excess food or, on the other hand, lots of dedicated exercise to change your body composition.

Regardless, these body shapes are correlated with certain levels of fat mass and muscle mass. Knowing which category you fall into can also help you set realistic goals for body composition and performance.

Try This

Find your starting point and work with a fitness professional to have your body fat percent measured.

Questions to Consider

1. Why should you care more about body composition than body weight?

2. Why might lifting weights change your waist size but not your body weight?

A Healthier Way to Measure Body Composition

Over the past 25 years, the body weight that Americans perceive to be ideal has steadily increased by over 10 pounds. Today, the average woman weighs 157 pounds but would like to weigh 140 pounds, while the average man weighs 193 pounds but would ideally weigh about 185 pounds. The trouble is, body weight gives us absolutely no indication of how much fat or how much muscle a person carries on their frame. This relative proportion is critical as it's related to our overall health, and how our body moves and behaves, and how we look and feel aesthetically.

I'm sure you've seen weight loss advertisements or even television series that showcase men and women who are able to lose hundreds of pounds over only a few weeks time. The contestants step up onto a scale to show the audience how much weight they have lost each week, with success being weight loss and failure being little or no loss. But no one ever quantifies those losses. Do they lose fat? Or do they lose muscle too? For some people, tracking body weight is an appropriate tool to keep them on track with their goals, but for others it may be misleading.

For example, in my research, in addition to tracking body weight, we also often track muscle mass and fat mass changes. We track these before, during, and after an exercise and nutritional intervention of several weeks or months. One of the most glaring examples of weighing misuse was when a participant—an overweight, middle-aged woman—came to me and told me she was going to drop out of the program because she was having no results.

This was a total shock because I had personally measured her success in the study. She had improved her upper and lower body strength, and had increased her ability to complete high-intensity cardiovascular exercise. She told me she was feeling better than she had in the past 10 years, and a blood chemistry panel showed that her cardiovascular and metabolic health was improving, too. As far as body composition, she had steadily lost fat mass and gained muscle during her first 6 weeks working out with us. She was an absolute image of success. But what did her scale read? Failure.

The only metric she had used to determine her progress was body weight. Despite her belief that her clothes fit better, and that her belt needed to be tightened, and that she was getting compliments from her family and friends about her physique, she didn't care, because the number on the scale had not yet changed. You see, she had lost several pounds of body fat but also gained a near equal amount of muscle, so she weighed exactly the same, despite the fact that the composition of the weight had changed dramatically. And this is the point: How can we better quantify success with weight management? After this lecture, you will have a better, healthier idea of what's happening to your body during weight loss, what benchmarks are typically used to indicate success, and why success goes far beyond simply what the scale tells you.

We'll start with a concept called body mass index, often abbreviated as BMI. Now, BMI compares your body weight in kilograms to your height in meters squared. A note of caution here: measures like BMI or body weight may be relevant only in certain situations. The usefulness of BMI is not great when considered on an individual-to-individual basis. In practice, BMI is most appropriate for large sample populations, like considering the status of a state or a country, or in clinical situations to quantify the risk for a patient who is clearly overweight and overfat at the same time.

So, if you are the same height as your best friend and you weigh a bit more, you will also have a slightly higher BMI. And BMI assumes any extra weight is due to greater fat weight, so in this case your higher BMI is associated with more negative health outcomes. But, as we've already discussed, that may be a problem with this measure. Let me explain. There are four main categories of BMI, which, again, is your weight in kilograms divided by your height in meters squared: underweight, which is less than 18.5; normal weight, which is 18.5 to 24.9; overweight, which is 25 to 29; and obese, which is classified as a BMI over 30.

Research has consistently shown a positive association between a high BMI and a greater risk of cardiovascular, pulmonary, and metabolic disease. If you are curious about your own body mass index, calculate it, or look online for a free website that can give you the information. The trouble is that BMI, once again, only considers your body weight and body height, and does not account for the proportion of muscle mass or fat mass, which is the composition of your body weight.

Take, for example, a typical NFL running back. These men are very strong, and have lots of lean muscle mass and very little body fat. They are professional athletes and do not look overweight or overfat; most will have a six-pack of abs. Assuming this running back is just about 6 feet tall and a touch over 230 pounds due to all of his muscle mass, his BMI would be over 31 kg/m². According to the BMI standards I just mentioned, our professional, healthy, lean athlete would be considered obese, even though common sense tells us otherwise. And, if you calculate BMI for the average U.S. woman, she is 5'6" tall and weighs 156 pounds, and subsequently has a BMI of 25.2, which, as you now know, is considered overweight. This example demonstrates that certain measures like BMI or body weight may be relevant only in certain situations.

Let's move on to better measures, measures of body composition, which is different from body weight and body mass index. As you now know, body composition is the relationship between the different types of tissue that comprise your body—in other words, how much muscle and how much fat make up your body weight. So, if you compare yourself again to your friend of equal height, and you weigh more, but we know that the extra weight is from increased muscle mass, this likely indicates better health despite a higher BMI.

To account for fat-free mass and not just total body weight, the fat-free mass index was developed. It is similar to BMI but it takes your fat-free mass, or muscle mass, again in kilograms, divided by your height in meters squared. This index can quantify your body composition more accurately when you know that you have extra weight that is mostly from muscle. It is not always a better index but it is a different index, and, like any index, will be more or less useful depending on the specific need of the information.

While the fat-free mass index is not used nearly as much as body mass index, a few research papers have attempted to come up with normal fat-free mass index values for men and women. A paper in 2002 in an *International Journal of Obesity and Related Metabolic Disorders* found the average fat-free mass index for young women is about 15 kg/m^2, and for young men is 19 kg/m^2. But keep in mind that these values change slightly after age 35, showing that fat mass is gained as we age, most likely due to a sedentary lifestyle. The number of options scientists have developed to better quantify fat and muscle indicates the importance of knowing them.

Now, let's look at the specific reasons why these indices are important to consider, and more specific information about body fat and muscle. For starters, it can be helpful for knowing your health status and risk of certain kinds of diseases, like cardiovascular disease, pulmonary disease, and metabolic disease like type 2 diabetes. It is well established that if you have a lot of fat deposition, particularly around your waist and belly near your major organs, that your chance of developing these types of diseases increases dramatically. Secondly, knowing your current body composition gives you greater clarity about your starting point if you decide that you need a change. You will better be able to track your body's changes over time and have a bigger picture of success.

Let's get a little bit more specific about body fat and muscle mass, and what they're actually describing. In terms of body composition, your total body fat includes essential and storage body fat. Essential fat includes fat in your organs such as your heart, liver, kidneys, intestines, muscles, and bone marrow. This type of fat is required for normal physiological functioning and is different greatly between men and women—in fact, it accounts for most of the major body fat differences between sexes. Women have around 12% essential fat compared to men who have about 3% essential fat.

Why do you think women might have a bit more essential fat? Well, mostly due to their biological function for reproduction. Women need extra fat stores during pregnancy. Regardless of whether a woman has children or not, she will most often have slightly more fat than a man. For this reason, it is important not to compare your body fat percentage to friends of the opposite sex. Now, it is fun to get competitive with a friend or a significant other, but realize that the optimal body fat percentage is vastly different between men and women.

So, to reiterate, men have about 3% essential fat, and women have about 12% essential fat, but these numbers are still drastically low. There's another type of fat that is also required for normal body function and this is called storage fat, which is fat stored, and it can be used for energy. It includes the visceral fat, or deep fat, around your organs, and the fat just underneath your skin, which is called subcutaneous fat. Storage fat can insulate your body, helps to maintain body temperature, and provides vital protection for your organs. The amount of storage fat is more similar between men and women, usually just 2%–3% percent higher in a woman. So, health issues come in when our storage fat become excessive. Body fat is important for supporting daily function and health, but excess amounts will contribute to overweight and overfat conditions.

Okay, so the other component of body mass that is not made up of fat is called fat-free mass or lean body mass. These terms often are used interchangeably; however, they are technically different. Fat-free mass is only muscle mass that you have, while lean body mass also includes your muscle mass, bone mass, connective tissue like ligaments and tendons, your internal organs, and any essential fat stored in these tissues. In practice, body composition is often described as a two-compartment model, meaning fat mass and fat-free mass or lean body mass. And, if you know these values, it can help avoid getting stuck in the rut of only measuring and talking about body weight. It will also give you much more information about your overall health.

By now you are probably saying to yourself, "How much body fat should I have?" Well, these standards have been established. Typically, body fat levels are broken into optimal health and optimal fitness. These terms are very similar, but in general, health refers to the optimal level for reduced risk of disease, and fitness takes it a step further to the optimal level for physical fitness. We should all strive for at least optimal health, and then optimal fitness. For women, optimal health is a body fat range of 18%–30% and optimal fitness is 16%–25%. For men, optimal health is 10%–25% and optimal fitness is 12%–18%. Consider your own goals to determine which range you should fall into. Then, the next step is to determine your current body composition.

So, how do we measure body composition? Many methods of assessing body composition exist, including direct and indirect measurements. Direct measurements include the dissolution of the body and physical dissection, meaning to truly know your body composition, you will have to wait until after you have passed away and then donate your body to science, and this obviously is not a viable option. But, lucky for us, multiple indirect methods are available to assess body composition and are fairly easy to get access to. One note though: because each method is indirect, each will have its own inherent error based on the accuracy compared to the direct method. That error threshold is usually somewhere between 1% and 4%.

So, depending on the modality, if you are measured at 30% body fat with a method that has plus or minus 4% error, your true body fat could really be anywhere between 26% and 34% body fat. And while this is somewhat disappointing, these assessment tools are great for tracking changes over time, so long as the machine and the technician are the same that are doing the measuring. The skill of the technician can also make a big difference in the measurement that is made in some instances.

Some of the more expensive and laboratory-based methods include: dual-energy X-ray absorptiometry, or DEXA; hydrostatic or underwater weighing; air-displacement plethysmography, or what is commonly known as the Bod Pod; skinfold measurements using skinfold pinches; bioelectrical impedance analysis using an electrical current; and even some advanced clinical methods like computerized tomography, or CT; or magnetic resonance imaging, or MRI.

Now this may sound like a lot of jargon, but with each technique we are able to assess body density through your body volume, like in water with underwater weighing, or your body volume in air, like with the Bod Pod, or via some sort of imaging technique like DEXA, CT, or MRI, among others. Because many of these methods are difficult to actually perform, I'll keep this part of our discussion to methods that are a bit more common. For most of these tests, you can either ask your local gym personnel to administer them, or search for a human performance or exercise science laboratory at a local college or university near you.

First, hydrostatic weighing, also called underwater weighing, involves getting into a large tub of water, going underneath, and fully exhaling. Yes, I said fully exhaling. This is definitely uncomfortable—we typically hold our breath underwater to avoid drowning. But with underwater weighing, it's important to expel as much air from the lungs as possible to get an accurate measurement. This technique is based on Archimedes principle, which states that an object immersed in fluid—in this case, you in a water tank—loses an amount of weight that is equivalent to the weight of the fluid displaced by the object's volume. In plain English, when you go underwater, you displace water. By weighing you both underwater and on dry land, we can calculate your body volume and density.

Because muscle is more dense than fat, those with more muscle mass will have a greater body density, and those with more fat will have less body density. Think about it: those who have more fat are able to float more easily in the pool than those who have more muscle mass. Ultimately, an equation using measured body density will estimate your body fat percentage, and hydrostatic weighing is often considered the gold standard for estimating body composition. However, the equations come with assumptions about sex, race, ethnicity, age, and lung volume. Ultimately, this technique is a great tool but can be difficult to get a truly accurate measurement and, importantly, not everyone is agreeable to being dunked underwater with no breath.

Well, to solve this problem, we use air-displacement plethysmography, or ADP. Air-displacement plethysmography uses something called the Bod Pod, and is another way to estimate body volume but uses air displacement rather than water displacement. The Bod Pod then relies on Boyle's law, which states that, at a constant temperature, volume and pressure are inversely related. So, just like with hydrostatic weighing, body volume is measured and then body density and body fat are estimated using standard calculations. And because you don't need to go underwater, many people find this technique more comfortable and accommodating.

While these two methods are considered two-compartment models—that is, they measure fat mass and fat-free mass only—other models do exist that consider a three-compartment model: fat mass, fat-free mass, and bone mineral density. The most common way to assess the three-compartment model is through a technique called dual-energy X-ray absorptiometry, or DEXA. You may have heard of this if your doctor ever wanted to check you for low bone mineral density or osteoporosis. This method is most often used in hospital settings or in research laboratories. To obtain this measure, you lie on a flat table as a scanning arm crosses above you to systematically image your body. Using a very low dose X-ray, about the amount you would get from a transatlantic flight, the DEXA calculates areas with more or less density, including your fat, muscle, and bone tissues. Other, more complex, expensive methods include computed tomography, or CT, and magnetic resonance imaging, or MRI, which you may often hear about for diagnostic imaging rather than measuring body composition.

The two most commonly used techniques are the skinfold method and something called bioelectrical impedance analysis. The skinfold method of assessing body composition is practical and widely used; you may have come across this method at some point or another. A caliper, or a plastic or metal pincher, is used to pinch the fat underneath your skin at specific sites on your body. Many times this method includes just three different sites. For women, this would be the back of your arm, your thigh, and your suprailium, which is just above your hip on the outside of your body. For men, the pinches are taken at your chest, your abdomen, and your thigh. And, ultimately, the percent body fat is calculated from your estimated body density using standard equations. Unfortunately, there may be considerable error using the skinfold method depending on the type of skinfold caliper and the experience of the technician taking the measurements.

But the most commonly used body composition analysis tool by gyms and clinics is something called bioelectrical impedance analysis. We actually use these in our lab from time to time, especially in field studies. You've probably seen these hand-held devices that you hold onto like a steering wheel and grip both handles. There are also floor models that you stand on like a scale, and there are high-grade BIAs where you lie on your back with small electrodes attached to your hands and your feet. With bioelectric impedance analysis technology, we use electricity to assess body composition. And because much of your body is comprised of water, and muscle mass is particularly high with water, almost 70%, an electrical current can pass through quite easily. Remember, water is conductive.

On the other hand, fat contains little water and will blunt the electrical current, slowing down the signal. The BIA uses a very low-level electrical current—you can't even feel it—and usually just two points of contact. Within the handheld model, this would run from your left hand to your right hand, and based on the relative amounts of fat and muscle you have, the BIA will calculate the speed of the current and ultimately estimate fat-free mass and fat mass.

Great: easy, right? Well, because this tool relies on total body water, you'd be right in thinking that your hydration status, or how much water you've had to drink, will influence the results of this measurement. In practice, the BIA tends to work well for most people to accurately gauge body fat levels, but it also may give very lean people a higher body fat measurement, or very obese people a lower value than anticipated. Therefore, if you fall at the extremes of either leanness or fatness, the BIA may not be the best modality for you.

Nevertheless, this tool can be used to track body fat levels over time, so long as the same pre-testing protocol is followed. For example, eating and drinking habits should be similar before testing, and you need to know other facts, such as activity level and alcohol consumption in the days prior, as both are known to influence hydration status. So, from this outline of testing modalities, we have a little more background on the complex measurement of body composition. Remember, though, all of these methods can only estimate your relative fat and lean components.

But just how much body fat you have is not the whole picture. It turns out that where you store your fat may be more important than how much fat you have. Typically, fat is stored either around your abdomen in an apple shape called android fat, or around your hips and buttocks, the typical pear shape called gynoid fat. Now, depending on where you store your fat, you can often predict your risk of future health complications.

The android or apple-shaped pattern of body fat indicates a lot of fat stored around your organs, which is called visceral fat, in addition to fat also underneath your skin, which is called subcutaneous fat. Think about it: would you want a large mass of fat around all of your vital organs? Probably not. This fat distribution is much more common in men and is associated with more disease risk than the pear-shape fat distributions. Specifically, a central or android fat distribution can increase the likelihood of narrowed artery walls, high blood pressure, and abnormal blood lipids, glucose, and insulin.

The pear-shape or gynoid fat deposition is typically thought of as the female pattern of weight gain. Now this may actually be protective against disease for women. However, after menopause, when estrogen production tapers off, women tend to shift more towards the android obesity that is associated with men.

This is really important. It shows us that it is not only how much fat we have that we need to care about, but also where we carry this fat. Because of this relationship, other measurements were developed to quickly and easily allow physicians to crudely estimate body composition, as well as to determine the risk based on where fat is located. This measurement is called your waist-to-hip ratio and your waist and hip circumferences. As the name implies, the size of your waist—the smallest part of your abdomen—in relation to your hips—the greatest protrusion from the buttocks—carefully paint the picture of your fat distribution.

There is a standardized set of values that can identify your risk based on both measurements. For example, your disease risk increases with a total waist circumference measurement of more than 35 inches—or 88.9 centimeters—for women, and more than 40 inches—or 101.6 centimeters—for men. And this is for just for your waist, regardless of your hip circumference. Similarly, a waist-to-hip ratio of greater than 0.86 for women or greater than 0.95 for men indicates an increased risk for disease. The closer to 1 or above, meaning a bigger belly than buttocks, gives you the apple shape. In both cases, improvements in body composition are recommended to avoid these associated health problems.

Just remember to place your measuring tape in the right place to get an accurate value. As one of my professors once told me, your waist is the first part of you that enters the room. All too often I'll see people measuring their waist and hips after moving and shifting their fat around to try to get a healthier profile. While this is interesting to watch, it does you no favors to have an inaccurate measurement.

Another way that body shape is often described is according to somatotype or physique shape. The three clearly defined shapes include ectomorphs, like long distance runners or basketball players who are naturally thin with longer limbs and smaller joints; mesomorphs, who are naturally muscular with broad shoulders and narrow waists like Serena Williams; and endomorphs that are more round and soft with thicker joints like Oprah Winfrey.

Most people can identify with one of these categories, even if they are a hybrid or a mixture of two groups. Just keep in mind that the type of body shape you may naturally be hiding or morphed by years of beating up your body with excess calories, foods, or on the other hand, lots of dedicated exercise to change your body composition. Regardless, these body shapes are correlated with certain levels of fat mass and muscle mass, and knowing which category you fall into also can help set realistic goals for body composition and performance.

Now, we need to spend a minute with one myth that persists around this topic, which is that muscle weighs more than fat. This myth is just like saying that 1 pound of bricks weighs more than 1 pound of feathers. Of course, if you have 1 pound of each, then they both weigh 1 pound. But here's the difference: muscle has more density than fat. This is the key to understanding why two people can weigh exactly the same at the same height but look entirely different.

Recall the underwater weighing method for measuring body composition; the more muscle mass someone has, the more dense they are, and the more they weigh underwater. However, the more fat mass someone has, the less dense they are, and they more likely they are to float in water.

Let's take a look at 5 pounds of fat and 5 pounds of muscle. Now, they weigh exactly the same, but the amount of muscle is smaller than the same amount of fat. The muscle is about 1/3 or 1/2 smaller than the fat because of its increased density. This explains why my research participant needed to tighten her belt despite seeing no change in her body weight. So, don't be fooled by this myth any longer—when you add muscle, you might weigh the same, but you could look entirely different.

Now you know the difference between body composition and weight. You also know that your body composition is a far better indicator of health, success, and even performance than simply body weight measured on your bathroom scale. So start here: take a good self-inventory. Do you feel healthy? Are you ever gasping for breath after activities that you used to do easily? Do you have any noticeable android or central fat levels? Has your doctor told you of any health issues due to excess body fat? Answer these questions and then work to set challenging but realistic goals.

For a very active person, the goal could be to complete a 10K or half-marathon race, or maybe to be able to do a set number of unassisted push-ups or pull-ups. For these sorts of people, a lower percent body fat will be reasonable with their overall lifestyle. For others, the goal may be just to keep disease at bay, lose a small amount of weight, or to maintain exactly what you've got. Remember, the goal may not be the same as your best friend's; it will always be personal and specific to you. Now, once your goal is determined, and you have a plan to get there with the help of a professional, then an ideal body fat level can be paired with that goal.

In the coming lectures, you will learn some strategies to begin taking on goals like this. You will also learn about how foods are digested and absorbed to ultimately provide energy, and how they can be manipulated to improve your body composition. Try this: find your starting point and work with a fitness professional to have your body fat percent measured.

How Food Is Digested and Absorbed

Every bit of the food you eat has a dramatic impact on your body composition, health, and how you feel. The bulk of this lecture will focus on the details of digestion and absorption. It will also touch on how the aging process can interfere with normal digestion absorption—and how that can affect body composition. You'll also learn about nutrient partitioning, which is the manipulation of both nutrient content and nutrient timing of your diet for specific physiological reasons.

Digestion and Absorption

How does the food you eat enter into your body for storage as glycogen (stored carbohydrate), fat, or protein? Many processes must happen inside your body to prepare food for use or storage.

Before the food you eat can be used for energy, it needs to be broken down inside the body into individual nutrients. This is digestion. Following digestion, the body must take up, or absorb, the individual nutrients to either use them or store them for later. This is called absorption.

Foods and beverages provide your body with nutrients that it needs to sustain itself. The nutrients for our body are split into two main categories: macronutrients and micronutrients.

Macronutrients, consisting of carbohydrates, fats, and proteins, are used by your body's cells to create energy. Micronutrients—vitamins, minerals, and water—do not provide calories, or energy, but they are required for many physiological processes in the body, including digestion and absorption.

Once you take a bite of food, the first section of the gastrointestinal (GI) tract that it hits is the mouth. The food then travels down the esophagus and enters the stomach to be chemically and mechanically broken down into smaller fragments.

After the stomach, these food fragments enter the small intestine, followed by the large intestine. Whatever nutrients and materials the body does not use up until this point are excreted through the rectum and anal canal.

Along the route, your pancreas, gallbladder, and liver all help digest and absorb the food by producing various enzymes (specialty proteins that help reactions occur) and enzyme solutions that help break down and transport foods.

Almost all nutrients within the food you eat must be digested before they are absorbed. Various physical and chemical activities from the mouth, stomach, pancreas, and small intestine are responsible for digestion.

Once all of the nutrients are broken down into their simplest forms, they are then taken up into the cells of the GI tract to be transported throughout the entire body. This process is known as absorption.

Most of the carbohydrates, fats, and proteins that you consume are generally absorbed within 30 minutes after reaching the small intestines. Any intestinal material that is not absorbed by the time it reaches the end of the last portion of the small intestine passes through something called the ileocecal valve and then into the large intestine.

Overall, it can take anywhere from 12 to 70 hours for food remnants to pass all the way through the colon, and waste products are eventually excreted as fecal matter through the anal canal.

Your body composition overall is highly influenced by the digestion and absorption of nutrients from the food you eat.

Carbohydrates

Through digestion, more complex carbohydrates are eventually broken down into individual units, known as monosaccharides. The three monosaccharides are glucose, galactose, and fructose, with the most common being glucose.

Most nutrients are absorbed somewhere along the length of the small intestine, through the brush border—where all of the intestinal digestive enzymes are produced and stored—into the intestinal cells. Carbohydrates are absorbed very efficiently and are usually cleared out of the small intestine more quickly than fats or proteins.

Glucose is absorbed into the intestinal cells by a protein complex called the sodium-glucose transporter. This is an "active" process, meaning that energy, or adenosine triphosphate (ATP), is required to make this happen.

After glucose is absorbed into the intestinal cell, it is then transported out of the cell and into the bloodstream. Some of the glucose simply diffuses into the blood, but a carrier protein transports much of the glucose from the intestinal cell into the blood.

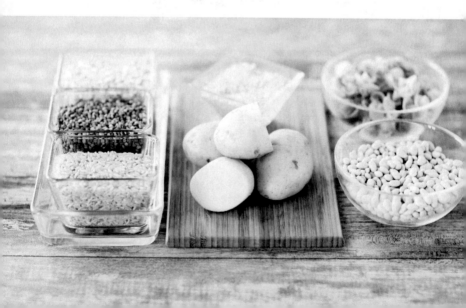

■ Once glucose enters the blood, it goes directly to the liver. This is called portal circulation. The liver is the main site of glucose metabolism, so it gets first choice on what to do with the incoming glucose: use it, store it, or let it move on.

■ Any glucose that is not metabolized and used in the liver passes through to systemic, or whole-body, circulation. From here, glucose travels to various other tissues, where it can be taken up through a facilitated transport process, using other transport proteins before it is used within that tissue.

Fat

■ Digestion of fat begins in the mouth by the action of an enzyme called lingual lipase. Only very small amounts are broken down in the stomach. The bulk of triglyceride (or fat) digestion occurs in the small intestine.

■ Before fats are broken into their component parts, they must first be emulsified by bile. Bile is produced in the liver but stored in the gallbladder.

■ Once fat is present in the small intestine, a hormone called cholecystokinin (CCK) is secreted, and then bile is released through the bile ducts into the small intestine, and the emulsification process begins.

■ Once emulsified, pancreatic lipase acts on the fats and further breaks them into smaller units that can be absorbed and transported for use.

■ Unlike carbohydrates, fats are a little tricky when it comes to their absorption and transportation. They are naturally insoluble in water. Because of this, they cannot move through the brush border or the blood as individual lipid units.

■ To solve this problem, broken-down fat particles mix with bile salts and form a water-soluble substance called a micelle, which then interacts at the brush border of the small intestine. Fat particles move out of the micelle and into the intestinal cell, and the water-soluble bile salts continue down through the small intestine until they are reabsorbed and sent back to the liver.

After the broken-down fat particles—which include free fatty acids, monoglycerides, and some cholesterol and phospholipid particles—are in the intestinal cell, they actually combine back together to their larger original triglyceride form. Then, they are transported.

Fats are not only broken down differently than carbohydrates; they also travel differently. Fats must travel through the lymph system instead of the blood. The lymphatic system is a network of vessels that transports nutrients to the cells and collects cell waste products.

In a slow process, fats move out into the lymphatic vessels and eventually into the blood, where they freely travel to tissues to deliver the fats for use or storage. Some fat will be used by your muscle cells to produce energy, and some will be deposited into your fat cells.

There are many things that affect how fats are used and stored, including when you last ate, what your overall calorie intake for the day and exercise habits are, and how physically fit you are.

Because the transportation process for fats is relatively slow, it could take anywhere from 30 minutes to 3 hours after you eat a high-fat meal for your blood lipids to reach the highest level. About 5 to 6 hours after the meal, however, the fats will have been delivered to the designated tissues, and your blood levels should return to normal.

Protein

The structure of protein is very complex. The reason that digestion of protein makes more demands on the body's metabolism is because of the complexity of protein.

Proteins stay fully intact until they get to your stomach. Large proteins are broken down into individual amino acids in the stomach by very acidic stomach juice. Proteins that are still intact after leaving the stomach are broken down further in the top portion of the small intestine. The end products of protein digestion are free amino acids, which are absorbed into the intestinal cell.

Proteins are absorbed in a process more similar to carbohydrates than fats. This process occurs along the entire small intestine.

Amino acids, just like glucose, require a sodium-dependent carrier to get into the intestinal cells. There are several uses for particular amino acids within the intestinal cell. However, amino acids that are not used within the intestinal cells themselves are transported out of the cells into the blood and make their first stop at the liver.

About 50 to 65 percent of all ingested amino acids are metabolized in the liver. The rest of the amino acids are used in other tissues, particularly the skeletal muscles, kidneys, and brain.

Micronutrients

Macronutrients provide the body with energy. Micronutrients, on the other hand, do not provide energy. Despite this, micronutrients are vital to make all of the digestive processes occur, along with hundreds of other reactions and processes within the body.

Water-soluble vitamins—vitamin C and all B-complex vitamins—are absorbed into and transported through the blood. With the exception of vitamin B_{12}, water-soluble vitamins are not stored in the body for long periods of time. They are either used fairly quickly in the body or are excreted in the urine, so we need to get them daily from the food we eat.

Fat-soluble vitamins—vitamins A, D, E, and K—are absorbed and transported much like fats. Unlike water-soluble vitamins, excess fat-soluble vitamins can be stored in the body for a decent amount of time.

For this reason, fat-soluble vitamins deficiencies are much less common than water-soluble vitamin deficiencies.

Anorexia of Aging

For the most part, the GI tract of a healthy individual works like a well-oiled machine. Along with the digestive system itself, the endocrine and nervous systems play a major role in regulating digestion, absorption, and transportation of nutrients.

Unfortunately, as people start to age, some functions of these systems begin to slow down. The main cause for these changes is the degeneration of the enteric nervous system, which is the nervous system of the GI tract. This can lead to serious GI complications.

Along with biological and nervous system complications, elderly individuals might experience what has come to be known as "anorexia of aging." This refers to a physiological age-related reduction in appetite and energy intake, which leads to significant weight loss and muscle wasting.

Basically, as you age, there might come a time when you just don't feel hungry very often. While this might lead to weight loss, this is not a good thing; oftentimes muscle mass is lost, too. Ultimately, low muscle mass prevents mobility.

Your best bet to avoid or slow this age-related reduction in appetite is to simply make sure that you are leading a healthy lifestyle. See your doctor regularly, exercise, and nourish yourself with foods that contribute to your health.

Nutrient Partitioning

Nutrient partitioning is the term used to describe how the food you eat is stored or partitioned into a specific storage area, such as muscle or fat. At the most basic level, the more of one type of food you eat—

carbohydrates, fats, or protein—the more of that fuel you will burn for energy.

Exercise is the most important and powerful tool to help you use the foods you eat to improve body composition. If you are active, you will tend to use the foods you eat to power exercise. But if you are sedentary, your body will tend to partition the foods you eat to being stored as fat, instead of being used and stored for a healthy purpose.

Try This

Pay attention to the foods you eat and how they make you feel and perform.

Questions to Consider

1. Why is nutrient digestion and absorption important to body composition?

2. What is the biggest determinant of nutrient partitioning?

How Food Is Digested and Absorbed

Have you ever wondered if breakfast really is the most important meal of the day? You probably have heard this phrase over and over for your entire life. But why is it the most important meal? And what happens if we just, well, skip it? Well, breakfast is an extremely important meal because it gives you the energy you need to start the day. You literally are breaking the overnight fast. And eating breakfast has also shown to contribute many health benefits such as weight control, improved physical and cognitive performance, and improved metabolic biomarkers. But is breakfast really the most important meal of the day? Let's face it, chances are that you know someone who seems to be very healthy but doesn't really take the time to eat breakfast.

Well, it turns out that researchers can't agree either, and several observational studies have reported that people who skip breakfast tend to weigh more overall. And this observation may go against the common thought. For example, if you want to lose weight, eating two meals instead of eating three meals means you're eating fewer calories, doesn't it? Well, not necessarily.

One theory is that breakfast skippers tend to get hungrier faster and therefore eat more calories later on throughout the day than regular breakfast eaters. The theory goes like this: skipping breakfast results in spending the rest of your day making up those missed calories at the end, resulting in overcompensating, and eventually leading to excess, unwanted weight gain. However, most of these reports have come strictly from observational studies, with little data from an experimental cause and effect setting. This means that many other factors could contribute to the weight gain, aside from just not eating breakfast.

So, in contrast to the common belief that skipping breakfast always leads to weight gain, randomized, controlled research trials have actually shown that these common theories and myths about breakfast are hard to confirm. For example, when two groups of overweight and obese individuals were randomly assigned to either eat breakfast or refrain from breakfast, there was no effect on the amount of weight lost in each of the groups. Another randomly controlled trial with lean individuals showed that skipping breakfast did not cause weight gain, nor did it lead to changes in resting metabolic rate, or the number of calories that subjects burned at rest that are required to sustain their basic physiological functions. Also, the overall daily caloric intake was the same whether the lean subjects ate breakfast or not, and this means that, in this study, skipping breakfast did not lead to eating more over the next few meals.

Now one interesting difference, though, was that both afternoon and evening blood glucose levels were more stable in the group who ate breakfast as compared to those who fasted until noon, and stable blood glucose is usually a great sign for good metabolic functioning. In fact, if blood sugar is consistently high, this can lead to a host of other issues including insulin resistance and even diabetes.

Long story short is that there is no clear-cut answer in the research saying that breakfast is the key to gaining or losing weight or improving body composition. And oftentimes I'm asked, "Should I eat breakfast" and my answer is, "Well, do you like breakfast?" I do this because what I've seen is that the key to making lasting improvements in body composition comes from working small exercise and nutrition habits into someone's lifestyle, rather than flipping their lives upside down from the start. And one main point to consider is that, on the outside, if you eat breakfast or skip it, or you eat often or just once a day, every bit of food you eat has a dramatic impact on your body composition, and your health, and how you feel.

Let's talk about what exactly happens to the food that you eat. How does it enter into your body for storage as glycogen or stored carbohydrate, as fat or as protein? Well, many processes must happen inside your body to prepare the food you use for storage or to be burned as energy. Now, before the food you eat can be used as energy, it needs to be broken down further inside the body into the individual nutrients, and this process is called digestion. And then, following digestion, the body must take up or absorb the individual nutrients to either use them or store them for later. This is called absorption.

The bulk of this lecture will focus on the details of digestion and absorption, and we'll touch on how the aging process can interfere with normal digestion and absorption, and how that can affect body composition overall. We'll also talk about nutrient partitioning, which is how we use foods and how we can partition them into storage as fat or into storage as muscle based on our physical condition.

Now, foods and beverages provide your body with nutrients that it needs to sustain itself—that's pretty common. The nutrients from our body, though, are split into two main categories: we have macronutrients and we have micronutrients. The macronutrients consist of carbohydrates, fats, and proteins, are these are used by your body's cells to create energy. But the micronutrients, including vitamins, minerals, and water, do not provide calories or energy, but they are required for many physiological processes in the body, including digestion and absorption.

You'll hear much more about the macronutrients and the micronutrients later in this course, but for now, to fully understand the digestion and absorption process, we will start with a brief overview to trace the food from the time it enters your mouth all the way through to when it exits as waste.

Once you take a bite of food, the first section of the gastrointestinal tract, or the GI tract, that it hits is the mouth. And obviously the food then travels down the esophagus and enters into the stomach to be chemically and mechanically broken down into smaller fragments. And then, after the stomach, these food fragments enter the small intestine followed by the large intestine. Whatever nutrients and materials the body does not use up along that process, they are excreted through the rectum and the anal canal.

Now along the route, your pancreas, gall bladder, and liver all help digest and absorb the food by producing various enzymes, and these are specialty proteins that help reactions occur in your body, and the enzyme solutions they make also help with the breakdown and transport of foods. So, that's the brief overview. Keep these major organs in mind as we dive now into some more detail.

Almost all nutrients within the food you eat must be digested before they are absorbed, and various physical and chemical activities from the mouth, the stomach, the pancreas, and the small intestine are responsible for digestion. Once you take a bite of your food, your teeth and your jaw muscles take care of the chewing of the food and mixing it with saliva to make the food easier to swallow. Water in your saliva, along with two major digestive enzymes called alpha-amylase and lingual lipase, begin to dissolve and chemically digest your food. Yes, technically, digestion begins in your mouth.

Once the food is mixed with saliva, we now refer to it as a bolus. The bolus leaves your mouth and travels through the pharynx and into your esophagus. The esophagus has a sphincter at the top called the esophageal sphincter, and this separates the oral cavity from your pharynx. Then, a wavelike neuromuscular movement known as peristalsis occurs progressively to move the bolus of food down your esophagus. And then another sphincter called the gastroesophageal sphincter separates the esophagus from the stomach, and this is where your food is headed next. So, this entire esophageal process usually takes about 10 seconds until the bolus of food has moved from the top to the bottom of your esophagus and then enters into your stomach.

The stomach is the major site of chemical digestion where any larger food items remaining are broken down into individual nutrients. For example, large carbohydrates are broken into individual sugars, and large proteins are broken down into individual amino acids. This has to occur because whole carbohydrates, fats, and whole proteins are just too big to enter your body from your GI tract. So, it is the smaller building blocks of the larger macronutrients that are needed to actually enter your body from the GI tract.

So, while the mouth and the stomach are referred to as digestive organs, they do things a bit differently. The mouth mainly takes care of the physical breakdown of food through chewing, and the stomach takes care of the chemical breakdown of food using very specific enzymes. The first enzyme is called pepsin, and pepsin breaks down large proteins into smaller amino acids. The second enzyme is called alpha-amylase, and this enzyme may sound familiar to you, as it already came into play when our food was still in our mouth. Alpha-amylase breaks starches into simple carbohydrates, but not for long, because the acidic environment of our stomach actually stops the majority of the alpha-amylase activity. Now, the third enzyme to take note of in the stomach is called gastric lipase. This enzyme breaks down some fats into smaller components that are easy to absorb.

Along with these three main enzymes, several other hormones and secretions play a role in the chemical digestion activities of the stomach. So, the stomach is where partially digested food is mixed with stomach juices and enzymes to create a substance called chyme. Once food is fully mixed and the chyme is ready to be emptied out of the stomach, it moves through yet another sphincter called the pyloric sphincter and enters into your small intestine.

Now, the small intestine is your main site for finishing up the digestion process. It is also the main site that absorbs all of the nutrients that you've just broken down. Although its name says small intestine, this organ is far from small in both length and in importance. For example, if you were to unravel the small intestine into a straight line, it would stretch out to be about 20 feet long. Also, the surface area spreads out to be about 300 m². So, picture a 3-foot-wide walkway that is more than 3 football fields in length. This is the amount of space that your small intestines would take up.

This is a huge surface area, and it's a unique aspect of the small intestine, as it allows us to maximize digestion and absorption. The reason the small intestine has such a large surface area is due to circular folds known as the folds of Kerckring. Now, these folds have many fingerlike projections called villi that project off of these folds and into the lumen or the inner side of the small intestine, and hundreds of these intestinal cells line the villi in order to absorb and transport the nutrients. These cells are called enterocytes. These microscopic structures called microvilli are tiny, hair-like projections that make up the villi themselves.

Now, these small microvilli make up an important section of the small intestine known as the brush border. It is within the brush border where all of the intestinal digestive enzymes are produced and stored. Almost all of the digestive activity in the small intestine occurs in the brush border. Now, once all of the nutrients are broken down into their simplest forms, they are then taken up into the cells of the GI tract to be transported throughout the entire body. This process is known as absorption.

Most of the carbohydrates, fats, and proteins that you consume are generally absorbed within about 30 minutes after reaching the small intestines. Any material that is not absorbed by the time it reaches the end of the ileum, or the last portion of the small intestine, passes through something called the ileocecal valve and then into the large intestine or the colon. The large intestine is about 5 feet long, and all of the remaining food items or intestinal material that enters the colon is still in a liquid form. But by the time it reaches the end of the colon, also called the sigmoid colon, the material is solid or semi-solid. This is because the large intestine is the main site for water reabsorption and for the reabsorption of electrolytes.

Overall, it can take anywhere from 12–70 hours for the food remnants to pass all the way through the colon, and waste products are eventually excreted as fecal matter through the anal canal. Now, your body composition overall is highly influenced by the digestion and absorption of the nutrients from the food you eat.

So what's next? After the nutrients are taken up into the small intestine's cells, where do they go? Do they just hang out there or do they move somewhere else? Well, there are actually several answers to this question, several extremely detailed answers. Let's begin with carbohydrates.

Through digestion, more complex carbohydrates are eventually broken down into individual units known as monosaccharides. The three monosaccharides are glucose, galactose, and fructose, with the most common being glucose. Now, as we talked about earlier, most nutrients are absorbed somewhere along the length of the small intestine, through the brush border and into the intestinal cells. And carbohydrates are absorbed very efficiently and are usually cleared of the small intestine more quickly than fats or proteins. Remember I mentioned earlier that carbohydrates make less demand on the body's metabolism than proteins. Well, glucose is absorbed in the intestinal cells by a protein complex called the sodium-glucose transporter. This is an active process, meaning that energy, or adenosine triphosphate—ATP—is required to make this happen.

After glucose is absorbed into the intestinal cells, it is then transported out of the cell and into the bloodstream. Now some of the glucose simply diffuses into the blood but a carrier protein called GLUT-2 transports much of the glucose from the intestinal cell into the blood. Once glucose enters the blood, it goes directly to your liver. This is called portal circulation. The liver is the main site of glucose metabolism, so it gets first choice on what to do with the incoming glucose—it can use it, store it, or simply let it move on. And any glucose that is not metabolized or used by the liver passes through to systemic or whole body circulation. From here, glucose travels to various other tissues where it can be taken up through a facilitated transport process using other transport proteins before it is used within that tissue.

Next we have fat. Now, digestion of fat begins in the mouth by the action of the enzyme called lingual lipase, and only very small amounts are broken down in the stomach. The bulk of triglyceride—or fat—digestion occurs in the small intestine. So, before fats are broken into their component parts, they first must be emulsified by bile. Bile is produced in your liver but stored in your gallbladder and, essentially, fats have to enter the aqueous environment of the small intestine. But fats are hydrophobic, or water fearing, so emulsification by bile helps fat break apart into smaller lipid droplets that can exist in the small intestine before being broken down. You may have heard of emulsification if you've tried to mix an oil and a vinegar salad dressing—they always separate. But if you add an emulsifier, you can get them to mix and play nice together. It's that bile that allows fat to play nice in the small intestine.

So, once fat is present in the small intestine, a hormone called cholecystokinin or CCK is secreted. And then bile is released through the bile ducts into the small intestine, and the emulsification process begins. Once emulsified, the pancreatic lipase acts on the fats and further breaks them into smaller units that can be absorbed and transported for use. Now, unlike carbohydrates, fats are a little tricky when it comes to their absorption and transportation. They are naturally insoluble in water, and because of this they cannot move through the brush border into the blood as an individual lipid unit.

To solve this problem, broken down fat particles mix with bile salts and form a water-soluble substance called a micelle. This micelle then interacts at the brush border of the small intestine. Fat particles move out of the micelle and into the intestinal cell, and the water-soluble bile salts continue down through the small intestine until they are reabsorbed and sent back to your liver.

So, after the broken down fat particles, which includes free fatty acids, monoglycerides, and some cholesterol, and phospholipid particles in the intestinal cell, or enterocyte, they actually re-form or combine back together into a larger original triglyceride form. Now you might ask, what's the point of breaking the fats down just to have them put back together again? Kind of sounds pointless, doesn't it? Well, the only way that fats can be absorbed out of the small intestine is in their smallest, most broken down form, but now they need to be transported.

As we noted earlier, fats are not only broken down differently than carbohydrates, they also travel differently. Fats must travel through the lymph system instead of the blood. The lymphatic system is a network of vessels that transports nutrients of the cells and collects cell waste products. The only way fats can travel out of the intestine and into the lymph is by combining into particles known as chylomicrons. Now, the re-formed fats combine with fat-soluble vitamins like vitamin A, D, E, or vitamin K, and a protein layer to form the full chylomicron. The chylomicron serves as the carrier for all digested fats that come from the food you eat.

When these chylomicrons are formed, they leave the intestinal cell and move into the lymphatic system. In a slow process, these fats move out into the lymphatic vessels and eventually into your blood where they freely travel to tissues to deliver fats for use or for storage. Some fat will be used by your muscle cells to produce energy, and some will be deposited into your fat cells. There are many things that can affect how fats are used and stored including when you last ate, your overall calorie intake for the day, your exercise habits, and how physically fit you are. I'll discuss this much more, later in the course.

Now, because this transportation process for fats is relatively slow and somewhat individualized, it could take anywhere from 30 minutes to 3 hours after you eat a high-fat meal for your blood lipids to reach the highest level. After about 5–6 hours from your meal, however, the chylomicrons will have delivered the fats to the designated tissues and your blood levels should return back to normal.

Now, our last macronutrient to discuss is protein. The structure of protein is very complex. Remember we talked about the digestion of protein making more demands on your body's metabolism. Well, that's because of the complexity of protein. Proteins stay fully intact until they get into your stomach, and large proteins are broken down into individual amino acids in the stomach by the very acidic stomach juice. Proteins that are still intact after leaving the stomach are broken down further in the top portion of the small intestine.

The end products of protein digestion are free amino acids, which are absorbed into your intestinal cells. Now, proteins are absorbed in a process more similar to carbohydrates than that of fats, and this process occurs along the entire length of the small intestine. Amino acids, just like glucose, require sodium-dependent carriers to get them into your intestinal cells.

There are several uses for particular amino acids within the intestinal cell; however, amino acids that are not used within the intestinal cells themselves are transported out of those cells and into the blood and make their first stop at your liver. About 50%–65% of all of the ingested amino acids are metabolized in your liver. The rest of the amino acids are used in other tissues, particularly the skeletal muscles, your kidneys, and the brain. In fact, these amino acids are used by skeletal muscle, for example, to directly repair muscle, or maintain muscle mass, or even help with growth of muscle, especially if it's combined with the proper exercise routine.

It is this skeletal muscle mass that has a huge influence on your muscle mass and your body fat ratio. The entire process of digestion and absorption is important to understand because it can determine how the food you eat makes you feel, and the food you eat is ultimately stored as body fat or glycogen or used as energy.

Now that we have discussed macronutrients' digestion, absorption, and transportation in detail, I want to touch briefly on the micronutrients. So, while it's the macronutrients' job to provide the body with energy, micronutrients, on the other hand, do not provide direct energy. However, they're vital in order to make all of the digestive processes occur, along with hundreds of other reactions and processes within the body. So the micronutrients are involved with energy production, but they just do not directly provide energy.

The water-soluble vitamins—vitamin C and the B-complex vitamins—are absorbed and transported through the blood. With the exception of vitamin B_{12}, which can be stored in your body for several years, water-soluble vitamins are not stored in your body for long periods of time. They are either used very quickly in the body or excreted in the urine, so we need to get them from the food we eat.

Fat-soluble vitamins, which are vitamins A, D, E, and K, are absorbed and transported very similarly to fats. They need to be packaged into the micelles to be absorbed and transported by chylomicrons throughout the lymph. Unlike water-soluble vitamins, excess fat-soluble vitamins can be stored in the body for a decent amount of time, and for this reason, fat-soluble vitamin deficiencies are much less common than water-soluble vitamin deficiencies.

So, back to the question about breakfast. As you can now understand, quite a bit happens inside your body after you take that first bite of your breakfast. For the most part, the GI tract of a healthy individual works like a well-oiled machine. Along with the digestive system itself, the endocrine and the nervous system play a major role in regulating digestion, absorption, and transportation of the nutrients. And the GI tract is really amazing. I mean, unfortunately, as people start to age, some functions of these systems begin to slow down, and the main cause for these changes is the degeneration of something called the enteric nervous system, and this is the nervous system specifically for the GI tract.

The enteric nervous system controls muscle contractions in the esophagus, and the stomach, and the colon, and when it degenerates, the movements of food and food-like products through the GI tract usually slows down. This can lead to serious GI complications including dysphagia, which is a swallowing difficulty; GI reflux; and even constipation. Gastric acid secretions can also be minimized with age, leading to bacterial overgrowth and inflammation.

So, along with biological and nervous system complications, elderly individuals may experience what has come to be known as anorexia of aging. No, this doesn't mean the elderly person has developed a psychological eating disorder. Anorexia of aging is referring to a physiological age-related reduction in appetite and energy intake, which ultimately leads to significant amounts of weight loss and muscle wasting. Basically, as you age, there may come a time when you just don't feel hungry very often. While this may lead to weight loss, this is not a good thing; oftentimes massive amounts of muscle mass is lost, too, and ultimately, low muscle mass prevents mobility.

Well, your best way to avoid or slow this age-related reduction in appetite is to simply make sure you are leading a healthy lifestyle—sounds pretty easy. But do some basic things like see your doctor regularly, exercise, and nourish yourself with foods that contribute to your health.

I want to touch on one final topic of interest that you may have heard about. This is called nutrient partitioning and the term is used to describe how the food you eat is stored or partitioned into a specific area like muscle or fat. So the question is this: "Can I eat a particular way to digest and absorb foods for the specific purpose of improving body composition?"

At the most basic level, the more of one type of food you eat—say, predominantly carbohydrate—the more of that fuel you will burn for energy. And the same thing would go for fat—the more that you eat, the more that you will use. What you really need to know is this: exercise is the most important and powerful tool to help you use your foods that you eat to improve your body composition. If you're active, you will tend to use the foods you eat to power your exercise, but if you are sedentary, your body will tend to partition the foods you eat to being stored as fat. So, no matter if your diet is mostly carbohydrates, fats, or proteins, if you're sedentary, only so much of your food will be used and stored for a healthy purpose before getting stored simply as body fat.

In fact, recently, Dr. Edward Archer, from the Nutrition Obesity Research Center at the University of Alabama at Birmingham, produced a short video on this specific topic and explained further how exercise is what drives the nutrients we eat towards a useful end, rather than being stored simply as excess body fat. You see, if you don't exercise, you essentially always have a full gas tank—you never really tap into those fuels to create any sort of deficit. So when you eat, no matter if it's a small meal or a large meal, there's less of an opportunity for your body to actually use the incoming fuels, and, as a result, you'll probably store them as body fat. But, when you exercise— like lifting weights, or walking, or working out vigorously to any extent—your body has the best chance to use the food you eat in a positive way.

Some people use nutrient partitioning strategies to try and fuel the body at the most optimal times to avoid excess weight and excess fat gain. Well, this is still a bit controversial, but we'll talk more about it later. For now, just know that exercise is the key to creating an internal environment in your body where the digestion and absorption of the foods you eat is optimal for powering your muscles, avoiding excessive fat storage, and ultimately improving your body composition.

So, back to breakfast: is breakfast really the most important meal of the day? Well, that's for you to find out. Over time your body will let you know what it needs—if it needs you to eat breakfast, it will tell you. If you listen to your body, it will respond in a positive way. You will feel healthy and ready to take on the day. If you don't listen to your body and don't provide the nutrients it needs at the right time, it will also respond. For example, if you're like me, then you probably have overeaten on occasion and then feel sluggish and tired.

We get great clues about the food needs we have and our overall health all the time, we just need to know what to listen for. All of this occurs because, essentially, you are what you eat—really. And my hope is that having a better understanding of the digestion and absorption process will help you to tune in more effectively to what your body is telling you.

Our body's cells, which make up who we are, are formed and nourished by the foods we eat; this is what we'll talk about next. So, try this: pay attention to the foods you eat and how they actually make you feel and perform. That's my plan—it's time for a snack.

Nutritional Needs and Cellular Function

I t is very easy to associate the food you eat with external, appearance-driven end points like body weight. But it's important to understand how the food you eat affects you on the inside, because your internal functioning directly influences how you feel, how you look, and your overall health. The nutrients you eat are an ingrained part of every cell and tissue that makes you what you are and who you are. In this lecture, you will learn which nutrients are needed to keep your cells healthy and what these nutrients actually do inside your body.

Cells in the Human Body

The cell is the smallest structural and functional unit of any organism. It is what every living being is made out of.

Our cells vary immensely in size, function, and chemical makeup. Each cell is a minute version of a human life. Each cell in our body must move, grow, consume food, excrete waste products, react to the environment it lives in, and reproduce.

Cells in the human body are constantly communicating to make the entire organism function. They communicate in response to your environment, what you touch, and how you move.

Cells bond together to make tissues; tissues make up our organs; our organs make up all of our organ systems; and our organ systems combine to make up the organism, which, in this case, is our body.

If your cells are not healthy, then they will not work properly. If the cells don't work properly, then the tissues won't work properly. If tissues aren't working, then the systems will begin to fail. Eventually, you will most likely experience increased fatigue, decreased physical capacity, improper nutrient use, and partitioning, which might ultimately lead to poor body composition as well as serious health consequences.

By keeping your cells healthy and fed with the proper nutrients, you are keeping your whole self healthy.

The average adult human body is made up of about 30 trillion cells. When the old cells become damaged, new ones are made to replace them. The nutrients we get from our food are used to make these new cells. This is the main reason why nutrition plays such a major role in cellular health and, therefore, in overall optimal functioning.

Also, certain nutrients from the food we eat can protect cells from early damage and provide the cells with the fuel needed to produce energy for our bodies.

Cell Components

The outermost component of the cell is the cell membrane. It is the boundary that separates the internal components of the cell from the outside environment. It keeps all of the cellular contents safe so that they can function properly without being damaged.

The cell membrane is referred to as "semipermeable," meaning that it has the ability to filter out important nutrients from damaging waste products. The membrane allows various nutrients to pass through the wall and sends the wastes out to be removed from the body. The permeability of this membrane also allows the cells to communicate clearly with one another.

All of the dietary macronutrients—carbohydrates, fats, and proteins—are found in the cell membrane. The most abundant form of fat found in the cell membrane is the phospholipids, which have a hydrophobic, or water-fearing, tail and a hydrophilic, or water-loving, head. This love-hate relationship with water is what gives the membrane its unique structure and stability.

Another type of fat-related compound found in the cell membrane is cholesterol. The cholesterol improves the mechanical stability of the membrane and helps regulate the fluidity.

The second major nutrient found in the cell membrane is protein. Proteins play a small role in forming the structure of the membrane, but they mostly contribute to the membrane functions. They direct proper operation within each individual cell and also the healthy functioning of your entire body.

Lastly, carbohydrates are also found in the cell membrane, but in smaller amounts compared to fats and proteins. Carbohydrates contribute to membrane structure and are present in the form of glycoproteins and glycolipids, which are protein and lipid molecules that have a glucose or sugar residue attached. These molecules also typically function to support cellular signaling.

The next important cellular structure that is essentially built from our foods is the nucleus. The nucleus is the largest organelle, or specialized structure, within the cell, and it contains the cell's DNA.

The nuclear envelope surrounds the nucleus. This two-layer membrane is composed primarily of lipids and proteins. It also contains minerals that are needed for activities within the nucleus.

The nucleus can be referred to as your "genetic storehouse" because it contains all of your personal information within its nuclear membrane walls in the DNA.

DNA is the blueprint for every one of the body's proteins. The proteins that make up your tissues, organs, chemical messengers, and more originate from the coding of DNA and the quality of food that we eat.

For this reason, it is vital that the nucleus has a solid structure to keep the DNA safe from damage that occurs from normal metabolic and oxidative stresses and aging. Nutrition also plays an important role in protecting your DNA.

Another cellular structure is the mitochondria. Known as the "powerhouse" of the cell, the mitochondria are responsible for energy production. All of the nutrients from your food are turned into energy within the microscopic mitochondria of your cells.

Just like the cell membrane and nuclear membrane, the mitochondrial membrane is made up of fats and proteins. The mitochondrial membrane has an inner and outer membrane, both of which play important roles in energy processes. The mitochondria also use many micronutrients to assist with producing energy.

The structural and functional integrity of the mitochondrial membrane is critical to your health. If the mitochondria structure and/or function is compromised, energy production from that cell will be compromised. This mitochondrial dysfunction can contribute to several chronic diseases, including diabetes, heart disease, and Parkinson's disease.

Omegas

Unsaturated fats are necessary for strong cell membranes. The membrane is semipermeable thanks to the fluid structure of the fats. However, saturated and trans fats are much more rigid than unsaturated fats. They don't function the same way as the unsaturated fats, and they cause membranes to be much more rigid than what is optimal, potentially limiting the functionality of cells.

Diets that are too high in one type of fat—for example, trans fats—might lead to rigid and brittle cell membranes that cannot communicate as well as if they were composed of a better mix of fat types. In general, diets high in unsaturated fats will promote healthy cell membranes.

Two categories of unsaturated fats to take particular note of are omega-6 fatty acids and omega-3 fatty acids.

Omega-6 fatty acids are highly concentrated in walnuts, almonds, and various types of vegetable oils, including corn, soybean, safflower, cottonseed, sunflower seed, and peanut oil.

Rich sources of omega-3 fatty acids include fatty fish, such as salmon, tuna, cod, and trout. Some seeds and nuts also contain omega-3 fatty acids, such as flaxseed, but to a much lower extent.

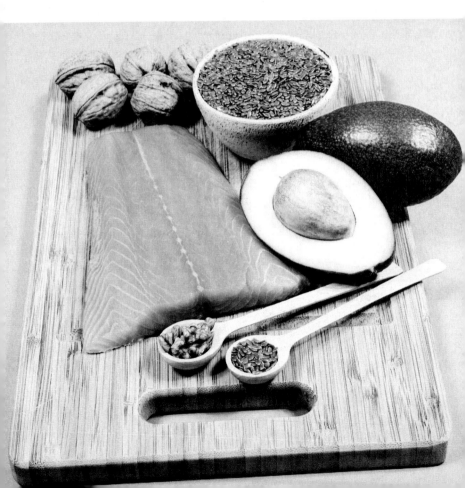

Both omega-6 and omega-3 fatty acids are essential for good health; however, they both play very different roles. Omega-3 fatty acids have an anti-inflammatory effect in the body, whereas omega-6 fatty acids have a pro-inflammatory effect.

While some amount of inflammation can help protect the body from infection and injury, too much inflammation can lead to heart disease, metabolic syndrome, diabetes, Alzheimer's disease, arthritis, and many different types of cancer. As opposed to omega-6 fatty acids, omega-3 fatty acids are known to lower the risk of these diseases by decreasing the amount of inflammation within the body.

Other nutrients required to maintain healthy cell membranes include high-quality proteins, fat-soluble vitamins (vitamins A, D, E, and K), and vitamin C. Whole grains, vegetables, fruits, and lean poultry and fish will provide you with all of these nutrients and will keep your cell membranes in top shape.

Because the cell nucleus and your DNA are also made up of nutrients, the quality of food you eat can greatly impact their structure and function as well. Unfortunately, despite the barrier provided by the nucleus, DNA can be damaged from any excess potentially harmful substances (often called toxins) circulating around in the body.

Damage to DNA can also occur from reactive oxygen species or excessive oxidative stress, which can be produced as by-products from the energy we produce from food or even from excessive exercise.

If reactive oxygen species make their way into the nuclear membrane, they can potentially alter normal DNA functioning. If this occurs, the proteins that the particular DNA strand produced will no longer be available to your body. This will lead to poor functioning in your body and could lead to various disease states.

One way to protect this from happening is by eating quality sources of polyunsaturated fats. You can focus on getting these fats from sources like fatty fish, flaxseeds, walnuts, and even soybeans.

Other nutrients that are needed to protect DNA include high-quality protein, antioxidants, and vitamins. The easiest way to get these nutrients into your diet is to consume foods like lean meat, eggs, dairy, colorful vegetables, whole grains, and fruits.

B Vitamins, Iron, Sulfur

The mitochondria can use the nutrients we eat and turn them into energy for everything we do. However, not all foods are created equal when it comes to efficiency of energy production.

Most of the energy that the mitochondria produce comes from fats and glucose (carbohydrate) either stored in your body or from your diet. This energy ultimately ends up in the form of adenosine triphosphate (ATP).

The process of making ATP from our foods is very complex. The obvious nutrients that are needed for these processes to occur are the energy-yielding macronutrients: carbohydrates, fats, and proteins. However, essential nutrients that are often overlooked when talking about energy production are the B vitamins, iron, and sulfur.

The B vitamins work to transfer electrons through the electron transport chain, which produces a massive amount of ATP in your mitochondria. Iron and sulfur are important components of the protein structures within the major energy-producing systems of your cells and are used to simply transport oxygen around your body.

If iron and sulfur are not available from the diet to the mitochondria, energy production will suffer. Just as with the cell membranes and the nuclear membranes, nutritional support for healthy mitochondria function comes from eating foods with a lot of nutrients that are minimally processed. Things like green leafy vegetables, complex carbohydrates, and lean proteins are a great start.

Exercise Levels

Some factors that have nothing to do with food can also impact our cellular health and function. For example, excessive exercise can actually cause some damage. Exercise naturally increases the production of free radicals, which are molecules that have an unpaired electron in their outer shell. The missing electron in these molecules causes them to be unstable and highly reactive.

To regain stability, the free radical molecule works to steal electrons from healthy cells in your body. When this happens, the free radical leaves a healthy cell damaged and unable to perform its usual functions.

This free radical damage does not stop with one cell. Once one free radical attack occurs, it sets off a domino effect. The newly damaged cells move on to other healthy cells as they attempt to become neutral again. Excessive free radical damage has been associated with accelerated aging, cancer, diabetes, and coronary artery disease.

Luckily, our bodies have the ability to fight free radical attacks by forming three natural antioxidants: glutathione, catalase, and superoxide dismutase. These substances donate extra electrons to free radicals and prevent them from damaging healthy cells.

The major problem with exercise occurs when it is too extreme, causing the production of free radicals to exceed the body's ability to produce antioxidants. This does not mean that you should shy away from all intense exercise, however, because your diet can help ward off this exercise-induced oxidative stress—a diet that includes lots of fruits and vegetables that are full of antioxidants.

Being still and sedentary can also have a negative impact on cellular health and integrity. Sedentary lifestyles are associated with increased cardiovascular disease, atherosclerosis, overweight/obesity, diabetes, accelerated aging, and more. Oxidative stress plays a major role in these dysfunctions. Sedentary lifestyles can lead to increased oxidative stress and vascular dysfunction.

Leading a physically active life (but not excessively active or sedentary) will help keep our cells healthy, happy, and functioning to the best of their ability.

Try This

Try eating more omega-3 fatty acids to decrease your ratio of omega-6 to omega-3 fatty acids.

Questions to Consider

1. What is really meant by "you are what you eat"?

2. Provide an example for where specific foods you eat are used for your cellular functioning.

Nutritional Needs and Cellular Function

I t's very easy to associate the food you eat with external, appearance-driven end points like body weight, but it's important to think about and understand how the food you eat affects you on the inside, too. This is important because your internal functioning directly influences how you feel, how you look, and your overall health, which includes a healthy body composition.

What you eat will ultimately make up portions of your cells, skin, hair, blood transportation systems, muscle, fat, and more. The nutrients you eat are not just being transported around throughout our digestive systems and in the blood like we've talked about, they are also an ingrained part of every cell tissue that makes us who we are and what we do. So, while the phrase 'you are what you eat' is probably a bit overstated or at least oversimplified, it is, in large part, true. Our bodies are to a significant extent composed of the foods that we eat. Let me explain.

Early nutrition recommendations focused strictly on the function of the human body. The main question for scientists and nutritionists was, "Which nutrients, and in what amounts, are needed keep the human body functioning to prevent it from any obvious disease?" Nutrition recommendations were basically made on a trial and error basis. Well, trial and error still has a place in nutrition, but nutrition science has evolved to be more than simply adjusting the amounts of nutrients we need to prevent disease. Nutrition science is now driven by a belief that eating should be about living to the very best that you can—living optimally, not just merely avoiding illness.

Researchers have discovered that not only do the nutrients from food affect how we function, but food affects how every single process inside our cells functions as well. And in order to understand this, and how each of us is made up of the same nutrients that are in the foods we choose to eat, we must begin with the basics. This takes us all the way down to the individual, microscopic cell.

The cell structure is the smallest structural and functional unit of any organism; it is the very thing that every living being is made out of. Our cells vary immensely in size, function, and chemical makeup. Each cell in our body must move, grow, consume food, excrete waste products, react to the environment it lives in, and reproduce. Cells in the human body are constantly communicating in order to make the entire organism function. They communicate in response to our environment, what you touch, and how you move.

So, cells bond together to make tissues, and tissues make up our organs, and our organs make up our organ system, and our organ system combine to make the entire organism, which, in this case, is your body. If your cells are not healthy they will not work properly, and if the cells don't work properly then the tissues won't work properly, and if tissues aren't working then the systems will begin to fail. You can see how this can easily snowball out of control. Eventually, you will most likely experience increased fatigue, decreased physical capacity, improper nutrient use, and nutrient partitioning, which ultimately lead to a poor body composition as well as some serious health consequences. By keeping your cells healthy and fed with the proper nutrients, you are keeping your whole self healthy.

Consider this: the average adult body is made up of about 30 trillion cells. When old cells become damaged, new ones are made to replace them, and the nutrients we get from our food are used to make these new cells. This is the main reason why nutrition plays such a major role in cellular health, and therefore in our optimal functioning. Also, certain nutrients, like the food we eat, can protect our cells from damage, and provide cells with the fuel needed to produce energy for our bodies.

Just think about your cells and their need to be replaced constantly. Then think about the type of food you choose to eat. Are you choosing foods that would help make the healthiest cells possible? Help make the healthiest body composition? The best environment to be active and stay active? This now leads me to the main question for this lecture: "What nutrients are needed to keep our cells healthy, and what do these nutrients actually do inside your body?"

To answer this question, let's take an even deeper dive into the cell by looking at some of the individual cell components, and discover where the nutrients that you eat fit in. Let's start with the outermost component, the cell membrane.

The cell membrane is the boundary that separates the internal components of the cell from the outside environment. It keeps all the cellular contents safe so that they can function properly without being damaged. The cell membrane is referred to as semi-permeable, meaning that it has the ability to filter out important nutrients from damaging waste products. The membrane allows various nutrients to pass through the wall and sends the waste products out to be removed from the body. The permeability of this membrane also allows the cells to communicate clearly with one another, as we mentioned previously. The membrane must be fluid and mobile, rather than too rigid and too tight, to allow for optimal functioning and adaptation to the internal environment. Here's the thing: all of the dietary macronutrients—carbohydrates, fats, and proteins—are found in the cell membrane.

The most abundant form of fat found in the cell membrane is the phospholipids, which are made of a glycerol backbone, a phosphate molecule, and two fatty acids. Yes, fat is needed for proper cell structure and function. The phospholipids have a hydrophobic or water fearing tail and a hydrophilic or water loving head. This love-hate relationship with water is what gives the membrane its unique structure and stability.

Imagine what a drop of oil looks like and acts like in water. This is what a cell looks like and acts like in the blood, but at a microscopic level. The unique geometry of the phospholipid, with the hydrophilic heads and the hydrophobic tails, causes them to spontaneously align into bilayers, like a sandwich, where the bread would be the phospholipid heads and the inside of the sandwich would contain the phospholipid tails. This way, the phospholipids are positioned with the hydrophilic or water loving phosphate heads facing outwards, and the hydrophobic water fearing hydrocarbon tails of the fatty acids aligning on the inside of the bilayer. So, the hydrophilic heads in a cell's plasma membrane face both the water based outside the cell and the water-based cytoplasm on the interior of the cell.

Another type of fat-related compound found in the cell membrane is cholesterol. The cholesterol improves the mechanical stability of the membrane and helps to regulate the fluidity. If the diet is too low in cholesterol, cell membrane structure can be compromised. We will discuss this more in just a few minutes.

The second major nutrient found in the cell membrane is protein. Proteins play a small role in forming the structure of the membrane, but they mostly contribute to the membrane functions. They direct proper operation within each individual cell, and also the healthy functioning of your entire body. You see, the proteins you eat have numerous functions in your body that go way beyond the popular thought that they only need to be eaten to help with muscle function, quality, and size.

At the cellular level, proteins serve as pumps, gates, receptors, and enzymes or catalysts for biochemical reactions. They're responsible for the advanced communication that occurs between your cells, and they provide attachment sites for various molecules. Cellular communication occurs at all times for various reasons. They communicate to take up nutrients from your bloodstream, to excrete waste products from the body, to signal chemical reactions, and more. All of this communication is completed by the proteins that are embedded in your cell membrane.

Proteins serve as channels by opening and closing when the cell receives a particular signal. They also can act as information transporters for what is going on outside the cell and within other surrounding adjacent cells. Without this sophisticated communication network, the cells throughout your body will not work together, and bodily functions will start to fail. Think of it like a game of Telephone. As soon as one message is not transmitted or received properly, the entire message is messed up, with the end result being the wrong message or no message, ultimately creating an environment that is likely not optimal for body composition, health, or performance.

Lastly, carbohydrates are also found in the cell membrane, but in smaller amounts compared to fats and proteins. Carbohydrates contribute to membrane structure and are present in the form of glycoproteins and glycolipids that are protein and lipid molecules that have a glucose or sugar residue attached to it. These molecules also typically function to support cellular signaling. Now that we understand how the nutrients in our food form and sustain our cell membranes, let's move on and focus to inside the cell.

The next important cellular structure that is essentially built from our foods is the nucleus. The nucleus is the largest organelle, or specialized structure, within the cell and it contains the cell's DNA. The nuclear envelope surrounds the nucleus. This two-layer membrane is composed primarily of lipids and proteins. It also contains minerals that are needed for activities within the nucleus itself. The nucleus can be referred to as your genetic storehouse, because it contains all of your personal information within its nuclear membrane walls in the DNA.

Now, DNA is a blueprint for every single one of the body proteins. The proteins that make up your tissues, your organs, and your chemical messengers and more originate from the coding of DNA and the quality of the food that we eat. For this reason, it's vital that the nucleus has a solid structure to keep the DNA safe from damage that occurs from normal metabolic and oxidative stresses including aging itself. Nutrition also plays an important role in protecting your DNA. In order to understand why the food you eat is important to your DNA, we need to quickly go over the makeup of it.

DNA is one of two very important nucleic acids, with the second being RNA. These are made of a nitrogen base, a 5-carbon sugar unit, and a phosphate molecule. RNA and DNA work together to provide the codes for your cells to produce new proteins and new cells themselves. You can see how what you eat influences your DNA. Think about how important the protein you get from your diet is, now that you know all of the different roles that proteins can play in your body.

The final cellular structure that we will discuss is the mitochondria. You may remember the mitochondria as the powerhouse of the cell from your high school biology days. This nickname was given to the mitochondria because it is part of the cell that is responsible for energy production. All of the nutrients from your food are turned into energy within the microscopic mitochondria of your cells. In fact, later in this course I'll go through how the food you eat turns into energy for you to use to alter body composition or to power a workout.

Each cell that you have contains anywhere from several hundred to over 2000 mitochondria, depending on the amount of energy that cell needs to function optimally. Your heart and your skeletal muscles are very hardworking organs that need a lot of energy, and cells within these organs may have up to 40% of their space occupied by mitochondria.

Again, just like the cell membrane and the nuclear membrane, the mitochondrial membrane is made up of fats and proteins. The mitochondrial membrane has an inner and an outer layer, both of which play important roles in energy processes. The inner membrane is made up of about 75% protein. These proteins function in the final stage of energy production in something called the electron transport chain. The mitochondria also use many micronutrients to assist with producing energy. The B-vitamins are particularly important micronutrients in the energy production processes of the mitochondria.

It's important to keep in mind that the structural and functional integrity of the mitochondrial membrane is absolutely critical to your health. If the mitochondria structure and/or function is compromised, energy production from that cell will be compromised. This mitochondrial dysfunction can contribute to several chronic diseases, including diabetes, heart disease, and Parkinson's disease, just to name a few.

Now, let's try to put all of this together into a more practical understanding. The structures of your cells are made up of fats, proteins, carbohydrates, vitamins, and minerals. The foods we eat every single day are made up of fats, proteins, carbohydrates, vitamins, and minerals. Do you hear any similarities or is this just a coincidence? Definitely not. You can see now why it is often said that you are what you eat. The foods you eat have a major influence on your cellular function because they ultimately become your cells.

Now, there are some very specific nutrients that can impact your internal cellular functioning. Let's start with unsaturated fats. Unsaturated fats are necessary for strong cell membranes. Remember I mentioned before that the membrane is semi-permeable? Well, that's thanks to the fluid structure of the fats. However, saturated and trans fats are much more rigid than unsaturated fats. They don't function the same way as the unsaturated fats, and they cause membranes to be much more rigid than is optimal, potentially limiting the functionality of the cells.

Diets that are too high in one type of fat—for example, trans fats—might lead to a rigid, brittle cell membrane that cannot communicate as well as if they were comprised of a better mix of fat types. This is one reason why many nutritionists recommend eating all types of fats so that one type doesn't predominate in the diet and end up altering the optimal functioning of those cells. In general, diets high in unsaturated fats will promote healthy cell membranes.

Two categories of the unsaturated fats to take particular note of are the omega-6 fatty acids and the omega-3 fatty acids. Omega-6 fatty acids are highly concentrated in foods like walnuts, almonds, and various types of vegetable oils, including corn, soybean, safflower, cottonseed, sunflower seed, and peanut oil. These are all types of oils that are in a majority of any processed, boxed, pre-packaged foods that you probably have in your kitchen pantry. Rich sources of omega-3 fatty acids include fatty fish such as salmon, tuna, cod, and trout. Some seeds and nuts also contain omega-3s, like flaxseed, but to a much lower extent. Both omega-6 and omega-3 fatty acids are essential for good health; however, they play very different roles.

Omega-3s have an anti-inflammatory effect in the body, whereas the omega-6s have a pro-inflammatory effect. This pro-inflammatory effect of omega-6 fatty acids may sound bad; however, some inflammation is actually necessary to some extent. Some amount of inflammation can help protect the body from infection and from injury. For example, if you roll your ankle, inflammation sets in to immobilize your ankle so you can begin to heal. Same thing goes for a cut—the inflammation shows that an immune response is underway to help fight off any pathogens that might make you sick. But, as you probably know, too much inflammation can lead to other things like heart disease, metabolic syndrome, diabetes, Alzheimer's disease, arthritis, and many different types of cancer. Conversely, omega-3s are known to lower the risk of these diseases by decreasing the amount of inflammation within the body.

In the current Western diet, the omega-6 to omega-3 ratio has skyrocketed because of the high intake of vegetable oils rich in omega-6 fatty acids. In order to protect the cells from damage, this ratio needs to be decreased. To lower the omega-6 to omega-3 fatty acid ratio, you need to decrease your intake of processed vegetable oils that are high in omega-6 fatty acids, as well as increase your intake of fatty fish, flaxseeds, chia seeds, and fish oil, which are all rich in omega-3 fats.

Other nutrients required to maintain healthy cell membranes include high quality proteins, fat-soluble vitamins like A, D, E, and K, vitamin C, whole grains, vegetables, fruits, and lean poultry and fish will all provide you with these nutrients to keep your cell membranes in top shape.

Next, what about the cell nucleus and your DNA? Naturally, it makes sense that, since these cellular components are also made up of nutrients, the quality of your food you eat can greatly impact their structure and function as well. But the DNA never leaves the protective barrier of the nucleus, so this means that your DNA is safe from harmful substances that you may eat, right? Well, not really, and here's why.

Unfortunately, despite the barrier provided by the nucleus, DNA can be damaged from any excess potential harmful substances, often called toxins, circulating around in the body. Now, toxins is a term that is far too widely used by so-called nutrition experts, but you can produce molecules that damage your DNA. For example, these molecules can come from excess trans fats and high amounts of omega-6 fatty acids, compared to omega-3 fatty acids in your diet.

Also, there is some concern, albeit controversial, about pesticides that we may consume from processed and conventionally grown foods. There appears to be a relationship between these sorts of foods and some cellular damage over time. I don't think we should be overly worried because we have many natural processes to help stop or repair any damage, and just washing your foods that you purchase can go a long way in reducing that risk.

But damage to DNA can also occur from reactive oxygen species or excessive oxidative stress, which can be produced as a by-product from the energy, or ATP, we produce from food or even from excessive exercise. If reactive oxygen species makes their way into the nuclear membrane, they can potentially alter normal DNA functioning. If this occurs, the proteins that the particular DNA strand produced will no longer be available to your body. I think you can see how this will lead to poor functioning in your body, and, in worst case scenario, could lead to various disease states. But here's the beautiful part: one way to protect this from happening is, once again, by eating quality sources of polyunsaturated fats. You can focus on getting these fats from sources like fatty fish, flaxseeds, walnuts, and even soybeans.

Other nutrients that are needed to protect DNA include high quality protein, antioxidants, and vitamins like vitamin E and C, the carotenoids, folate, and vitamin B_{12}. The easiest way to get all of these nutrients into your diet, though, is to consume foods like lean meats, eggs, dairy, colorful vegetables, whole grains, and fruits. If you do this, you will have the best chance at protecting your DNA from excessive damage.

Last, let's look at what foods most efficiently keep our cellular energy production working well. As you'll learn about in great detail in the next lecture, the mitochondria can use the nutrients we eat to turn them into energy for everything we do. However, not all foods are created equal when it comes to efficient energy production. Most of the energy that the mitochondria produce comes from fats and glucose, or carbohydrate, that's either stored in your body or comes in from your diet. This energy ultimately ends up in the form of adenosine triphosphate, also known as ATP.

The process of making ATP from our foods is very complex. The obvious nutrients that are needed for these processes to occur are the energy-yielding macronutrients: carbohydrates, fats, and proteins. However, essential nutrients that are often overlooked when talking about energy production are the B-vitamins, iron, and sulfur. The B-vitamins work to transfer electrons through the electron transport chain, which ultimately produces massive amount of ATP in your mitochondria. Iron and sulfur are important components of the protein structures within the major energy-producing systems of your cells, and are used to simply transport oxygen around your body.

If iron and sulfur are not available from the diet for the mitochondria, energy production will suffer, and, just as with the cell membranes and the nuclear membranes, nutritional support for healthy mitochondrial function comes from eating foods with a lot of nutrients that are minimally processed. Things like green leafy vegetables, complex carbohydrates, and lean proteins are a great start.

One thing to also understand is that some factors that have nothing to do with food can also impact your cellular health and function. For example, excessive exercise can actually cause some damage. And keep in mind that excessive is the key word here. Now, you may be scratching your head a bit and saying, "I thought that exercise was good for your health. How could it cause damage?" It seems contradictory, but it's actually true. Exercise naturally increases the production of free radicals, which are molecules that have an unpaired electron in their outer shell. This missing electron in these molecules causes them to be unstable and highly reactive.

But, to regain stability, the free radical molecule works to steal electrons from healthy cells in your body. And when this happens, the free radical leaves the healthy cell damaged and unable to perform its usual functions. This free radical damage doesn't stop with just one cell; once one free radical attack occurs, it sets off a domino effect, and the newly damaged cell moves on to other healthy cells as they attempt to become neutral again. A single chain reaction can lead to thousands of damaged cells just from one intense bout of exercise, and excessive free radical damage has been associated with accelerated aging, cancer, diabetes, and coronary artery disease.

Now, don't let this scare you too much, and don't stop exercising because these potential free radical attacks might occur, because, luckily, our bodies have the ability to fight free radical attacks by forming three natural antioxidants known as glutathione, catalase, and superoxide dismutase. These substances donate extra electrons to free radicals and prevent them from damaging healthy cells. The major problem with exercise occurs when it's too extreme, causing the production of free radicals to exceed the body's ability to produce antioxidants.

For example, a study conducted at Hebrew University in Israel in conjunction with the National Institutes of Health in Maryland looked at this exercise-induced oxidative stress. Thirty-one men completed a 6-month, 5 days per week training schedule that involved two very extreme 30- and 50-mile marches while carrying an extra 77 pounds—or 35 kilograms—of weight. Well, not surprisingly, after these long marches, there was significant cellular damage. There was also significant increase in liver enzymes, indicating more work being done by your liver and possibly liver injury.

So, here it was clear that excessive exercise led to increased oxidative damage, causing cellular damage. This study was in men but my lab has also seen excessive cell damage in ultra-endurance athletes of both sexes. This, again, does not mean you should shy away from all intense exercise, because your diet can help ward off this exercise-induced oxidative stress. Once again, the answer is a diet that includes lots of fruits and veggies that are full of antioxidants such as vitamin C, and vitamin E, vitamin A, and selenium. A great newly researched postexercise supplement to reduce oxidative stress is tart cherry juice—it's loaded with antioxidants.

Now, before you think that sitting on the couch is a way to avoid even worrying about excessive exercise damage, you need to keep in mind that being still and sedentary can also have a negative impact on cellular health and integrity. You see, it is well known that sedentary lifestyles are associated with increased cardiovascular disease, atherosclerosis, overweight and obesity, diabetes, accelerated aging, and more. And it's amazing just how long we sit every single day.

Yet again, reactive oxygen species are involved here. Oxidative stress plays a major role in these dysfunctions, and what people may be unaware of is that not only does excessive exercise cause this stress, but complete physical inactivity also causes this. In fact, researchers from Germany compared the effects of physical inactivity, or doing nothing, with voluntary running in mice. And after 6 weeks of remaining completely inactive and doing no physical activity, there was a significant increase in markers of cellular damage, vascular dysfunction, and an increased production of the antioxidant superoxide dismutase that was likely produced to prevent the excessive damage that was going on. Overall, the results of this study, and several others, suggests that sedentary lifestyles can lead to increased oxidative stress and vascular dysfunction.

The logical conclusion we can draw from these two extreme cases—extreme exercise and complete inactivity—is that leading a physically active life, but not excessively active or sedentary, will help keep our cells healthy, happy, and functioning to the best of their ability. Ultimately, this sort of cellular environment is exactly what you want for optimal functioning. This is where you will have the best chance of using the food you eat to provide fuel and nourishment, rather than excessive storage as body fat. This means that your cellular health is involved in creating a chance for you to optimize your body composition.

Now, before we close out our discussion on cellular function and how nutrition is so much a part of cellular health, I want to briefly touch on a fairly new scientific research area called nutritional genomics. Nutritional genomics is the study of how our genes interact with environmental factors, and, most specifically, the bioactive compounds of food.

As you have learned, your DNA holds all the information necessary for the development and function of your body. The genes within the DNA are responsible for coding for all of the proteins that carry out your cellular functions. As the study of nutritional genomics evolves, scientists may one day be able to help individualize your nutritional needs more efficiently than ever before. With this knowledge, you could one day even choose foods that have medicinal and health benefits that are specific to you.

For example, it is well known through nutritional genomics research that cocoa and red wine both contain bioactive substances that can help reduce the risk of heart disease. However, the components of cocoa may not be beneficial for lowering your risk of heart disease, but they may lower mine. And, conversely, the effects of red wine may not be advantageous to my health, but they may be for yours, all because of the differences in our genetic makeup. The same things could even be said for why certain compounds like caffeine or even certain medications work better for some people than for others.

More information will come from that nutritional genomics research in years to come, but right now we know that the foods you eat serve as the building blocks for your cells, and you can understand now why it's said that you are what you eat. Simply put, your body is only as healthy as the foods you eat. Just like a car, if you put low-grade fuel into your car, your gas mileage would not be as high as it would if you filled your tank with premium. However, once you start to fill your gas tank with premium-grade fuel, over time your gas mileage will begin to soar, the engine will run clean, and you will get a lot more life out of your car. And, just like your car, your body needs premium-grade fuel to run as efficiently as possible. Sure, it can run on poor food choices, but not optimally, and not efficiently.

Our bodies work to replace billions of cells each day, and the nutrients we eat are the building blocks for these new cells. If the cells are built correctly, our bodies will have no issue growing, developing, and flourishing. If the cells are built with errors or with low-grade materials, our body is at risk for developing disease and ending life early. A healthy diet, accompanied by physical activity, is the recipe for healthy genes, healthy cells, and ultimately your best body composition and health possible. So try this: try eating more omega-3 fatty acids to decrease your omega-6 to omega-3 fatty acid ratio.

Bioenergetics: Converting Food to Energy

I n this lecture, you will learn how we produce energy from the food we eat and which food choices might be best based on your activity level. Knowing how to use your energy systems to your advantage is a huge asset when wanting to change your body composition. After digesting and absorbing the food you eat, it is amazing how it is used to provide energy for everything you want to do, including changing your body composition.

Bioenergetics and Metabolism

- Bioenergetics is the process of converting the components of the foods we eat—such as carbohydrates, fats, and proteins—into a usable form of energy. Bioenergetics relates directly to your overall metabolism, which is the sum of all energy transformations that occur in your body.

- We produce energy by converting the food we eat into adenosine triphosphate (ATP), which is often called the "energy currency" of the body because in a sense we "pay" for all of our biological actions with ATP.

- To release the energy from ATP, it is broken apart in a process called hydrolysis, using an enzyme called ATPase. ATP is broken apart into smaller components to produce adenosine diphosphate (ADP), a single phosphate, and energy.

- Food is eaten and eventually converted to energy (ATP), carbon dioxide, and water. And the ATP is used to produce work for all of your metabolic needs and daily activities. Heat is also produced in the process of making energy.

Essentially, you simply changed the chemical composition of the food you eat into other forms of useable energy and heat. This follows the first law of thermodynamics, which states that energy is neither created nor destroyed, but only changed in form.

ATP is the stored chemical energy that links the energy-producing and energy-requiring functions within all cells. This energy fuels all forms of biological work, such as digestion of food and muscle contractions.

Making and Replacing Stores of ATP

We have three energy systems that make and replace our stores of ATP for us. In all three systems, a phosphate group is added to an adenosine diphosphate (ADP) molecule in a process called phosphorylation to create adenosine triphosphate (ATP). That phosphate is added to ADP and then stored as ATP until the energy from ATP is needed for activities, such as exercising.

Each energy system has a specific role and works at the highest rate based on how hard or intensely you are working. Each system has a different way of providing ATP, but they are used on a continuum and overlap quite a bit.

In addition, certain parts of each of the three energy systems can also work to provide ATP in the other two energy systems. In this way, you get the most ATP out of whatever you are doing and whatever fuel source—carbohydrates, fats, or proteins—you are using to provide energy.

By understanding these energy systems, you will gain the ability to decide what to eat, or what certain nutrients may be best to support whatever you are doing. This allows you to better understand how to eat what you can use best for energy production, limit storing excess body fat, and improve success in fat loss.

The three energy-producing systems are the creatine phosphate system, the glycolytic system, and the oxidative system. All of these systems are at work for us to provide energy, but one system is typically used more than the others during different exercise and rest scenarios.

The creatine phosphate system works hardest for us during maximal-intensity exercise. In this system, you will create ATP by first combining a phosphate with stored creatine, which is a combination of amino acids, to form creatine phosphate. Then, the enzyme creatine kinase breaks off the phosphate from creatine phosphate and allows it to combine with ADP. This forms more ATP and free creatine.

This process is anaerobic, meaning that it occurs without oxygen. This does not mean that you aren't taking in oxygen by breathing; it just means that ATP can be produced without the presence of oxygen in the cells.

The creatine phosphate energy system works quickly but does not last for long; about 30 seconds is all you'll get (depending on your fitness level), but it is the most rapid method to regenerate ATP.

The second energy system is the glycolytic system, also called anaerobic glycolysis, which relies on carbohydrates as a fuel source to make energy. The glycolytic system lasts longer than the creatine phosphate system—but probably not more than about two minutes while you are working hard. Once again, you produce ATP without the need for oxygen in your cells.

Glycolysis is the breakdown of carbohydrates or glucose to make ATP. Glucose is in any type of carbohydrate that you eat or drink, such as a sports drink or piece of bread. Once the glucose is in your blood, you need to get it into your cells to break it down to either make ATP or store it as glycogen for later use.

You can use stored glycogen or the glucose from food that you've recently eaten to make ATP. In both cases, you first need to get the glucose into your cells. There is an elaborate system of proteins called GLUT transporters that assist with this. The glycolytic energy system is one you rely on a lot during any kind of physical activity.

The third energy system is the oxidative system, which relies on carbohydrates, fats, and in some cases protein to provide ATP. The oxidative system is the long and slow system, which kicks in after about 90 seconds to 2 minutes of activity and can last almost indefinitely—as long as the intensity of activity is low to moderate. It's aerobic, unlike the other two energy systems, so it uses oxygen.

The oxidative system is active for most of your day: while sitting at a computer, walking around, and even just watching television. Carbohydrates and fats are the primary fuel sources used to provide ATP in the oxidative system, but this system can also metabolize some protein for energy production. This does not typically happen, though, unless someone has been exercising for a very long time (longer than two to three hours) or for someone who has not eaten in a long time.

You never *only* use fat or *only* use carbohydrates. The reality is that the fuel used to provide ATP in this energy system is typically a combination of fuels and not an all-or-none kind of action.

Fitness and the Respiratory Exchange Ratio

The fitter you are, the better you become at using fat as a fuel source. Also, the fitter you are, the better you are at saving your stored glucose or glycogen until you really need it—such as when you pick up the intensity of your exercise. This is just one more reason to consider adding physical activity into your daily lifestyle: It will impact the fuel you use all day long.

As you exercise and your training status increases, you can increase the number of mitochondria that you have in the cells of the muscles at work. This called mitochondrial density, and you want it to be high. The mitochondria are the organelles within your cells that help you produce large amounts of ATP, so it makes sense that the more exercise you put into your lifestyle, the better you are at making energy.

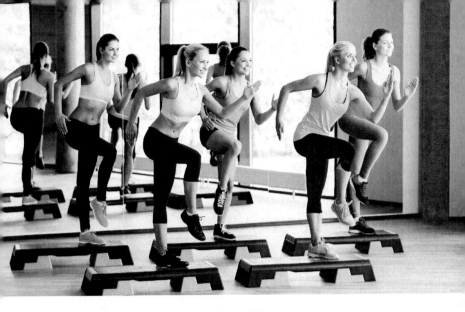

Another benefit is that you can increase the number of capillaries, or small blood vessels, you have to bring blood, oxygen, and other nutrients to working muscles. This is called capillary density, which you also want to be high.

Additionally, with exercise training, you actually increase the activity of enzymes called lipases that increase fat breakdown. Exercise also increases the hormones that are used to help initiate this breakdown.

By making exercise a part of your life, you increase your body's ability to effectively use fuels. You decrease your reliance on carbohydrates and use more fat for fuel, regardless of what you are doing all day. This means that at rest and during exercise, you are burning a greater amount of fat. Over time, this will impact your body composition.

The fat that is used to make ATP can come from stored fat tissue, such as the fat around your waist and hips, or from dietary fat that you've eaten. You even have fat stored in your muscles to use for energy; this type of fat is called intramuscular triglyceride (IMTG).

Interestingly, you'll find IMTGs in both very fit people and also out-of-shape people. But how these storage depots of fat are utilized is extremely different between the fit and unfit. For the out-of-shape people, these intramuscular fat stores can do harm and alter the proper cell signaling that should occur in response to various hormones. But in physically active people, the intramuscular fats tend to be used as an energy source, sparing glycogen and increasing fat use for activity.

So, while both fat and carbohydrates will be used in the oxidative system, the amount of fat used compared to how much carbohydrate used is highly dependent on a number of key factors, including when you last ate, when you last exercised, how fit you are, and what hormones are circulating in your blood.

The human body is amazing and adjusts to what you eat by burning more of that type of nutrient. This ability to shift easily from one fuel source to another based on the circumstance is called metabolic flexibility.

In a lab setting, we can determine which fuel source (fat or carbohydrate) you are using by measuring the amounts of carbon dioxide and oxygen in your breath at rest or during exercise. The ratio of carbon dioxide produced to oxygen consumed is called the respiratory exchange ratio (RER). When burning 100 percent fat for fuel, your RER is equal to 0.7, but when burning 100 percent carbohydrate for energy, your RER is 1.

Basically, the faster and harder you go, the greater percent of carbohydrate that will be used to make energy, or ATP. But there will always be a mix of carbohydrates, fats, and some proteins used to produce ATP. The more metabolically flexible you are, the better you will be at using all the energy sources at the exact right moment.

Aim to change your food intake and carbohydrate intake based on your activity level each day.

1. If you like to walk as your primary form of physical activity, what fuel are you most likely to use to provide energy? What source of food might you want to consider eating more of? Less of?

2. What activities might the first energy system, the creatine phosphate system, be used for in your typical daily routine?

3. How will understanding nutrient bioenergetics impact the choices you will make while trying to improve body composition?

Bioenergetics: Converting Food to Energy

N ow we need to learn about how we produce energy from the food we eat, and which food choices might be best based on your activity level. Well, bioenergetics is the process of converting the compounds of the foods we eat, like carbohydrates, fats, and proteins, into a usable form of energy. Bioenergetics then relates directly to your metabolism, and metabolism is the sum of all the energy transformations that occur in your body. This could be anything from activating certain proteins or helping your immune system to function properly. These processes all require energy.

Most people think that energy is, in this context, something you might get from coffee or from an energy drink. That is not what I'm talking about here, but we will talk about that later in the course. We produce actual energy by converting the food we eat into something called adenosine triphosphate, better known as ATP, and ATP is often called the energy currency of the body, because in a sense we pay for all of our biological actions with ATP. To release the energy from ATP, it is broken apart into smaller components in a process called hydrolysis using an enzyme called ATPase. ATP is broken into the smaller components to produce adenosine diphosphate, a single phosphate molecule, and energy.

So, food is eaten, eventually converted into ATP, carbon dioxide, and water, and, when ATP is used, to produce work for all of your metabolic needs and daily activities. And heat is also produced in the process of making energy. Essentially, you simply have changed the chemical composition of the food you eat into other forms of useable energy and heat. This follows what is known to you as the first law of thermodynamics, which states that energy is neither created nor destroyed, but only changed in form.

So, ATP is stored chemical energy that links the energy-producing and energy-requiring functions within all of our cells. This energy fuels all forms of biological work. Just think about processes that utilize ATP, like digestion and absorption, nerve transmission, blood circulating through your body, and muscular contractions.

One question you may have is: how do we make and replace our stores of ATP? Well, we have three energy systems to do this for us. In all three systems, a phosphate group is added to adenosine diphosphate, or ADP, in a process called phosphorylation to ultimately create adenosine triphosphate, or ATP. And what this means is that phosphate is added to ADP, and then it's stored as ATP until the energy in ATP is needed for activities like walking up the stairs, picking up a box, or exercising.

The really interesting part is that each energy system has a specific role and works at the highest rate based on how hard or how intense you are working. Each system has a different way of providing ATP, but it is important to realize that they are used on a continuum, and they do overlap quite a bit. In addition, certain parts of each of the three energy systems can also work to provide ATP in the other two energy systems. So, while this may sound confusing and problematic, it is actually a really cool way for you to get all of the ATP out of whatever it is that you are doing and whatever fuel source—carbohydrates, fats, or proteins—that you are using to provide the energy. And by understanding these three energy systems, what you will gain is the ability to decide what to eat, or what certain nutrients may be best to support whatever it is you are actually doing.

Think about it like this. If you are doing something that uses more carbohydrates to produce ATP, then you will know what to eat to optimize not only your performance but also your body composition. But then, on the other hand, if you are doing something in your daily routine that burns more fat for ATP or energy production, then there is less need to eat carbohydrates at that time. And this allows you to better understand what you should eat to optimize energy production, limit storing excess fat, and improve success for fat loss.

Now, I'll describe these energy systems in terms of how carbohydrates, fats, and proteins are used to make ATP. But, in reality, we don't go to the grocery store and buy carbohydrates, proteins, and fats individually, we buy and eat food, and foods are typically a combination of the three macronutrients. So, while this may be some of the nitty-gritty details of how you make energy, we will follow this lecture up with plenty of information that might be more readily applicable to your body composition goals. Sounds good, right? Well, let's get into it.

The three energy-producing systems are the creatine phosphate system, the glycolytic system, and the oxidative system. All of these systems work to provide us energy, but one system typically is used more than the others during different exercise and rest scenarios.

So for the first energy system, the creatine phosphate system, this works hardest for us during maximal intensity exercise. Just think about running fast for a few seconds or lifting a heavy object or weight—that's the creatine phosphate system. In this system, you will create ATP first by combining a phosphate with stored creatine—which is a combination of amino acids—to form creatine phosphate. Then, the enzyme creatine kinase breaks the phosphate off of creatine phosphate and allows it to combine with ADP. This forms more ATP and free creatine. This process is anaerobic; it occurs without oxygen.

Now, of course you are still breathing oxygen at the normal 21% that exists in the atmosphere, but these energy-creating processes are called anaerobic, meaning without oxygen, because ATP can be produced without the presence of oxygen in the cells. Think about when you run up a flight of stairs and you're out of breath. This would be a lack of oxygen in your cells, but the ability to get up the stairs, despite the lack of oxygen, is provided primarily by the creatine phosphate system. So the term anaerobic also tells us that this system is one that will work when you are doing intense activity or exercise. So the creatine phosphate energy system works quickly but it does not last for long—about 30 seconds is all you'll get, depending on your fitness level. But it is the most rapid method to regenerate ATP.

But, don't think that just because the creatine phosphate system is so short-lived that is isn't valuable—it is extremely useful to us. Think about anytime you need to do a very quick action, quickly jump out of the way of something, run quickly for a few steps, or lift something heavy. All of these require the creatine phosphate system. If you're really active, this system is also handy to give quick hard efforts when need to you run up a hill, pass someone in a race, or lift heavy weights.

Most exercise physiology textbooks will set a 30-second limit rule for this system, but the creatine phosphate system can be used at nearly any point of activity and repeated after a short break, even though the energy production only lasts for a few seconds. This is because of something called the size principle for muscle use, which says that you can recruit muscles for activity in an orderly and efficient fashion, from smallest to largest. So, some muscles will burn through their stored creatine phosphate but other larger muscle fibers will keep it until it is needed for a burst of high-intensity activity.

Interestingly, creatine stores are useful for everyone, not just power and strength athletes. Also, although creatine is made naturally in our bodies, we do get some from the foods we eat, mostly from meat. So, yes, vegetarians and vegans who primarily eat vegetables will likely have less stored creatine. But creatine can also be consumed as a supplement. In fact, it is the most widely studied sports nutrition supplement on the planet, and now research is showing the benefits of creatine supplement use for just about every population: young, old, healthy, and diseased. We'll discuss this and other supplements later in the course.

The second energy system is the glycolytic system, which is also called anaerobic glycolysis, and this system relies on carbohydrates as a fuel source to make energy. The glycolytic system lasts longer than the creatine phosphate system, but probably not more than about 2 minutes while you are working hard. It is also called anaerobic glycolysis because, once again, you produce ATP without the need for oxygen in your cells. Think of an athlete running a 400-meter dash. Or think of yourself doing short swimming intervals or treadmill exercise that you could only maintain for 1–2 minutes before needing a break.

Glycolysis, as the name implies, is the breakdown of carbohydrates or glucose to make ATP, and glucose is in any type of carbohydrate that you would eat or drink—it could be a sports drink, it could be a piece of bread, or even an apple. But once the glucose is in your blood, you need to get it into your cells to break it down to either make ATP or to store it as glycogen for later use. You can use stored glycogen or the glucose from food that you've recently eaten to make ATP. In both cases, you first need to get the glucose into your cells. Okay, luckily there is an elaborate system of proteins called GLUT transporters that assist with this.

The glycolytic energy system is one you rely on during any sort of physical activity. Again, the three energy systems work on a continuum where they all are working but kick in to a much greater extent when required by the intensity for what you are doing, whether typing on your computer, or lifting weights, or running a marathon.

So, during glycolysis, your body breaks down glucose to eventually produce molecules called pyruvate as well as ATP. It's interesting to note that glycolysis both uses up and produces ATP, so along this pathway the net amount of ATP produced is considered moderate at best. And don't forget, this energy system can only sustain activity for about 2 minutes. And the other end product of the glycolytic system, in addition to ATP, is pyruvate.

Under conditions where oxygen is limited, like during hard exercise, pyruvate will go on to form lactate, and lactate or lactic acid is often considered to be a bad thing. You have probably heard of people saying that lactate causes pain in your legs when exercising, for example. Well, truth be told, lactate is the good guy, not the bad guy of metabolism. Lactate is actually a storage depot for the excess hydrogen ions produced as a byproduct of this glycolytic energy system working to make you ATP.

You see, when you break down glucose to make some ATP, you also produce hydrogen ions. Well, if you are working out intensely, then the hydrogen ions will accumulate and build up, eventually causing a drop in your pH of the muscles. This drop in pH from the hydrogen ions is known as lactate acidosis, and it's painful. It is this acidity that makes you slow down or even stop for a breather during exercise. But here's why lactate is not bad. The lactic acid formed helps keep glycolysis functioning to make just a little more ATP, or to give you energy to perform more work for just a little bit longer before you have to slow down or stop.

One really neat thing about lactate is that it can also be transformed back into glucose for later use in this glycolytic energy system. The process of forming new glucose from non-carbohydrate sources—in this case from lactate—is called gluconeogenesis. Lactate leaves the muscle, it's converted back into pyruvate in the liver, and then re-formed into glucose; this process is called the Cori cycle. The newly formed glucose then makes its way back to the blood and then to the muscles to produce ATP in this glycolytic energy system.

Think of it this way: pretend you are doing hard exercise intervals, like running uphill. Eventually you will feel your legs begin to burn, which is just an indication that the energy is being produced and the acidity is increasing in your muscles. This again is caused by the hydrogen ions that are a product of glycolysis, and they ultimately combine with pyruvate to form lactic acid. Likely the pain associated with the acidity increasing in your legs will make you slow down. Now, having slowed down, you are able to actually use that built up lactate by transforming it back into glucose to provide more fuel to produce ATP in this energy system.

Because you slowed down and allowed yourself to catch your breath—that is, allowed oxygen to be available to your metabolic processes—you begin again to transform pyruvate, the end product of glycolysis, into another molecule called acetyl coenzyme A, or acetyl-CoA, rather than forming lactate. It is this acetyl-CoA that can then move into the third energy system to provide even more ATP. Acetyl-CoA is actually called the common intermediate for energy production because, in order to make lots of ATP in the third energy system, you must first form Acetyl-CoA, no matter if you are burning carbohydrates, fats, or proteins as your energy source. It is the common point for entry of all of these fuels to make energy in the oxidative system.

We've discussed the creatine phosphate system, the glycolytic system, so the third energy system is the oxidative system. This energy system relies on carbohydrates, fats, and, in some cases, protein to provide ATP. The oxidative system is your long and slow system, which kicks in after about 90 seconds to 2 minutes of activity and can last almost indefinitely, as long as the intensity of activity is low to moderate. It's aerobic, unlike the other two energy systems, so it uses oxygen.

As you know, with sufficient oxygen—from slowing down to breathe a little during vigorous exercise—the pyruvate will get transferred into acetyl-CoA rather than forming lactate in the glycolytic energy system. It is through the aerobic transformation of acetyl-CoA that glucose and fat continue to be metabolized with this third energy system: aerobic glycolysis or the oxidative system.

Here, the acetyl-CoA will now enter what is called the Krebs cycle or the citric acid cycle. In the Krebs cycle, and further down the metabolic pathway, you get to begin to produce much more ATP than was possible in the first two energy systems. This production of ATP is completed in the electron transport chain where oxygen is present. So, because oxygen must be present, this means that the system works when you are working at a low to moderate level of activity, or simply sitting still. For example, if you are walking, you'll be using the aerobic system to produce energy.

The way the electron transport chain works is by shuttling electrons down the electron transport chain to create a concentration gradient that ultimately works to produce ATP using an enzyme called ATP synthase. If glucose is being used in this third system to make ATP, you can make almost 40 molecules of ATP. Compare this to the 2–3 molecules of ATP made in the glycolytic system and you can easily see that much more ATP is made with the aerobic oxidative system. Here's another really cool aspect of metabolism: when fat is used in the oxidative system, this is where you really make a lot of energy.

Now, fat burning or fat oxidation requires more oxygen per ATP produced compared to energy production from glucose or glycogen, meaning, once again, you need to be resting or working out at a slow to moderate intensity to utilize fat as a fuel. However, fat provides 12 times more ATP than glucose, just at a slower rate. So now it is easy to see why fat is thought of as an almost endless source of energy. Fat provides lots of ATP and we have lots of stored fat on our bodies, even if you are very lean.

The oxidative system is active for most of your day—while sitting at a computer, walking around, or even when just watching TV. Again, carbohydrates and fats are the primary fuel sources used to provide ATP in the oxidative system, but this system can also metabolize some protein for energy production. This does not typically happen though, unless someone has been exercising for a very long time—say, longer than 2–3 hours—or for someone who has not eaten in a long time. Keep in mind, though, that you never only use fat or only use carbohydrates. The reality is that the fuel used to provide ATP in these energy systems is typically a combination of fuels and, again, not an all or none sort of action. For example, while you're at rest and just sitting around, about 2/3 of the ATP you make is from fat and 1/3 will be from carbohydrates.

What is really interesting is that the more fit you are, the better you are at using fat as a fuel. Also, the more fit you are, the better you are at saving your stored glucose or glycogen until you really need it, like when you pick up the intensity of your exercise. This is just one more reason to consider adding physical activity into your daily lifestyle; it will impact the fuel you use all day long.

You see, as you exercise and your training status increases, you can increase the number of mitochondria that you have in the cells of the muscles at work. This is called mitochondrial density and you want it to be high. The mitochondria are the organelles within your cells that help you produce large amounts of ATP. So it makes sense, right? The more you exercise, the more you put exercise into your lifestyle, the better you are at making energy.

Another benefit is that you can increase the number of capillaries or small blood vessels you have to bring blood, oxygen, and other nutrients to working muscles. This is called capillary density, which you also want to be high. What's more is that, with exercise training, you actually increase the activity of enzymes called lipases that increase fat breakdown. Exercise also increases the hormones that are used to help initiate this fat breakdown.

So, by maintaining exercise as part of your life, you increase the ability to use fuels effectively by your body. And here's the key: you decrease your reliance on carbohydrates and use more fat as a fuel, regardless of what you're doing all day long. This means that at rest and during exercise you are burning a greater amount of fat, and over time this will no doubt impact your body composition. The fat that is used to make ATP can come from stored fat tissue, like around your waist and hips, but it can also come from dietary fat that you've eaten. You even have fat stored in your muscles to use for energy, and this type of fat is called intramuscular triglycerides or IMTG.

Interestingly, you'll find intramuscular triglycerides in both very fit and also in out of shape people, but how these stored depots of fat are utilized is extremely different between the fit and the unfit. For the out of shape people, these intramuscular fat stores can actually do harm and alter proper cell signaling that should occur in response to various hormones. But in physically active people the intramuscular fats tend to be used as an energy source, sparing glycogen and increasing fat use for activity.

So, while both fat and carbohydrates will be used in the oxidative system, the amount of fat used compared to how much carbohydrate is used is highly dependent on a number of key factors. These factors include things like: when did you last eat? When did you last exercise? How fit are you? And what hormones are circulating in your blood?

All of these aspects of how fuel is used to alter body composition will be covered in this course, but for now just know that the human body is absolutely amazing and adjusts to what you eat by burning more of that type of nutrient. For example, in a healthy person, you should be able to use more fat for fuel when you eat more fat, when you have not eaten for a long time, or during prolonged periods of exercise. This ability to shift easily from one fuel source to the other, based on the exact circumstance, is called metabolic flexibility.

Interestingly, researchers are now investigating people who are unable to switch easily between fuel sources, those who might be classified as metabolically inflexible. What we know now is that being sedentary, overweight, or obese is associated with less metabolic flexibility. Essentially, someone who is obese may have more trouble burning fat as a fuel than someone who is physically active and lean.

One really cool part about metabolic flexibility is that, in a lab setting, we can actually measure what fuel source—fat or carbohydrate—you are using. This is done by measuring the amounts of carbon dioxide and oxygen in your breath at rest or during exercise. The ratio of carbon dioxide produced to oxygen consumed is called the respiratory exchange ratio, or RER. When burning 100% fat for fuel, your RER is equal to 0.7. But, when burning 100% carbohydrate for energy, your RER is 1.0.

So, when walking slowly, you'll be using primarily fat to produce ATP because this is aerobic and would use the oxidative energy system. And, as a result, your RER would be at or very close to 0.7. But, as you increase the intensity of your walk to a jog or to a run and move into the glycolytic energy system, you'll use much more carbohydrate as the primary fuel source. Here, your RER would be at or near 1.0.

Basically, the faster and harder you go, the greater percent of carbohydrate that will be used to make energy or ATP. But keep in mind that there will always be a mix of carbohydrates, fats, and proteins used to produce energy. The more metabolically flexible you are, the better you will be at using energy sources at the exact right moment.

So now you can see that when you are doing low intensity effort—walking, working while sedentary, or watching TV—you would not need a large amount of carbohydrates; it simply doesn't make sense metabolically. But when you decide to be physically active—exert yourself to strengthen your heart, lungs, and muscles—then you might be better off eating carbohydrates on those days. In this way, you can take advantage of your metabolism and use the inherent metabolic use of fuels that is called bioenergetics. In this way, you'll be less likely to store what you eat as excess body fat and improve your nutrient partitioning, particularly when food is not eaten in a huge serving size.

So, the point of this lecture was not to overwhelm you with metabolic and biochemical pathways, but rather to demonstrate how the food we eat is broken down to provide energy for us in everything we do and enjoy doing. It should be clear now that your body composition could be changed quite a bit by just understanding the three energy systems and what the primary fuel source is for each one of them.

To recap, if most of your day is spent in a sedentary way—sitting at a computer, in a car, or on a couch—then the reliance on carbohydrate for energy is very small, so for this individual it might make sense to consider cutting way back on overall carbohydrate intake. However, for someone who is quite active all day—standing and walking most of the day, actively engaged in exercise, and using intense exercise frequently—then it would make sense to eat a higher amount of carbohydrates.

It might help to think of your fuel use and energy systems like a car with a series of gas tanks in it. This is an analogy that is often used in exercise physiology courses. Tank 1 would be very small but would produce ATP quickly, although you soon would run out of fuel. So then you move on to tank 2, where you can go a bit longer because the tank is bigger. These first two tanks will deplete much of your stored creatine phosphate and your stored carbohydrate to use as a fuel. These get used up—not all the way of course, but a good bit of them do—before moving on to tank 3, which is the largest tank but the slowest tank. This tank uses fat for the largest part of its fuel supply. So, in order to make a real dent in tank 3, the fat tank, you must first have to slow down and burn through tank 2 or use a lot of fuel. Then you can rely on tank 3 for the long haul.

So you can see that knowing how to use your energy systems to your advantage is a huge asset when wanting to change your body composition. After digesting and absorbing the food you eat, it's just amazing how it is used to provide you with energy for everything you want to do, including changing your body composition. Try this: aim to change your food intake and carbohydrate intake based on your activity level each day.

Carbohydrates: Composition, Storage, and Use

I n this lecture, you will learn why carbohydrates—fruit, pasta, whole grains, corn, peas, and breads—don't have to be scary or off-limits. You will also learn how carbohydrates impact your body composition and health, why there might be certain carbohydrates to eat at certain times of the day, and how exercise fits into the puzzle. In the end, you will have a firm grasp of the many types of carbohydrates that exist, how and why they might impact your body composition differently, and when you can eat a high-carbohydrate meal with less fear of storing it as fat.

Glucose and Ketosis

Glucose is the preferred fuel source by your brain and nervous system, as opposed to protein or fat. The body needs glucose for some actions, and it is estimated that we make about 50 grams of glucose per day in a process called gluconeogenesis. This amount is quite low, and for people who are physically active and like to exercise, the amount of carbohydrate needed will likely be more.

The current acceptable macronutrient distribution range from the Institute of Medicine for carbohydrate is between 45 and 65 percent of your total calorie intake, with no less than 130 grams of carbohydrate per day to meet our basic physiological needs. Because 1 gram of carbohydrate yields 4 calories, you will need roughly 500 calories per day from carbohydrates just to meet minimal needs.

However, more and more research is showing that we might be able to consume far less than 130 grams per day as long as dietary fat and protein are increased in the diet.

Fortunately, when you eat very little carbohydrate, you can still function from the production of ketones, which are simply a by-product of excess fat breakdown as a result of a low-carbohydrate diet. This excess fat breakdown is called ketosis.

Recently, ketone use for energy has been the topic of much research and debate. Some experts support nutritional ketosis for weight loss and health. Nutritional ketosis is induced when a person is put on a low-carbohydrate diet to encourage the breakdown of excess fat. Other experts recommend the traditional model of a higher-carbohydrate, low-fat diet for weight management and health.

The research is clear that some glucose is required for life, and even more is likely needed if you decide to become extremely active. However, most scientists agree that the United States is an "over-carbed" nation. They recommend that steps be taken to identify which carbohydrates are best to eat at what times during the day to provide the best health and performance benefits and to minimize negative changes to body composition.

How active you are, what size you are, and what your specific goals are will dictate how much carbohydrate you should have in your diet.

Of the three macronutrients (carbohydrates, fats, and proteins), carbohydrates are traditionally thought of as the most important fuel for exercise, particularly during high-intensity exercise.

The carbohydrate foods that we eat can range from quite simple, like sugar, to more complex forms, like starches and fibers. This ultimately determines how quickly we digest, absorb, and use them to fuel our activity or store them as fat in our muscles, liver, or fat tissue.

Types of Carbohydrates

- We classify carbohydrates by their structure, from simplest to most complex. These include monosaccharides, disaccharides, oligosaccharides, and polysaccharides.

- In all of these types of carbohydrates, the term "saccharide" means "sugar." The prefixes "mono-," "di-," "oligo-," and "poly-" refer to how many sugars are linked together—1, 2, 3 to 9, and 10 or more, respectively.

- The length of the carbohydrate chain is one factor that determines the rate of carbohydrate breakdown. The shorter the chain, the faster this rate becomes. In terms of overall health, you want a slower rate of breakdown to avoid any large variations in blood sugar and insulin concentrations. Insulin is one hormone that is responsible for inhibiting our ability to use fat as a fuel.

- Another interesting factor that determines the rate of carbohydrate breakdown is the shape of the carbohydrate. Starch, which is

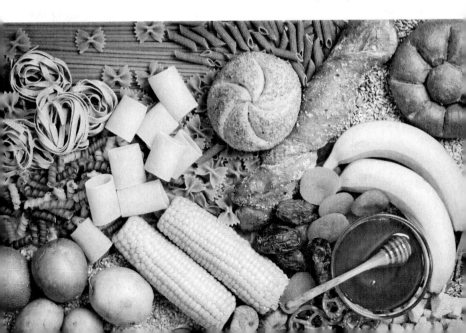

carbohydrate from plant sources, can have two basic forms: amylose (a straight, long chain molecule that is digested slowly) and amylopectin (which is highly branched and rapidly digested). Glycogen is also highly branched and is the form of carbohydrate that we store in our bodies.

In the context of body composition, we typically just think about the carbohydrates we eat as something that either makes us fat or doesn't. However, we also have to remember that carbohydrates provide us with fuel to ultimately produce energy, especially when we try to exercise at a high intensity.

Another source of carbohydrate that has clear health and body composition benefits is fiber. Dietary fibers are from plants and are not digested or absorbed by humans, so having these in your diet will slow the rate of carbohydrate digestion, which is usually a good thing.

Dietary fibers are found in foods like bananas, oatmeal, beans, whole grains, and dark leafy greens.

Fiber might help you feel more satiated or full for a longer period of time, lower your blood cholesterol and fat levels, and improve overall gut health. That means you might eat less by including fiber in your meals.

Digestion

The process of carbohydrate breakdown starts in your mouth with an enzyme called salivary amylase. It breaks the long sugars apart into smaller units to be absorbed. These small simple carbohydrates move through the cell lining of the small intestine and into the blood in capillaries that lead to the portal vein.

The portal vein takes blood to the liver, and the liver takes what glucose it needs for its own energy requirements and also what it needs to store as glycogen.

The remaining glucose continues to circulate in the blood. No matter what carbohydrate you eat, ultimately it will be in your blood as glucose because your body favors glucose for production of energy, or ATP.

The fructose you eat is stored as liver glycogen, and once the liver stores all the glycogen it needs from fructose, fructose then serves to increase fat synthesis. Clearly, this might not be the best thing for overall health.

The end result of carbohydrate breakdown is glucose being directed into circulation and ultimately to the cells that need it throughout your body.

Glycemic Index, Glycemic Load, and Insulin Index

There is a limit to how much glucose the body can use, and when those uses are met, the body responds by storing the energy in other forms, such as fat.

The glucose in your blood is used by cells to produce energy, especially by your nervous system and red blood cells.

Glucose can be stored as glycogen for later use, or the fat cells can remove glucose from the blood to form glycerol that is needed for triglyceride, or fat, storage.

Our bodies work best for us when blood glucose remains at a constant level without large fluctuations throughout the day. To a large extent, blood glucose levels can determine our mood and energy levels.

When blood sugar is elevated for a prolonged period of time, numerous detrimental health and body composition outcomes may occur, particularly for people who are hypo- or hyperglycemic. The good thing is that we have an index that tells us how quickly a food you eat will raise your blood glucose levels: the glycemic index.

By knowing the glycemic index of common foods that you eat, you will have an idea of what your blood glucose response will be after you eat that food. The higher your blood glucose, the higher the hormone insulin is in your blood.

Insulin is highly involved with the storage of carbohydrates in your cells. Insulin also blunts fat burning in most cases. It plays a critical role in this important function of balancing blood glucose levels.

If you have high insulin levels for a prolonged period of time, losing fat will likely be much more difficult to do. High levels of insulin also might interfere with your ability to achieve optimal health and performance.

Foods like bread, pastries, and bagels have a high glycemic index and therefore spike your blood sugar. On the other hand, foods like apples, cherries, beans, and nuts tend to have a much lower glycemic index.

The glycemic index provides a snapshot of good information but needs to be balanced with some other basic nutrition principles. One mechanism that has been developed to overcome some of the shortcomings of the glycemic index is called the glycemic load.

The glycemic load is the glycemic index of a particular food multiplied by the actual amount of food that you eat. Similar to a high glycemic index, a high glycemic load of a carbohydrate food means that your blood glucose values will increase quickly.

This glucose response is used to predict what should happen to insulin levels. The problem is that there is not always a direct correlation between a high glycemic index or a high glycemic load food with a high insulin response.

For this reason, research from *The American Journal of Clinical Nutrition* has provided an insulin index of common foods. So, rather than eating and measuring how high glucose gets in your blood, we would measure how high insulin gets in response to specific foods.

The glycemic index, glycemic load, and insulin index are useful tools, but other methods for choosing carbohydrates should also be considered. Ideally, we need a way to monitor the carbohydrates that we eat so that they serve the greatest benefit to us while also minimizing any negative impact to our body composition and health.

Balancing Blood Glucose

Lower-glycemic-index, lower-glycemic-load, and lower-insulin-index foods have the best potential to improve your body composition, keep you healthy, and avoid large spikes in blood glucose and insulin.

On the other hand, many prepackaged foods and other refined carbohydrates will quickly get into your bloodstream and over time have the greatest chance for causing some negative health consequences, including insulin resistance, where your body has to produce more and more insulin just to have the same effect it normally should have.

So, unprocessed carbohydrates like vegetables, which are high in fiber and nutrient density, should be the staple of your carbohydrate intake, compared to overly processed carbohydrates and added sugars. Eating this way regularly should improve your fiber and micronutrient intake and increase your feeling of fullness, or satiety, for a longer period of time after eating.

Another step in keeping blood glucose levels balanced is to exercise. At the end of exercise, your body is primed to store glucose as glycogen. Additionally, the exercise has increased your body's insulin sensitivity, meaning that you are more responsive to less of this powerful hormone. Theoretically, then, the best time to consume any carbohydrate-heavy meals would be after vigorous exercise, because you are metabolically prepared to handle them best at that point.

Try This

Aim to eat your most starchy meal of the day, such as pasta, after your hardest workouts.

Questions to Consider

1. What sources of carbohydrate in your diet would be best for optimizing your body composition?

2. How many added sugars do you eat on a typical day?

Carbohydrates: Composition, Storage, and Use

You've heard the message: carbohydrates make us fat. You've probably even seen this emphasized and overemphasized again in the popularity of diet books on sale today. If you do a quick search online for carbohydrate books, you'll see over 4 million results pop up instantly. You'll see books like *The Ultimate Carbohydrate Counter*, and *The Ultimate Low-Carb Diet Cookbook*, and the entire series of books by Dr. Atkins. So, is this accurate? Have our traditional guidelines to eat high carbohydrate levels been completely misguided—or worse, harmful? Maybe carbohydrates are to blame for the now 2.1 billion people—and that is 30% of the world—that are obese.

The short answer is that carbohydrates, particularly sugary deserts, sodas, and even sports drinks, cause dramatic changes to your hormones and can prime your body to store fat. These foods have what we call added sugars. If you didn't know it, sugar is one form of carbohydrate, and added sugars means that sugar was added in the preparation of the food, and this is different from the sugar that is naturally in the food. It is the difference between sugars in a candy bar compared to the sugar you would find in fruit.

Most people don't think they eat many added sugars. The trouble is, sugars are hidden in many of the foods we eat, like candy, crackers, and many boxed goods, because sugar provides a flavor that most people like. In fact, most of the foods we eat are pre-packaged; they have sugars. To find out, just have a look at the Nutrition Facts label and you'll be able to see a section called sugars. This is most likely from added sugars.

Added sugars have been shown to increase inflammation in our vascular system and are linked with diabetes, and are recently shown to increase your risk of death from cardiovascular disease. So, how much added sugar is acceptable? Well, unfortunately, the current recommendations vary a lot. The Institute of Medicine recommends that less than 25% of your total calorie intake come from added sugars. But the World Health Organization recently lowered their recommendation of added sugars from less than 10% to less than 5% of total daily calorie intake.

In real life, it can be hard to determine how much this actually is in terms of real food. For example, the American Heart Association recommends less than 100 calories or 25 grams of added sugar for women, and less than 150 calories or 38 grams of added sugar for men. Considering that 1 teaspoon is equal to roughly 4 grams of sugar, a woman would be able to afford about 6 teaspoons of added sugar and a man can eat about 9 teaspoons of added sugar. Just to illustrate, 12 ounces of one popular soda has about 39 grams of sugar, or just over 9 teaspoons. This exceeds the highest recommendation for the entire day for men and women.

Does this seem like a lot? Well it is, but some people use the same amount of added sugar just in their morning coffee. Also, if you look at the labels for any packaged foods you eat, this number of added sugar will quickly rise above recommended values. And keep this in mind: the recommended value is given just to avoid major health issues; it certainly is not about how to look and feel your best. Another tricky part about this part of nutrition is that sugar can hide very well—it goes by many other names, such as cane syrup, molasses, sucrose, maltodextrin, and others. If you see multiple names of sugars like these on a food label, you might want to think about another choice. You can also look for food labels that say no added sugar.

Believe it or not, over 70% of U.S. adults take in more than 10% of their daily calories from added sugar, from things like boxed goods, baked items, cereals, and sodas. Luckily, there are some easy ways to minimize your intake of added sugar. One of the easiest changes to make is simply to avoid drinking excess sugar. If you can avoid sugary sodas, juices, and energy drinks, you can easily save a ton of added sugar and added calories.

So, you might ask yourself what types of carbohydrates exist. Well, carbohydrates include things like fruit, pasta, whole grains, corn, peas, and breads. But do they all have the same impact on our bodies? For example, is fruit considered a carbohydrate just like pasta? Do candy bars affect us the same way as a bowl of oatmeal or a serving of green beans does? Well, in this lecture on carbohydrates, you will learn why carbohydrates don't have to be scary or off-limits. You will also learn how carbohydrates impact your body composition and health, why there are certain carbohydrates to eat at certain times of the day, and how exercise fits into this puzzle. In the end, you will have a firm grasp of the ways that carbohydrates exist, and how and why they may impact your body composition differently, and when you can eat a high carbohydrate meal with less fear of storing it as fat.

The first thing to keep in mind is that glucose is the preferred fuel source by your brain and your nervous system as opposed to protein or fat. The body needs glucose for some actions and it is estimated that we actually make about 50 grams of glucose per day in a process called gluconeogenesis. This amount is quite low, and for people who are physically active and like to exercise, the amount of carbohydrate needed will likely be more. Well, the current Acceptable Macronutrient Distribution Range from the Institute of Medicine for carbohydrate is between 45% and 65% of your total calorie intake, with no less than 130 grams of carbohydrate per day to meet our basic physiological needs. And because 1 gram of carbohydrate yields 4 calories, you will need roughly 500 calories per day from carbohydrate just to meet minimal needs.

However, more and more research is beginning to accumulate showing that we may be able to consume far less than 130 grams per day, so long as the dietary fat and protein are also increased in the diet. Fortunately, when you eat very little carbohydrate, you can still function from the production of ketones, which is simply a by-product of excessive fat breakdown as a result of a low-carbohydrate diet. This excess fat breakdown is called ketosis.

Recently, ketone use for energy has been the topic of much research and debate, and currently, in 2015, some experts support nutritional ketosis for weight loss and health. Nutritional ketosis is induced when a person is put on a very low-carbohydrate diet to encourage the breakdown of excess fat.

Other experts recommend the traditional model of a higher carbohydrate, low-fat diet for weight management and health.

In any case, the research is quite clear that some glucose is required for life, and even more is likely needed if you decide to become extremely active. However, most scientists agree that the U.S. is an over-carbed nation. They recommend that steps should be taken to identify what carbohydrates are best to eat at what times during the day to provide the best health and performance benefits, and to minimize negative changes to body composition.

We know that how active you are, what size you are, and what your specific goals are will dictate how much carbohydrate you should have in your diet. And of the three macronutrients—carbohydrates, fats, and proteins—carbohydrates are traditionally thought of as the most important fuel for exercise, particularly during high-intensity exercise like running fast, cycling fast, and lifting heavy weights.

A few examples of common carbohydrate-rich foods that you are familiar with are grains, pastas, potatoes, and rice. But carbohydrates are also found in fruits and vegetables. And sugar itself is also a very simple form of carbohydrate, meaning it is rapidly digested and absorbed by your body. These foods are all considered carbohydrates due to their similar chemical structure. Carbohydrates are all composed of carbon, hydrogen, and oxygen atoms in a 1:2:1 ratio.

The important point is that the breakdown of these atoms ultimately provides ATP, or the energy needed for all human functions. So the carbohydrate foods that we eat can range from quite simple, like sugar, to more complex forms, like starches and fibers. This ultimately determines how quickly we can digest, absorb, and use them to fuel our activity and store them as fat in our muscles, liver, and fat tissue.

We classify carbohydrates by their structure, from simplest to most complex, and these include monosaccharides, disaccharides, oligosaccharides, and polysaccharides. In all of these types of carbohydrates, the term saccharide means sugar, from the Greek word *saccharum*. The prefixes mono, di, oligo, and poly refer to how many sugars are linked together. So mono would be 1 sugar, di would be 2 sugar molecules, oligo would be 3–9 molecules, and poly would be 10 or more sugar molecules bound together. The simplest form of carbohydrate is the monosaccharide, which consists of only one sugar molecule. You've probably have heard of these because they are household names like glucose and fructose, which is derived from fruit sugar.

When monosaccharides are combined, a disaccharide is formed, such as sucrose—fructose and glucose bound together—also known as table sugar. Longer chains of monosaccharides can also combine to form oligosaccharides, which are commonly found in vegetables, and even longer chains called polysaccharides. If you've ever heard of starch, glycogen, or fiber you're hearing about polysaccharides.

The point is that the length of the carbohydrate chain is one factor that determines the rate of carbohydrate breakdown. Obviously, the shorter the chain, the faster this rate becomes. In terms of overall health, you actually want a slower rate of breakdown to avoid any large variations in blood sugar and insulin concentrations. Insulin is one hormone responsible for inhibiting our ability to use fat as a fuel.

Another interesting factor that determines the rate of carbohydrate breakdown is the shape of the carbohydrate. Starch, which is a carbohydrate from plant sources, can have two basic forms. Amylose is a straight, long chain molecule, which is digested slowly. Amylopectin, on the other hand, is a highly branched and rapidly digested molecule due to the increased surface area of the molecule due to the branched structure. And glycogen is also highly branched, and it's in the form of carbohydrate that we store in our bodies.

In the context of body composition, we typically just think about carbohydrates that we eat as something that either makes us fat or doesn't. However, we also have to remember that carbohydrates provide us with fuel to ultimately produce energy, especially when we try to exercise at high intensity. Through a process called glycogenolysis, or the breaking apart of glycogen, glucose fuels active muscles during exercise. About 100 grams of glycogen are stored in your liver with another 300–900 grams stored in your skeletal muscles, and just a minor amount circulating in your blood. So if you weigh 150 pounds, or 68 kilograms, you will store somewhere around 500–1000 grams of glycogen or roughly 2000 or maybe up to 4000 calories of fuel as carbohydrate.

Another source of carbohydrate that has clear health and body composition benefits is fiber. Now, dietary fibers are from plants and are not digested or absorbed by humans, so obviously having these in your diet will slow the rate of carbohydrate digestion, which is usually a good thing. The only exception would be for some athletes during exercise—this is when an athlete needs food that can be digested and absorbed quickly. Dietary fibers are found in foods like bananas, oatmeal, beans, whole grains, and dark leafy greens. Fiber may help you feel full or satiated for a longer period of time, and might help lower your blood cholesterol levels and your blood fat levels, and maybe even improve overall gut health. That means you might eat less by including fiber in your meals.

You may be wondering, "How much fiber should I eat?" Well, the minimum recommendation of fiber from the Institute of Medicine is to eat about 14 grams of fiber per every 1000 calories that you eat. This is about 25 grams per day for women and 38 grams per day for men. However, it's useful to note that these numbers were set to prevent health issues and not necessarily to live optimally. Anyway, fruit like a banana has 5 grams of fiber and 1 cup of baked beans has about 15 grams of fiber.

Now, I think it's interesting to talk about mono, di, and polysaccharides along with starches and fibers, but we don't really eat like this—we eat real food. So, while it's important to know about the different types of sugars and how fast or how slow they get into our bloodstream, first we must understand how the food we eat, like a piece of bread or an apple, are broken down from this complex form into smaller monosaccharide subunits and eventually put into our bloodstream as glucose.

The process of carbohydrate breakdown starts in our mouth with an enzyme called salivary amylase. It breaks the long sugars apart into smaller subunits to be absorbed, and these small, simple carbohydrates move through the cell lining of the small intestine and into the blood in capillaries that lead to the portal vein. The portal vein takes the blood to the liver, and the liver takes what glucose it needs for its own energy requirements and also what it needs to store as glycogen. The remaining glucose continues to circulate in the blood, and no matter what carbohydrate you eat, ultimately it will be in your blood as glucose because your body favors glucose for production of energy or ATP.

The fructose you eat is actually stored as liver glycogen, and once the liver stores all the glycogen it needs from fructose, fructose then serves to increase fat synthesis. Clearly, this may not be the best for overall health. The end result of carbohydrate breakdown is glucose being directed into circulation and ultimately to the cells that need it throughout your body.

So, you are probably asking how all of this relates to body composition. There is a limit to how much glucose the body can use, and when those uses are met, the body responds by storing the energy in other forms, such as fat. The glucose in your blood is used by cells to produce energy, especially by your nervous system and red blood cells. Glucose can also be stored as glycogen for later use, or the fat cells can remove glucose from the blood to form glycerol that is needed for triglyceride or fat storage.

What is important to understand is that our bodies work best for us when blood glucose remains at a constant level without large fluctuations throughout the day, and to a large extent, blood glucose levels can determine our mood and our energy levels. Just think about the last time you were really hungry. You might find yourself irritable, angry, and moody. We like to call this hangry, and I know that at my house it's clear when somebody needs some food—fast.

Anyway, much of this mood change is determined when your blood glucose dips too low or gets too high. After an overnight fast, we are able to maintain our blood glucose values using glycogenolysis, or the breakdown of glycogen to make glucose, and gluconeogenesis, the creation of new glucose from non-carbohydrate sources in the liver.

Glycogenolysis provides about 65%–75% of the glucose released into your blood, and gluconeogenesis provides the remaining 25%–35% of the glucose released by the liver. Interestingly, once you store glucose as muscle glycogen, it cannot be converted back into blood glucose—it is in essence locked in your cells and it must be used for energy. So, only liver glycogen can help maintain your blood glucose concentrations, not muscle glycogen, and some carbohydrate foods can have a dramatic impact on how high your blood glucose will rise after a meal. Some foods only have a minor effect on blood glucose, which, naturally, your body would prefer as it likes things to stay constant.

When blood sugar is elevated for a prolonged period of time, numerous detrimental health and body composition outcomes can occur, particularly for people who are hypo or hyperglycemic. The good thing is that we have an index that can tell us how quickly a food you eat will raise your blood glucose levels; you may have even heard of it. It's called the glycemic index.

The glycemic index gives us an idea of how quickly 50 grams of a specific food can raise your blood glucose levels compared to 50 grams of table sugar, which is given a glycemic index value of 100. Now, why is this important? Well, by knowing the glycemic index of common foods that you eat, you will have an idea of what your blood glucose response will be after you eat that food. The higher your blood glucose, the higher the hormone insulin is in your blood. If you know about diabetes, you know about insulin. The hormone is highly involved with the storage of carbohydrates into your cells. Insulin also blunts fat burning in most cases. It plays a critical role in this important function of balancing blood glucose levels.

If you have high insulin levels for a prolonged period of time, losing fat will likely be much more difficult to do. High levels of insulin also may interfere with your ability to achieve optimal health. Now, you might imagine that foods like breads, pastries, and bagels would have a high glycemic index and therefore spike your blood sugar. Well, you're correct. But, on the other hand, foods like apples, cherries, beans, and nuts tend to have a much lower glycemic index. So it is quite easy to see why many nutrition experts recommend eating foods that primarily have a low glycemic index value.

However, if you based your entire diet on the glycemic index, that isn't optimal either. This is because: one, you don't always eat 50 grams of a particular food, which is, as you know, what the entire glycemic index is based on; and two, we typically don't eat just one nutrient at a time—you would eat a meal of mixed carbohydrate, fat, and protein. Therefore, if you had a high glycemic index food such as a handful of pretzels, this wouldn't cause much of a problem if you combine them with lower glycemic foods like a serving of vegetables and a lean protein.

Interestingly, how you prepare foods in the kitchen can influence the glycemic index of the food as well. For example, simply boiling carrots will raise their glycemic index. It is also important to recall that the glycemic index of a food doesn't tell you much about the quality of that food. For example, the American Diabetes Association stresses that many nutritious foods have a higher glycemic index than foods that we typically think of as junk food. For example, some candy bars have a similar glycemic index value to green peas. So, if you're monitoring the glycemic index of foods only, then you need to be cautious about eating green peas as you would be about eating some candy bars.

But do you really eat the same serving size in weight of peas as easily as you would from a candy bar? Well, probably not. You see, it's quite easy to eat 50 grams of some foods, but rather hard to eat 50 grams of others—celery, for example. So it is clear that the glycemic index provides a snapshot of good information, but needs to be balanced with some other basic nutrition principles.

One of the mechanisms that has been developed to overcome some, but not all, of the shortcomings of the glycemic index is called the glycemic load. The glycemic load is the glycemic index of a particular food multiplied by the actual amount of food that you eat. Similar to a high glycemic index, a high glycemic load of a carbohydrate food means that your blood glucose values will increase quickly.

This glucose response is used to predict what should happen to insulin levels. The trouble is there is not always a direct correlation between a high glycemic index or a high glycemic load food with a high insulin response, and for this reason research from the *American Journal of Clinical Nutrition* has provided an insulin index of common foods. So, rather than eating and measuring how high your glucose gets in your blood, we would measure how high insulin gets in response to specific foods.

So, the glycemic index, glycemic load, and insulin index are all useful tools, but other methods for choosing carbohydrates should also be considered. Ideally what we need is a way to monitor carbohydrates that we eat so that they serve us to the greatest benefit while also minimizing any negative impact to our body composition and health.

So, how do we eat carbohydrates and not have it become a problem? Well, there are a few strategies for approaching this goal. It is clear that a lower glycemic index, lower glycemic load, and lower insulin index foods have the best potential to improve body composition, keep you healthy, and avoid large spikes in blood glucose and insulin. On the other hand, many pre-packaged foods and other refined carbohydrates like cereal, many breads, candy, and soda will quickly get into your blood stream and, over time, have the greatest chance for causing some negative health consequences, things like insulin resistance, where your body has to produce more and more insulin just to have the same effect it normally should have.

So, unprocessed carbohydrates like vegetables, which are high in fiber and nutrient density—meaning it has many beneficial nutrients compared to the calories that it contains—should be a staple of our carbohydrate intake compared to overly processed carbohydrates and added sugars. Eating this way regularly should improve your fiber intake, your micronutrient intake for things like vitamins and minerals, and increase your feeling of fullness or satiety for a longer period of time after eating.

Another step in keeping blood glucose levels balanced is to exercise. How exactly does this work? Well, getting glucose from your blood and into your muscles and into your fat cells for energy requires the help of the hormone insulin secreted from your pancreas. Cells use a small transporter protein to help glucose enter cells, and this glucose transporter is called GLUT-4 and it becomes active when insulin is present, like after a high sugar snack. GLUT-4 is part of a large family of GLUT transport proteins that exists in different body tissues.

But muscle contractions that occur with exercise also help shuttle blood glucose into your cells without insulin. So, during and after exercise, you have a greater ability to use blood glucose to produce energy, and after exercise to store glucose as muscle glycogen. You see, after exercise you have used up at least some of your stored muscle glycogen. This depletion of stored glycogen and the exercise activity itself ramp up the activity of an enzyme called glycogen synthase, which is used to make glycogen in your cells.

So, at the end of exercise, your body is primed and prepared to store glucose as glycogen. What's more is that the exercise increased your body's ability to be insulin sensitive, meaning you are more responsive to less of this powerful hormone. Theoretically then, the best time to consume any carbohydrate-heavy meals would be after vigorous exercise, because you've metabolically prepared to handle them the best that you can.

I find it interesting that researchers have investigated what happens to a high carbohydrate pasta meal both after rest and after exercise. As you might expect, after rest the high carbohydrate meal stopped the ability of these participants to burn fat. The authors wrote that this was because of the large insulin increase, which stops fat burning. But after moderate intensity exercise—just 60% of maximal effort—eating the high carbohydrate pasta meal did not lower their ability to burn fat and no body fat was gained. So, the best time to eat a meal with a lot of carbohydrates to preserve your healthiest body composition is most likely right after you exercise.

As you can tell, there is quite a bit to know when it comes to how carbohydrates can impact your body composition and health. They are required for many physiological mechanisms, including providing our brains and nervous system with energy. And, although carbohydrates in excess will likely disrupt health and body composition, carbohydrates don't have to be off-limits. We can choose to minimize added sugars in our diets; we can choose to eat low glycemic index and glycemic load carbohydrates like vegetables and less processed grains that are ultimately full of nutrients and fiber.

This will help give us a better overall diet quality and may help keep us feeling full for a longer period of time compared to a diet with only high glycemic sugary foods. It also looks like our bodies may best use carbohydrates after moderate to vigorous exercise sessions. It's after exercise when eating carbohydrates would be most likely to restock your glycogen stores so you are ready to exercise again the next day and are least likely to store them as fat.

Carbohydrates can and should be tailor-made to fit your activity level and body composition because carbohydrates play an important role in our overall nutritional intake. We don't have to fear them, but we should choose them wisely, eat appropriate portion sizes, and be smart about when to eat them. Try this: aim to eat your most starchy meals of the day, like pasta, after your hardest workouts.

Fat: Not the Nutritional Bad Guy

This lecture focuses on the many different valuable and necessary physiological roles that fat has in the human body. While fat has been maligned as the nutrition "bad guy" for a long time, there is new evidence indicating that eating fat is likely not all that bad for health or body composition, as long as fat intake is not combined with high sugar/refined carbohydrate intake; fat is consumed in a more balanced manner between saturated, monounsaturated, and polyunsaturated fats; and total calorie intake remains aligned with your nutritional and body composition goals.

What Is Fat?

▪ Just as carbohydrates are composed of monosaccharides linked together, fats are composed of fatty acids. This is the simplest form of fat. And fat goes by a few names. You might hear about fat as a lipid or even a phospholipid. All of these are considered fats, and in general, they are all composed of carbon, hydrogen, and oxygen atoms, just like carbohydrates.

▪ However, the carbon chain in fats is much longer than the carbon chain in a carbohydrate. This longer carbon chain is a unique feature of fats and plays a pivotal role in energy production. All fats also contain nine calories per gram, making them the macronutrient that provides more calories per gram than any carbohydrate or protein, which both provide only four calories per gram.

▪ Fatty acids are found in the food you eat. There are two types of fatty acids that you've heard of already: saturated fatty acids and unsaturated fatty acids.

Fatty acids vary by the length of their carbon-to-carbon chain and the number of hydrogen atoms that surround the carbon chain. That's the definition of saturated or unsaturated fat: They are either saturated with hydrogens or not.

When fatty acids are joined together, you get a triglyceride. Triglycerides are lipids with three fatty acids that are attached to a glycerol backbone. Triglycerides are the major storage form of fat in the body and the major form of fat in your diet.

On a food label, you will often see saturated and unsaturated fats highlighted. You might also see monounsaturated, polyunsaturated, and trans fats listed.

Saturated fats are saturated with hydrogens and have no double bonds in the carbon chain. These fats—like animal fats in meat and butter—are usually solid at room temperature.

When saturated fats are the predominant source of fat in the diet or just eaten in excess, they have been associated with increased blood levels of total cholesterol. And high cholesterol levels have been correlated in some research to increased risk of heart disease.

However, new research questions the common recommendation that we need to lower our saturated fat intake from our diets.

Some experts now suggest that high saturated fat in combination with high intake of sugar and other processed carbohydrates might be the real problem for our health and body composition. In fact, saturated fat might be less of a problem than originally thought, as long as carbohydrate intake is not excessive and a balanced fat intake is in place.

A balance of fat intake occurs when unsaturated fats are also in your diet. Unsaturated fats contain one or more double bonds along the carbon chain, meaning that, unlike saturated fat, they are not completely saturated with hydrogen molecules.

- There are two types of unsaturated fats: monounsaturated fats and polyunsaturated fats. Monounsaturated fats have only one unsaturated bond (also called a double bond), while polyunsaturated fats have more than one unsaturated (double) bond.

- An easy way to identify an unsaturated fat is that it is typically in liquid form at room temperature. But if unsaturated fats are chilled or refrigerated, they will solidify.

- Examples of monounsaturated fat include olive oil, canola oil, peanut oil, and sesame oil. You will also find monounsaturated fats in foods like avocados, peanut butter, and many nuts and seeds.

- The polyunsaturated fats are also known as essential fatty acids, meaning that they are essential to eat because our bodies cannot make them naturally. Many foods have a mix of fat types, but some examples of polyunsaturated fats include soybean oil, canola oil, flax, tofu, soybeans, and fatty fish like salmon.

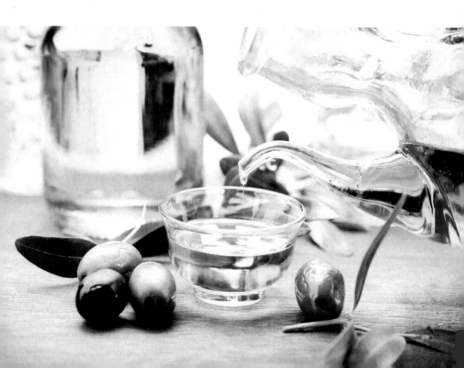

Polyunsaturated fats include both omega-6 and omega-3 fatty acids. These essential fatty acids are needed for immune function, vision, and cell membrane integrity, among other things.

Omega-6, Omega-3, and Trans Fat

Omega-6 fatty acids ultimately produce compounds that are involved with inflammation, blood vessel constriction, and immunity. All of these functions are important, and it's critical that they are well controlled.

Because omega-6 fats lead to inflammation when taken at high levels, they are known as pro-inflammatory agents. Eating too many foods with omega-6 fatty acids, such as heated vegetable oils and many boxed and packaged grocery items, can compromise health and optimal body composition, especially when not balanced with other types of fats, such as omega-3 fatty acids.

Omega-3 fatty acids are beneficial for health, due to their anti-inflammatory effects and effects on decreasing blood clot formation. Some omega-3 fatty acids keep cells less rigid and more fluid. In doing so, they promote blood vessel dilation, which lowers blood pressure and can decrease instances of heart attacks.

Omega-3 fatty acid consumption can also lower blood concentrations of triglycerides, cut the chances of rheumatoid arthritis, and even reduce some behavioral disorders. Some data even shows that low omega-3 intake is associated with both poor memory and mood disorders.

Because omega-3 fatty acids essentially have the opposite role of omega-6 fatty acids, a balanced intake of omega-6 and omega-3 will be needed for optimal health and physical function.

Americans tend to have very high omega-6 fatty acid consumption in comparison to omega-3 fatty acids in the diet. This is a problem because a high ratio is reported to promote things like cardiovascular disease, cancer, and inflammatory and autoimmune diseases. But a higher intake of omega-3 fatty acids seems to have the opposite effect and reduce the likelihood of cardiovascular disease, cancer, and inflammatory disorders.

If you can't lower your omega-6 intake, then be sure to reduce the gap in the ratio by eating more omega-3 fatty acids. For optimal health, decrease the amount of omega-6 fats that you eat and increase the amount of omega-3 fats that you eat.

The other type of fat is trans fat. Trans fats are often in the media, and legislation in the United States to completely ban trans fats from restaurants has been a big issue.

Trans fat is made in an industrial manufacturing process that adds hydrogen to previously liquid vegetable oil, making it a solid at room temperature. The fat is essentially artificially hydrogenated.

This is done to give foods a longer shelf life and might make certain foods taste better. Many restaurants will use partially hydrogenated vegetable oils to deep-fry foods because the oil does not need to be changed as frequently as other types of oils, resulting in a cost savings.

Many foods contain trans fats, including many baked goods, fried foods, potato chips, and margarine. A diet high in trans fats might increase your "bad," or LDL, cholesterol and decrease your "good," or HDL, cholesterol. It might also be associated with your risk of developing heart disease. But some trans fat occurs naturally in food, so it is not entirely avoidable.

How Much Fat Should You Eat?

Opinions vary when it comes to how much of each type of fat you should eat. The American Heart Association recommends that, for good health, the majority of the fats that you eat should be monounsaturated or polyunsaturated, rather than saturated fats and trans fats.

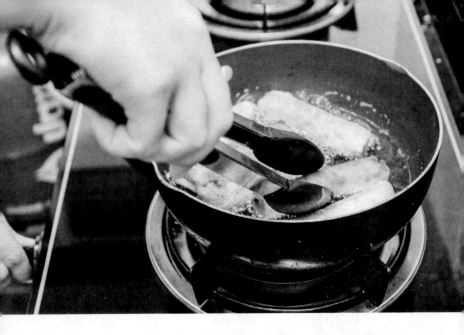

Others recommend eating about one-third of each type of fat—saturated, monounsaturated, and polyunsaturated fats—that includes a balance of omega-6 and omega-3 fatty acids.

The 2010 Dietary Guidelines for Americans recommends fat intake between 20 and 35 percent of your total calorie intake and recommends that saturated fat make up no more than 10 percent of these calories. They also recommend replacing "solid fats" with oils when possible and limiting foods with trans fats or hydrogenated oils as much as possible. The guidelines also recommend eating less than 300 milligrams of dietary cholesterol per day.

Fat is the most energy-dense macronutrient that we eat, because one gram of fat yields nine calories. Many people don't need to seek out additional fat to eat when considering total fat eaten per day, because fat is usually in many of the foods that we eat normally.

However, research is showing that it might be useful to make an effort to eat more high-quality fats in your diet, such as nuts, seeds, avocados, and fish. These foods provide a nice variety of saturated, monounsaturated, and polyunsaturated fats. And because fats help you feel full, these foods can be used to help reduce the total number of calories that you consume in a day.

Burning Fat

Fat provides the most abundant source of energy that we have. It fuels your body at rest and during activity that is light to moderate in intensity. During this type of exercise, a muscle's main source of fat supply is your fat (or adipose) tissue.

Muscles can also rely on fat that is stored inside of the muscle called intramuscular triglycerides (IMTG). The amount of IMTG used during exercise or activity will vary with fitness level. The more fit you are, the more fat you use.

This is a great adaptation to exercise. With fat stored in your muscle, it is already located where it needs to be so that it can be used as energy. The amount of IMTG will also vary with the intensity and duration of exercise, where longer and slower activity will rely more on fat use than short and fast activity.

To use fat as a fuel during exercise, your body needs to be able to break down stored triglyceride into free fatty acids to make ATP for energy. The intensity of the exercise will determine if fat will be used during exercise. The more intense the exercise, the less your body will be able to utilize the fat stores, and vice versa.

Fat oxidation (or burning) is regulated in part by how much glucose you have in your blood. So, eating lots of carbohydrates will increase blood glucose and decrease the breakdown of stored body fat (which is called lipolysis) and fat's use (or oxidation) for energy.

But fat oxidation is enhanced by exercise training. This occurs because exercise training can increase the number of mitochondria you have, as well as the capillary density. The increase in mitochondria will help the body process the fat at a higher volume, and the increase in capillary density will help increase the blood flow and oxygen delivery to the exercising muscle, which is required to burn fat.

Another interesting aspect of fat burning is the differences we see between men and women. Recently, it was reported that fat use relative to total body muscle mass was higher in women than in men. In general, women also tend to have a higher fat oxidation than men during exercise of low to moderate intensity. But women and men alike need to exercise to use fat and to eat in the best possible way to support fat use and optimal health.

Try This

Add at least two servings of fatty fish to your diet each week or begin to use a high-quality fish oil supplement.

Questions to Consider

1. What types of fat do you normally eat? What is in your kitchen now?

2. Does eating fat make you fat?

Fat: Not the Nutritional Bad Guy

D o you have that one friend who has to hunt down every avocado in sight or add nuts to every snack that they eat? Or maybe it's the friend who tries to avoid fat at all costs—no to butter, oils, mayonnaise, or other creamy spreads and dressings. Well, I have changed the way that I eat over the years based on conflicting research that I've come across in medical journals and from other reputable sources, and it's no secret that dietary fat is still a controversial topic in our culture. Does this sound familiar? "Eat butter for optimal health?" Or maybe it's this. "Avoid butter for optimal health."

We have seen similar controversial examples in the carbohydrate lecture already, but that really is the nature of this field, and to me it's really exciting. Our field, as with many sciences, continues to progress and evolve, and it's the latest research that can take your knowledge to the next level. Just imagine if you took a flight across the country. You wouldn't want all of the technology from 50 years ago; you would want the best new technology and advances in the field for a pleasant and safe journey. And so it goes with nutrition and exercise.

For example, how much fat should we have in our diet? Should we completely avoid dietary fat as many people once thought, or should we make fat a major component of what we eat? Can adding fat to our diets actually improve our body composition, or will eating fat just make us, well, fat?

For now, these questions are a bit premature, so let's first talk about what fat really is and what fat actually does for us physiologically. Fats have many different roles in our body that go way beyond just how we look. In fact, we need fat for optimal health.

Most people think of fat as what is underneath your skin. Here, it is an insulator acting to keep you warm. But fat is also found in your cell membranes, surrounding your internal organs, and in your muscles. It also helps cells to communicate with each other, because fats are a major component of cell membranes, cell receptors, and chemical signals in the blood. Certain fats are even used by your body to make other important compounds, including some very important hormones. For example, the cholesterol found in many fatty foods is required to produce your steroid hormones. This is very important for body composition because some of the steroid hormones, like testosterone, can have a big impact on muscle mass and fat mass for men and women.

It is often thought that the more fat you eat, the more fat you store on your body. But the truth is that excessive calorie consumption, whether from fat, protein, or carbohydrates will result in fat storage. The America Council on Exercise classifies the average healthy woman as having about 25%–31% body fat and the average healthy man with 18%–24% body fat. Fit individuals and athletes typically have even lower body fat than this. And, of all the functions of fat, its primary role is to provide you with an energy source or an energy reserve that is much greater than any other fuel that you can tap into.

For example, if you weigh 180 pounds, or 81 kilograms, and have 25% body fat, then approximately 45 pounds, or 20 kilograms, of fat is stored in your body. And because 1 pound of stored fat is thought to provide 3500 calories, then you essentially have about 160,000 calories of fat to use at any given time.

Now, assuming that you can burn about 100 calories per mile while walking, then, in theory, you could walk about 1600 miles on your stored body fat. That would get you from Atlanta to Denver. Of course there are a number of other factors that would challenge this, but it is important to understand what a large fuel source we have in the form of stored fat. It's far greater than stored carbohydrate that can only provide a theoretical 2000 calories or slightly more for energy.

Fats are actually used to fuel most of your cells in your body including contracting muscles in the arms and the legs. Fat provides 80%–90% of the fuel you use while at rest, like working at a computer all day, driving in your car, or watching TV. Almost 2%–4% of your body fat serves to protect and insulate vital organs like your heart, your liver, spleen, kidneys, brain, and your spinal cord. And the fat-soluble vitamins A, D, E, and K are dependent on fat in your diet for absorption and movement in your body. This is why you should take these vitamins with your meals.

In fact, if you have a diet very low in fat, then you can't absorb these key vitamins. This would then impact how well your body can use other nutrients in your diet. One advantage to fat is that it empties very slowly from your stomach, and due to this fact, eating fatty foods like nuts, seeds, or avocado can also decrease your hunger. In fact, many people report feeling fuller for longer by simply having fat included in their meals. So, fats actually have many roles, and because of this they must be included in a healthy diet. Now, let's dig into what fat actually is, the various types of fats that exist, and when we might be set up to either store fat on our bodies or burn it for energy.

Just as carbohydrates are composed of monosaccharides linked together, fats are composed of fatty acids. This is the simplest form of fat, and fat goes by a few names. You may hear about fat as a lipid or even a phospholipid. All of these are considered fats and, in general, they are composed of carbon, hydrogen, and oxygen atoms, just like carbohydrates. However, the carbon chain in fats is much longer than the carbon chain in carbohydrate. This longer carbon chain is a unique feature of fats and plays a pivotal role in energy production, but I'll get into that in just a few minutes. All fats also contain 9 calories per gram, making them the macronutrient that provides more calories per gram than carbohydrate or protein, which provide only 4 calories per gram.

Let's break the forms of fat down a bit. Fatty acids are found in the food you eat, and there are two types of fatty acids that you've heard of already: these are saturated fatty acids and unsaturated fatty acids. These are examples of two different types of fats. Fatty acids vary by the length of their carbon-to-carbon chain and the number of hydrogen atoms that surround the carbon chain. That's the definition of saturated or unsaturated—they're either saturated with hydrogens or not. And when fatty acids are joined together, you form a triglyceride. A triglyceride, as the prefix tri tells us, are lipids with three fatty acids that are attached to a glycerol backbone. Triglycerides are the major storage form of fat in the body and the major form of fat in your diet.

On a food label, you will often see saturated and unsaturated fats highlighted. You may also see monounsaturated, polyunsaturated, and trans fats listed. Well, let's define these types of fat a bit more now.

Saturated fats are saturated with hydrogens and have no double bonds in the carbon chain. These fats, like animal fats in meat, butter, and coconut oil, are usually solid at room temperature. When saturated fats are the predominant source of fat in the diet, or just eaten in excess, they have been associated with increased blood levels of total cholesterol. And high cholesterol levels have been correlated in some research to increased risk of heart disease.

However, not everyone agrees on this. In fact, new research no longer supports the idea that high cholesterol causes heart disease, although correlational data does exist. Some research also shows that excessive intake of saturated fat, without balancing it by also eating unsaturated fat, is correlated to other serious conditions like Alzheimer's disease, certain cancers, diabetes, and cardiovascular disease. But, again, new research questions the common recommendation that we need to lower our saturated fat intake from our diets.

Some experts now suggest that high saturated fat in combination with high intake of sugar and other processed carbohydrates may be the real problem for our health and body composition. In fact, saturated fat may be less of a problem than originally thought, so long as carbohydrate intake is not excessive and balanced fat intake is in place. A balance of fat intake occurs when unsaturated fats are also in your diet.

Unsaturated fats contain one or more double bonds along the carbon chain, meaning that, unlike saturated fat, they are not completely saturated with hydrogen molecules. There are two types of unsaturated fats, which are called mono and polyunsaturated fats. Monounsaturated fats have only one unsaturated bond—these are called a double bond—while polyunsaturated fats have more than one unsaturated double bond. And an easy way to identify an unsaturated fat is that it is typically liquid at room temperature. But if unsaturated fats are chilled or refrigerated, they will solidify. Examples of monounsaturated fat include olive oil, canola oil, peanut oil, and sesame oil. You will also find monounsaturated fats in foods like avocados, peanut butter, and even nuts and seeds.

Now, the polyunsaturated fats are also known as essential fatty acids, meaning that they are essential to eat because our bodies cannot make them naturally. Many foods have a mix of fat types, but some examples of polyunsaturated fats include soybean oil, canola oil, flax, tofu, soybeans, and fatty fish like salmon. Polyunsaturated fats include both omega-6 and omega-3 fatty acids. These essential fatty acids are needed for immune function, vision, and cell membrane integrity among other things.

Omega-6 fatty acids ultimately produce compounds that are involved with inflammation, blood vessel constriction, and immunity. All of these functions are important, and it's critical that they are well controlled. Because omega-6 fats lead to inflammation when taken at high levels, they are known as pro-inflammatory agents. So eating too many foods with omega-6 fatty acids, like heated vegetable oils and many boxed and packaged grocery items, can compromise health and optimal body composition, especially when not balanced with other types of fats like omega-3 fatty acids.

Omega-3 fatty acids are beneficial for health due to their anti-inflammatory effects and effects on decreasing blood clot formation. Some omega-3 fats keep cells less rigid and more fluid. In doing so, they promote blood vessel dilation which lowers blood pressure and can decrease instances of heart attacks. Omega-3 fatty acid consumption can also lower blood concentrations of triglycerides, cut the chances of rheumatoid arthritis, and even reduce some behavioral disorders. Some data even show that the omega-3 intake is associated with both poor memory and mood disorders. Interestingly, more and more evidence is emerging to support using omega-3 fatty acids in cases of traumatic brain injury to help with immediate and long-term outcomes for these patients.

Essentially, omega-3 fatty acids have the opposite role of omega-6 fatty acids. Because of this, you can see that a balanced intake of omega-6 and omega-3 fatty acids will be needed for optimal health and physical function. Americans tend to have very high omega-6 fatty acids consumption in comparison to omega-3 fatty acids in the diet because of the high content of omega-6s in many of the pre-packaged foods and vegetable oils that we eat. In fact, the typical Western diet is reported to be almost 20:1 for the omega-6 to the omega-3 ratio, but many experts suggest that the ratio should be more like 2:1 or 1:1 for optimal health.

This is a real problem because a high ratio is reported to promote things like cardiovascular disease, cancer, and inflammatory and immune diseases. But a higher intake of omega-3 fatty acids seems to have the opposite effect and reduce the likelihood of cardiovascular disease, cancer, and inflammatory disorders. If you can't lower your omega-6 intake, then be sure to reduce the gap in the ratio between eating more omega-3 fatty acids. The balance of the omega-3s in your diet is very important for optimal health, so it's a good idea to attack this from both sides: decrease the amount of omega-6 fatty acids that you eat, and increase the amount of omega-3 fatty acids that you eat.

The other type of fat we haven't discussed is trans fat. You may recall that trans fats are often in the media, and legislation in the U.S. to completely ban fats from restaurants has been a big issue. Trans fats are called trans due to the chemical structure of the molecule that surrounds the double bonds between the carbons in the fatty acid chain.

Let me explain this. Fatty acids that have a degree of unsaturation will have a double bond between the carbon atoms. This provides a chance for the fatty acids to exist in either a cis form, where hydrogen atoms are on the same side of the carbon chain, or in the trans form, where hydrogen atoms are on opposite sides of the carbon chain. These forms, the cis and the trans, alter the geometric shape of the fat. The trans figuration allows for more stable structure due to equal distribution of hydrogen molecules on both sides of the double bond.

Cis fats, with hydrogen atoms on just one side of the carbon atom chain, tend to fold upon themselves, while trans fats do not fold up very well, and this makes trans fats able to pack tightly together in the cell membranes and essentially make them rigid. Most naturally occurring fatty acids in foods are in the cis form, and most trans fats are man-made. Trans fats are made in an industrial manufacturing process that adds hydrogen to previously liquid vegetable oil, making it a solid or hard at room temperature. This fat is essentially artificially hydrogenated.

This is done to give foods a longer shelf life, and may make certain foods taste better. Many restaurants will use partially hydrogenated vegetable oils to deep-fry foods because the oil does not need to be changed as frequently as other types of oils, so there is a cost savings for restaurants to consider when they choose the types of oils that they cook with.

Many foods contain trans fats including many baked goods like cookies, fried foods, potato chips, and margarine. A diet high in trans fats may increase your bad LDL cholesterol and decrease your good HDL cholesterol. It may also be associated with your risk of developing heart disease, but some trans fat occurs naturally in food, so it is not entirely avoidable.

Now, you may wonder just how much of each type of fat you should eat. Well, opinions vary. The American Heart Association recommends that, for good health, the majority of fats that you eat should be monounsaturated or polyunsaturated, rather than saturated fats and trans fats. Others recommend eating about 1/3 of each type of fat—saturated fat, monounsaturated fat, and polyunsaturated fats—that include a balance of omega-6 and omega-3 fatty acids. I like to focus on eating high quality sources of fat like avocados, nuts, seeds, olive oil, and omega-3 fatty acids from fish and fish oil. Then I just let the rest of my fat take care of itself because it's already in many of the animal products and occasional treats that I have. This has worked well to balance my fat intake to roughly equal parts of mono, poly, and saturated fat intake.

So, now you understand that there are different types of fats that we can consume, and different ways in which we can store fat in the body or use it for energy. Fat is an enormous supply of fuel for us to tap into, and understanding fat use will clearly help improve body composition. The 2010 Dietary Guidelines for Americans recommends fat intake to be between 20% and 35% of your total calorie intake, and recommends that saturated fat make up no more than 10% of these calories. They also recommend replacing solid fats with oils when possible, and limiting foods with trans fats or hydrogenated oils as much as possible. The guidelines also recommend eating less than 300 milligrams of dietary cholesterol per day.

According to the U.S. Department of Agriculture, one large egg has about 186 milligrams of cholesterol, all of which is found in the yolk. So, two eggs would put you over the recommended limit. But, as we've discussed, this relationship between cholesterol and saturated fat in the diet may not correlate with cholesterol in your blood. Also, many vegetable oils are very high in omega-6 fatty acids, so that could be exactly the wrong recommendation to give to people. So, clearly these fat-related scientific topics continue to be hotly debated as of 2015.

No matter how you cut it, fat is the most energy-dense macronutrient that we eat, because 1 gram of fat yields 9 calories and many people don't need to seek out additional fat to eat when considering total fat eaten per day. That's because fat is usually in many of the foods you eat normally. However, research is now showing that it may be useful to make a real effort to eat more high quality fats in your diet like nuts, seeds, avocados, and fish. These foods, as you know, provide a nice variety of saturated, monounsaturated, and polyunsaturated fats. And because fat helps you feel full, these foods can be used to help reduce the total number of calories that you consume in a day.

One question that you may have now is, "How do I actually burn fat as a fuel? How do I use my stored fat to provide energy and ultimately improve my body composition?" Well, as I mentioned earlier, fat provides the most abundant source of energy that we have; it fuels your body at rest and during light- to moderate-intensity activity. And during this type of exercise, a muscle's main source of fat supply is your fat or your adipose tissue. Muscles can also rely on fat that is stored inside of the muscle called intramuscular triglycerides or IMTG. The amount of intramuscular triglycerides used during exercise or activity will vary with your fitness level, with the more fit you are, the more fat you'll use.

This is a great adaptation to exercise, actually. With fat stored in your muscle, it is already located where it needs to be in order to be used as energy. The amount of intramuscular triglycerides will also vary with the intensity and the duration of exercise, where longer and slower activity will rely more on fat use than short and fast activity. The trick is for your body to get the fat from your fat cells into the blood and then into your muscles in order to be burned or oxidized for energy in the mitochondria of your cells. To do this, fats enter something called the carnitine fatty acid transport system. This system works as a gatekeeper to allow fat into the cell's mitochondria.

But fat is not able to enter the mitochondria effectively when levels of glucose are high because another molecule called malonyl-CoA shuts down the carnitine transport system. This means that after a high carbohydrate meal—for example, a muffin—you literally impair the ability to transport fat into your cell's mitochondria to be used as energy. Likewise, some hormone changes occur with high carbohydrate intake that can also work against you being able to burn fat. So just be aware of what you eat and when you eat it; it can impact your body composition and performance dramatically. Anyway, once the free fatty acids released from the stored triglyceride are inside the mitochondria, these fatty acids are broken down to provide energy during a process called beta-oxidation, which just means fat is burned as a fuel.

What all this boils down to is that to use fat as a fuel during exercise, your body needs to be able to break down stored triglycerides into free fatty acids to make ATP for energy. The intensity of the exercise will determine if fat will be used during exercise. The more intense the exercise, the less your body will be able to utilize the fat stores and vice versa. As mentioned already, fat oxidation or burning is regulated in part by how much glucose you have in your blood, so eating lots of carbohydrate will increase blood glucose and decrease the breakdown of stored body fat, which is called lipolysis, and fat's use or oxidation for energy.

But fat oxidation is enhanced by exercise training, and this occurs because exercise training can increase the number of mitochondria you have, as well as the capillary density. The increase in mitochondria will help the body process the fat at a higher volume, and an increase in capillary density will help increase the blood flow and oxygen delivery to the exercising muscle, which is required to burn fat.

Exercise training will also increase the activity of the carnitine fatty acid transport system that essentially allows more fat to enter the increased number of mitochondria that you have from exercising. Interestingly, some supplements may also work through this transport system to help burn fat. We will talk more about this in an upcoming lecture. So, as you probably expected, exercise does help burn more fat, but of course it depends on the intensity and the duration of exercise, as well as that overall mix of foods that you have recently eaten.

Another interesting aspect of fat burning is the difference we see between men and women. Early studies of sex differences in fuel use during exercise were conducted during the late 1970s and early 1980s. Men and women were asked to run between 65% and 70% of their maximum intensity, and repeatedly fat use was not shown to be different between men and women when running at a set percent of their maximum. But in follow-up work, another study tracked the number of miles that the men and women ran per week, their years of exercise training, and their relative ability to use oxygen during exercise. And using this advanced design, some differences were found.

When the research participants ran at 63% of their maximum on the treadmill for 90 minutes, the women used significantly more fat than men during the exercise when matched for the different variables of training experience and muscle mass. Also, there weren't significant differences in blood levels of free fatty acids between men and women. This was all despite women having significantly higher blood glucose levels throughout the exercise session.

Others looked into 14 untrained, and 14 moderately trained, and 14 endurance trained men and women before and after cycling at 60% of their maximal oxygen consumption for 90 minutes. The researchers found that in all three training scenarios only the women were able to significantly utilize the fat stored in their muscle cells. This shows that, when compared to men, women are better at using stored fat in their muscles for energy. Also, women were better able to store fat in their muscles than men prior to exercise starting.

Recently, it was also reported that fat use relative to body muscle mass was higher in women than in men. This is not entirely surprising because it is well established that, on average, women have a significantly higher percentage of the type of muscle fiber that is best used to burn fat as a fuel. These fibers are known as type 1 oxidative muscle fibers. Women have about 68% of their muscle mass composed of type 1 fibers compared to men at about 55%, and these are the fibers that are used during slower and longer duration activities, the type of exercise that uses a lot of fat during the activity. In general, women also tend to have a greater capillary density, higher percent of type 1 muscle fibers, and a higher fat oxidation than men during low- to moderate-intensity exercise.

So you might ask then, "Well, why do men seem to lose weight more quickly if woman are actually better at using fat as a fuel?" The answer may be quite complicated but for simplicity sake, in my experience, men typically have more room to change, meaning they tend to start this journey at a higher fat mass than women in general. But let's not go too far yet. All this means is that women and men alike need to exercise to use fat, and need to eat in the best possible way to support fat use and optimal health. This is exactly what the rest of this course will cover.

Ultimately, fat has many different valuable and necessary physiological roles in the human body. And while fat has been maligned in the nutrition as the bad guy for a long time, there is new evidence indicating that eating fat is likely not all that bad for health or body composition, so long as: one, fat intake is not combined with a high sugar or refined carbohydrate intake; two, fat is consumed in a more balanced manner between saturated fat, monounsaturated fat, and polyunsaturated fat; three, total caloric intake remains aligned with your nutrition and body composition goals.

It is also very clear that exercise of low and moderate intensity helps oxidize or burn fat, but that we also need to increase our overall calorie burn from exercise, too. That could occur with either more exercise or by including high-intensity exercise that really gets your blood pumping. You'll learn much more about this topic soon.

In the end, there may be small differences in how fat is burned and how much fat is stored between men and women, but I wouldn't get too bogged down by that information. It is far better to stay focused on what you eat and how you choose to incorporate exercise into your life. So try this: add at least two servings of fatty fish to your diet each week or begin to use a high quality fish oil supplement.

Protein's Critical Role in Body Composition

E ating more protein might be the best nutritional strategy to manage body composition, given its influence on metabolism, satiety, and even maintenance of muscle mass. And the impact of a high-protein diet when combined with an exercise program can provide even better results for improving our metabolism and body composition. In this lecture, you will learn how protein does all of these positive things in our bodies and how you can use it to improve your body composition.

Protein and Metabolism

In terms of our body composition, eating protein can help boost your metabolism. In fact, there are a number of foods and supplements that are thought to boost your resting metabolic rate. But exercise and nutrition research suggests that you can do that by including more protein in your diet and by eating lean protein with every meal—such as chicken, turkey breast, fish, and lean beef. Plant protein sources—such as beans, legumes, some grains, and tofu—can be incorporated as well.

This strategy can be controversial, but much of the current research supports the fact that protein should make up about 20 to 30 percent of your diet. This is higher than the 10 to 15 percent that has been traditionally recommended.

This recommendation applies to healthy individuals free from kidney disease (because protein could be an added stress to someone with diseased kidneys). Protein is especially important when trying to lose weight.

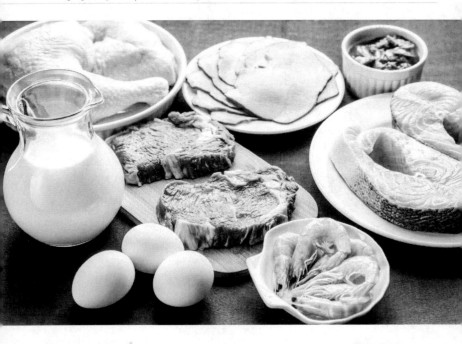

Protein Functions

- Similar to carbohydrates and fats, proteins contain carbon, hydrogen, and oxygen, but proteins also have a nitrogen molecule attached to their structure. It is this nitrogen found in protein that distinguishes it from the other macronutrients.

- Proteins are composed of amino acids that are linked together by peptide bonds. Twenty different amino acids exist, and they can all combine in unique ways to make new and different proteins in our bodies.

- But because so many different types of foods can provide you with protein, how can you tell if a specific protein or protein food is good-quality protein? One way to tell is by knowing the biological value of the protein. The higher the biological value of a protein, the higher its quality.

There are two types of proteins: essential and nonessential. They are either essential to include in our diets because our bodies don't make them, or they are nonessential because our bodies make them from other proteins, so we don't need to worry about eating them. There are 11 nonessential and 9 essential amino acids.

Essential amino acids are the ones we tend to worry about the most. When proteins contain all of the essential amino acids, they are called "complete" proteins and have a high biological value. These proteins are typically from animal sources and include meat, poultry, fish, eggs, milk, and cheese.

When food does not have all of the essential amino acids, they are called "incomplete" proteins and have a low biological value. These are lower-quality proteins that are missing at least one of the essential amino acids. A diet made up of incomplete proteins might eventually lead to protein malnutrition. Examples of incomplete proteins are usually found in plants, grains, nuts, and vegetables.

Classifying the amino acids like this is probably most important for people who do not eat animal products. This is because animal meats contain all of the essential amino acids, but plant products generally do not. This means that one or more of the amino acids will be missing, which could mean that you won't be able to make certain products that your body needs.

The good news is that most people don't eat only one source of plant food. And by combining various types of incomplete proteins, you can make up for any amino acids that were missing in your diet. This is called eating complementary proteins. The most common example of this is to eat rice and beans together.

One exception is soy, which is a plant product that *does* contain all of the essential amino acids, making it a complete protein.

Of the 9 essential amino acids, three are important because they are branched-chain amino acids, which can provide some fuel during long bouts of exercise or when we go long periods of time between eating. They might also help improve body composition.

The three branched-chain amino acids are leucine, isoleucine, and valine. These amino acids have a "branched" side chain that distinguishes them from other amino acids.

If you work out, consuming branched-chain amino acids might be beneficial in preventing muscle damage or helping repair damaged muscle tissue. This means that you might be less sore and uncomfortable after moderate to strenuous exercise if protein—such as milk, yogurt, or a protein shake—is consumed beforehand.

With regard to body composition, leucine gets the most attention of the three because it is considered to be the "trigger" to start muscle protein synthesis. In fact, research suggests that you not only want to eat some protein at each meal, but that you might also want to make sure that you are getting roughly two to three grams of leucine in the protein foods that you eat.

Over the past 5 to 10 years, there has been a huge increase in scientific papers that support using protein or amino acids to prevent the loss of muscle as a result of aging or extreme exercise. The scientific literature has repeatedly shown that a higher-protein diet helps with fat loss and improves body composition.

Nitrogen Balance

Some amino acids, such as the branched-chain amino acids and alanine, can be used to make ATP in your energy systems. In this way, it is estimated that protein contributes as much as 10 to 15 percent of your energy supply during intense prolonged exercise.

One common way to use amino acids for energy is to convert them to glucose in a process called the glucose-alanine cycle. This is one way to produce new glucose from non-carbohydrate sources, which is known as gluconeogenesis. This is how the amino acid alanine contributes to energy production.

Research shows that the more oxygen a person consumes, such as when breathing heavily from exercise, the greater the amount of leucine she or he uses as a fuel source.

In the process of eating protein, using it to make other proteins, and using it for energy, proteins are constantly being broken down (or metabolized) and built back up (or synthesized). This process is called protein turnover, and it is a never-ending process, which is why we must eat a sufficient amount of protein in our diets, particularly when we exercise a lot.

Nitrogen is the part of protein that distinguishes it from carbohydrates and fat on a chemical level. In the lab, we can measure nitrogen balance, which is the balance between nitrogen intake and nitrogen output. Protein foods can be analyzed for their nitrogen content, and this will take care of the "nitrogen in" part of the nitrogen balance equation. Doctors can then analyze nitrogen from body outputs, including urine, feces, sweat, skin, and hair.

When nitrogen intake is higher than output, you are in a positive nitrogen balance. In this scenario, you would likely be "anabolic" and in a muscle growth mode. If you are trying to maintain or build muscle mass, or lose fat, you want to be in a positive nitrogen balance.

When nitrogen intake is less than nitrogen output, you are in negative nitrogen balance. In this case, you would likely be sacrificing muscle to support your protein needs. This occurs during very long and intense workouts, if you don't eat for very long periods of time, or during the normal process of aging—if you don't pay attention to how much protein you eat.

- States of positive and negative nitrogen balance are drastically different and are both very important to your overall body composition.

- Factors that might affect nitrogen balance include protein quality and total calorie intake. High-quality animal proteins, such as eggs and dairy products, are best because of their amino acid content and high digestibility—that is, they are easy to digest and absorb.

- Plant proteins have lower digestibility—meaning that they are more difficult to digest and absorb and are low in some essential amino acids. In fact, a common recommendation for vegetarians is to increase protein intake by about 10 percent, just to account for this.

Exercise and Protein Needs

- The amount of protein in your diet can make a difference to overall body composition and health, but protein needs can change based on how much and what type of exercise you do.

- Endurance and resistance exercise can use or burn a lot of calories. This fact alone would require more protein in your diet, but exercise also puts a lot of strain on your body's protein stores.

- Protein breakdown increases when you exercise hard, and protein intake at an optimal level is required to maintain or improve muscle mass. Ultimately, you have the best chance at maintaining or improving muscle mass by choosing a diet with high rather than adequate protein levels.

Metabolism and Energy Balance

- There are three major components of total daily energy expenditure: resting metabolic rate, the thermic effect of activity, and the thermic effect of food. The largest percent of total daily energy expenditure belongs to our resting metabolic rate—close to 75 percent.

Your metabolism tends to slow as you age. The overall decrease in metabolism is only about one to three percent during the aging process, which really isn't much and can be offset with a few simple nutrition or exercise strategies—one of which might be eating more protein.

How does eating more protein help us adjust to a slowing metabolism? Your body digests a certain percentage of the macronutrients we eat—protein, carbohydrates, and fat—and protein is the least digested, because your body cannot oxidize, or burn, the nitrogen in protein sources of food.

In essence, your body works hard to digest and absorb protein, and this is probably why eating protein gives you the largest increase in metabolism when eating it. This is called the thermic effect of food. A

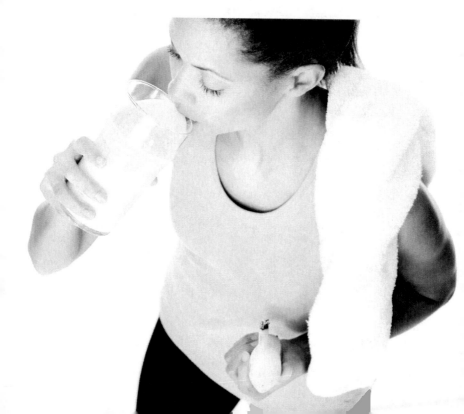

number of research studies have been designed to measure metabolism after a meal containing protein versus fat versus carbohydrate, and the majority of these indicate that the greatest increase in metabolism comes after eating protein.

In addition to the increase in metabolism we get from eating protein, it also makes us feel the most satiated after eating it. Here, the research is also clear: Low protein intake is linked to increased feelings of hunger and desire to eat again, while increased protein intake is linked to decreased feelings of hunger and less desire to eat again.

Even without exercise, research is showing that adding protein to the diet of overweight (but otherwise healthy) people can help improve body composition.

How Much Protein Do You Need?

The standard recommendation for protein is 0.8 grams per kilogram (0.36 grams per pound) of body weight per day, but we need more to have an optimal body composition response. The most recent research tells us we should be consuming up to about double the current recommendation.

Most women can aim for about one palm-sized portion of protein every time you eat. Most men can aim for two palm-sized portions of protein at each meal. This will, surprisingly, come close to your optimal needs for protein without having to count and weigh everything you eat.

These guidelines should be discussed with a qualified professional to get specific recommendations. You want information that best suits your lifestyle and health status.

Try This

Make sure you make protein a priority with every meal.

Questions to Consider

1. How much protein do you need to add to your diet to meet the "new" research recommendations?

2. What food sources of protein are in your diet, and which ones do you want to add to your diet? Why?

Protein's Critical Role in Body Composition

I n my opinion, protein is probably the most underrated macronutrient of all to help us control body composition. Carbohydrate and fat tend to get all of the attention as dieters try to eliminate one food or the other, but protein is extremely important for maintaining or even increasing muscle mass, losing body fat, increasing metabolism, and making you feel full for longer. You might think that you should only worry about protein if you want to add muscle and bulk up, but there are so many more aspects to protein than its ability to turn on muscle building, a process called muscle protein synthesis.

Proteins are all an integral part of your cell membranes, your cytoplasm, and your organelles like the mitochondria. They are also components of your tendons, and your skin, and your hair. They make up enzymes and assist in metabolic reactions. Proteins are essential elements in hemoglobin, the oxygen transport protein found in red blood cells, and plasma proteins, which are involved in transport of various substances in the blood. They are also very important in buffering acidity in your blood and in your cells. They assist in your body's natural immune system response, too. And many hormones, like insulin and growth hormone, are proteins as well.

Proteins are large components of muscle and they produce movement in your muscle tissue because they contract to help you bend your arm, or stand up, or just to get around. These proteins are called actin and myosin. Proteins can even be an energy source to provide ATP or the actual energy currency of your body used to produce work for all of your metabolic needs and daily activities. So, as you can tell, proteins are involved in just about every bodily process that we have.

In terms of your body composition, eating protein can help boost your metabolism. In fact, there are a number of foods and supplements that are thought to boost your resting metabolic rate. But research from my lab and from other exercise and nutrition scientists suggests that you can do that by including more protein in your diet and by eating lean protein with every meal, foods like chicken, turkey breast, fish, and lean beef. Plant protein sources like beans, legumes, some grains, and tofu can be incorporated as well.

This strategy can be controversial but much of the current research supports the fact that protein should make up around 20%–30% of your diet. This is higher than the 10%–15% that has traditionally been recommended. This recommendation applies to healthy individuals free from kidney disease, because protein could be an added stress to someone with diseased kidneys, and protein is especially important when trying to lose weight. But first, let's step back for a minute and go over some of the basics about protein.

Similar to carbohydrates and fats, proteins contain carbon, hydrogen, and oxygen, but proteins also have nitrogen, and it's attached to their structure. It is this nitrogen found in protein that distinguishes it from the other macronutrients. Proteins are composed of amino acids that are linked together by peptide bonds. There are 20 different amino acids that exist and they can all combine to make unique and new cells and different proteins in our bodies. But, because so many different types of foods can provide you with protein, how can you tell if a specific protein or protein food is a good quality protein?

Well, one way to tell is by knowing the biological value of the protein—the higher the biological value, the higher the quality. I need to explain what I mean by biological value here. There are two types of proteins: essential and non-essential. They are either essential to include in our diets because our bodies don't make them, or non-essential because our bodies make them from other proteins, so we don't need to worry about eating them. There are 11 non-essential and 9 essential amino acids. As you probably guessed, essential amino acids are the ones we tend to worry about most.

When proteins contain all of the essential amino acids, they are called complete proteins, and they have a high biological value. These proteins are typically from animal sources and include meat, poultry, fish, eggs, milk, and cheese. And when food does not have all of these essential amino acids, they are called incomplete proteins, and they have a low biological value. These are lower quality proteins that are missing at least one of the essential amino acids. So a diet made up of incomplete proteins may eventually lead to protein malnutrition. Examples of incomplete proteins are usually found in plants, grains, nuts, and vegetables.

Classifying the amino acids like this is probably most important for those of you who do not eat animal products. This is because animal meats contain all of the essential amino acids but plant products generally do not. This means that one or more of the amino acids will be missing, which could mean that you won't be able to make certain proteins that your body needs. The good news is that most people don't eat only one source of plant food, though, and by combining various types of incomplete proteins, you can make up for any amino acids that were missing in your diet. This is called eating complimentary proteins, and the most common example of this is to eat rice and beans together.

One exception is soy. Soy is a plant product that does contain all of the essential amino acids, making it a complete protein. Of the nine essential amino acids, three are important to point out because they are called branched-chain amino acids. Branched-chain amino acids can provide some fuel during long bouts of exercise or when we go long periods of time between eating. They may also help improve body composition.

The three branched-chain amino acids are leucine, isoleucine, and valine. As the name implies, these amino acids have a branched side chain that distinguishes them from the other amino acids. If you work out, it turns out that consuming branched-chain amino acids may be beneficial in preventing muscle damage and helping repair damaged muscle tissue. One study investigated the effect of eating foods containing branched-chain amino acid 60 minutes before a 90-minute aerobic exercise session at moderate intensity. These researchers wanted to see whether they had any impact on muscle damage after exercise.

What they found was that the biological markers of muscle damage and muscle soreness were lower when branched-chain amino acids were eaten before exercise compared to a placebo group that took no amino acids before exercise. This means that you may be less sore and uncomfortable after moderate to strenuous exercise if protein is consumed beforehand. Something like milk, yogurt, or a protein shake could do the trick. With regard to body composition, of the three—leucine, isoleucine, and valine— it's leucine that gets the most attention. This is because leucine is considered to be the trigger to start muscle protein synthesis.

In fact, research suggests that you not only want to eat some protein at each meal, but that you might also want to make sure that you're getting roughly 2–3 grams of leucine in the protein foods that you choose to eat. This is pretty easy to do. Most lean meats eaten in a normal palm-sized portion will provide 2.5–4.5 grams of leucine. You can also get about a half to 1 gram of leucine by drinking one cup of cow's milk. Also, eating beans or nuts will provide around 2–3 grams of leucine per cup. So, before a workout, you might think about a snack of milk, yogurt, beans and nuts, or a protein shake.

Over the past 5–10 years, I've seen a huge increase in scientific papers that support using protein or amino acids to prevent the loss of muscle as a result of aging or extreme exercise like marathon running, long-distance triathlon, or even ultra-distance events. The scientific literature has repeatedly shown that a higher protein diet helps with fat loss and improves body composition. But you may be wondering how protein does all of these positive things in our bodies, and how can you use it to improve your body composition.

Well, some amino acids, like the branched-chain amino acids and alanine, among others, can be used to make adenosine triphosphate or ATP in your energy systems. In this way, it is estimated that protein contributes as much as 10%–15% of your energy supply during intense prolonged exercise. Now, one common way to use amino acids for energy is to convert them to glucose in a process called the glucose-alanine cycle. This is one way to produce new glucose from non-carbohydrate sources, which is known as gluconeogenesis. This is how the amino acid alanine contributes to energy production. Research shows that the more oxygen a person consumes, like when breathing heavily from exercise, the greater the amount of leucine she or he uses as a fuel source.

So in the process of eating protein, using it to make other proteins, and using protein for energy, proteins are constantly being broken down or metabolized and built back up or synthesized. This process is called protein turnover. Now, this turnover process is never-ending, which is why we must eat a good amount of protein in our diets, particularly when we exercise a lot. One common question then is how much protein do we need to eat? In order to figure that out, it's important to talk about your nitrogen balance. Remember that nitrogen is part of the protein that distinguishes it from carbohydrates and fat on a chemical level.

In the lab, we can measure nitrogen balance, which is defined as the balance between nitrogen intake and nitrogen output. Protein foods can be analyzed for their nitrogen content, and this will take care of the nitrogen in part of the nitrogen balance equation. And doctors can then analyze nitrogen from body output including urine, feces, sweat, skin, and hair. And when nitrogen intake is higher than nitrogen output, you are in a positive nitrogen balance. So, in this scenario, you would be likely to be anabolic and in muscle growth mode. If you are trying to maintain or build muscle mass or lose fat, you want to be in a positive nitrogen balance.

When nitrogen intake is less than nitrogen output, you are in a negative nitrogen balance. You would likely be sacrificing muscle to support your protein needs in this case. This occurs during very long and intense workouts, if you don't eat for very long periods of time, or during the normal process of aging, if you don't pay attention to how much protein you eat. You can see that positive and negative nitrogen balance states are drastically different and are both very important to your overall body composition. Factors that may influence nitrogen balance include protein quality, like complete or incomplete, and amino acid content and total calorie intake. High-quality animal proteins like eggs and dairy products are best because of their amino acid content and their high digestibility—that is, they are easy to digest and absorb.

As I mentioned earlier, plant proteins have a lower digestibility, meaning that they are harder to digest and absorb, and are low in some of the essential amino acids. In fact, a common recommendation for vegetarians is to increase protein intake by about 10% just to account for this. And you should now understand that the amount of protein in your diet can make a difference to overall body composition and health. But protein needs can change based on how much and what type of exercise you do.

So, how does exercise affect our protein needs? Well, endurance and resistance exercise can use or burn a lot of calories; this fact alone would require more protein in your diet. But exercise also puts a lot of strain on your body's protein stores. These protein stores are known as the amino acid pool.

One study measured nitrogen balance in young and middle-aged distance runners. These runners were randomly assigned to a low-, moderate-, or high-protein intake from egg and milk proteins for 10 days, and nitrogen balance was measured in the final 5 days of each of the low-, moderate-, and high-protein diets. And whether the athletes were young or middle-aged, a low-protein diet made all the runners on that diet fall into a negative nitrogen balance. The moderate-protein intake, which was just above the current recommended dose of 0.8 grams of protein per kilogram of body weight, or 0.36 grams per pound of body weight, made about half of the runners go into a positive nitrogen balance, but the other half remained in a negative nitrogen state. But when a high-protein diet was given, the majority of runners were in positive nitrogen balance.

So, in runners, regardless of age, research shows that protein intake that is higher than current recommendations was best, in this study, to promote an environment that stops muscle wasting. In this study, the high-protein diet was 1.21 grams of protein per kilogram of body weight, or 0.6 grams per pound. If you weigh 145 pounds, or 66 kilograms, this would be about 80 grams of protein per day. But if you weigh 185 pounds, or 84 kilograms, this would be about 100 grams of protein per day. Now, just as a reminder, you simply divide your body weight in pounds by 2.2 to get your weight in kilograms.

But does the same thing happen if you lift weights instead of run? Well, the short answer is yes. Researchers used men who were new to lifting weights and sedentary men, and they ate a low-protein diet that was actually just above what is currently recommended at 0.86 grams of protein per kilogram of body weight per day, or a moderate-protein diet at 1.4 grams of protein per kilogram of body weight per day, or a high-protein diet at 2.4 grams of protein per kilogram of body weight per day. And they did this for 13 days each. They found that in men who did not exercise, the low-, moderate-, and high-protein diets all led to a positive nitrogen balance, but in the men who lifted weights, only the moderate- and high-protein diets led to a positive nitrogen balance.

So, once again, we see that for people who choose to exercise, which I hope is all of you, a higher intake of protein is needed to give yourself the best possible chance to maintain or increase your muscle mass. It's important to tell you, though, that there were no differences in protein synthesis between the moderate 1.4 grams of protein and the high 2.4 grams of protein per kilogram of body weight groups.

So, this tells us that around 1.4 grams of protein per kilogram of body weight, or 0.64 grams of protein per pound of body weight, may be optimal for promoting protein synthesis. So, again, if you weigh 145 pounds, or 66 kilograms, this would be about 92 grams of protein. And if you weigh 185 pounds, or 84 kilograms, this would be about 118 grams of protein per day. You could eat 90 grams in a typical day if you ate 2 large eggs at breakfast, 1 cup of Greek yogurt at lunch, a handful of almonds as a midday snack, and a 6-ounce chicken breast at dinner.

The takeaway here is that protein breakdown increases when you exercise hard, and protein intake at an optimal level is required to maintain or improve muscle mass. Ultimately, you have the best chance at maintaining or improving muscle mass by choosing a diet with high rather than adequate protein levels.

Now you can probably tell that protein is good for your muscles, but what does this do to your metabolism and energy balance? Well, first it's important to know that there are three major components of total daily energy expenditure. These include resting metabolic rate, the thermic effect of activity, and the thermic effect of food. And the largest percent of total daily energy expenditure belongs to our resting metabolic rate, close to 75%. And you may also remember that your metabolism tends to slow as you age. Now, the overall decrease in metabolism is only about 1%–3% during the entire aging process, which really isn't that much. As we age, we lose about 5% of our muscle mass every 10 years, so from age 40 to age 80 you could lose as much as 20% of your muscle mass, which would lower your overall calorie burn and metabolism.

But we can do something about it. For example, if your resting metabolism is 1800 calories per day, then the metabolic decrease over time could be somewhere around 20–60 calories in total. That's pretty easy to offset with just a few simple nutrition or exercise strategies, one of which just might be eating more protein. If you are used to eating minimal protein, as many adults do, then even doubling your intake from what is currently recommended is likely a great thing to try. So you would simply be sure to have a good protein source at each meal to base the rest of your meal around.

Now, how does eating more protein help us to adjust to a slowing metabolism? Well, an interesting fact about the macronutrients that we eat—which are protein, carbohydrates, and fat—is that they all have what is called a coefficient of digestibility. What this means is that if you ate a food that was 100% carbohydrate, you would digest about 97% of that food. However, if it was all fat, you would digest about 95% of that food. But if you ate 100% protein, you would only digest about 92% of that food. Your body digests a certain percentage of those three macronutrients, and protein is the least digested, compared to carbohydrate and fat. And that's because your body cannot oxidize or burn the nitrogen in protein sources of food.

In essence, your body works hard to digest and absorb protein, and this is probably why eating protein gives you the largest increase in metabolism when eating it. This is called the thermic effect of food. A number of research studies have been designed to measure metabolism after a meal containing protein versus fat versus carbohydrate, and the majority of these indicate that the greatest increase in metabolism comes after eating protein. So, by eating protein, you begin to increase your metabolism and your caloric burn.

Now, outside of the increase in metabolism we get from eating protein, it also makes us feel full or satiated after eating it. Here, the research is also clear: low-protein intake is linked to increased feelings of hunger and desire to eat again, while increased protein intake is linked to decreased feelings of hunger and less desire to eat again. And even without exercise, our research is showing that adding protein to the diet of overweight but otherwise healthy people can improve body composition.

For example, in overweight and obese adults, nutrition scientists demonstrated that a protein supplement providing 56 grams per day of whey protein with no other dietary alterations resulted in significantly lower body fat mass by 5 pounds, or 2.3 kilograms, over 23 weeks of doing this. This was compared to a carbohydrate supplement of equal calories given to another test group. So you can see that eating more protein may be the best nutritional strategy to manage body composition, given its influence on metabolism, satiety, and even maintenance of muscle mass. And the impact of a high-protein diet when combined with an exercise program can provide even better results for improving metabolism and body composition.

In fact, I collaborated on a research project with lead investigator Dr. Paul Arciero from Skidmore College and found that a diet high in protein, which was about 40%, combined with exercise training that included both resistance training and high-intensity interval training was optimal for reducing both body weight and body fat in obese men and women between 40 and 60 years old. This protein and exercise combination also helped to maintain or even improve muscle mass.

And, in 2014, we teamed up to see what sort of exercise was best with a higher protein diet. Our results were really interesting—we found that the greatest improvements in body composition of middle-aged overweight and/ or obese men and women when they ate a high-protein diet and included a high-quality variety of exercise in their weekly schedules. They completed 4 days of exercise per week: 1 day of weight training, 1 day of sprint interval training to really get the heart rate going, 1 day of stretching and yoga, and 1 day of slower endurance exercise. Dr. Arciero and I called this program the PRISE program, which stands for protein, resistance exercise, interval training, stretching or yoga, and endurance.

The PRISE group was compared to two other groups—one group had a higher protein diet, but no exercise program; and the other group had a high-protein diet but also lifted weights. Interestingly, all three groups lost fat and improved body composition. But, as you might imagine, lifting weights improved things further, and adding the variety of exercise was the best overall.

Now, back to that question I raised earlier: "Just how much protein do I need?" Well, the standard recommendation is 0.8 grams per kilogram, or 0.36 grams per pound, of body weight per day. So, if you weigh 150 pounds, which is 68 kilograms, that would give you a daily protein requirement of 55 grams of protein per day. This is equivalent to about 2 eggs for breakfast, which would give you roughly 12 grams, one chicken breast for lunch, which would give you about 40 grams, and one Greek yogurt, which would be about 10 grams of protein.

But, as we discussed, we need more to have optimal body composition as the response. The most recent research tells us that we should be consuming up to about double the current recommendation for protein. So, that would be around 1.6 grams per kilogram, or 0.73 grams per pound, of your body weight—or higher—if your goal is weight loss. Now, this will give you your best shot at maintaining your muscle mass while also losing fat.

So, if you weigh 150 pounds, or 68 kilograms, your new protein requirement would come in close to 110 grams of protein—or possibly more—per day. You would essentially add another lean cut of protein to a salad, and have a glass of milk and a large serving of vegetables. Now, most people don't like to remember these numbers and, honestly, getting bogged down with them makes adding more protein difficult to put into practice. So, for most women, the best option is to aim for about one palm-sized portion of protein every time you eat. And for most men, you can aim for two palm-sized portions of protein at each meal. This will surprisingly come quite close to your optimal needs for protein without having to count and weigh everything you eat.

I don't typically suggest weighing foods, but sometimes it does help in the short term. For example, you could weigh your foods to start out and get an idea of the weight and content of the foods you eat most often. But, after some time, using the hand method is much more convenient. One note, of course, is that these and any recommendations should be discussed with a qualified professional for you to get specific recommendations. You want information that best suits your lifestyle and health status.

But one point I want to make clear is that eating more protein will not change things so drastically that it will automatically make your body fat melt off or make your muscles big and strong. In short, it will not magically give you your optimal body composition. But eating protein at every meal, combined with the other strategies that you'll learn in this course, like exercising right, just might set you up with the ideal scenario to begin to see changes if you're searching for them. So try this: make sure to have protein as a priority with every meal.

High-Protein Diets and Anabolic Resistance

How much protein should you eat? In this lecture, you will learn about the amounts, timing, and type of protein that you might need to consume to lose body fat while maintaining muscle mass—even with a low-calorie diet. You will also learn about muscle growth and breakdown and how, as you grow older, you will need even more protein to support what is happening to your body. In general, diets that are higher than typically recommended in protein are safe and are an effective tool for improving body composition.

The Amount of Protein You Eat

- Many people still think that eating protein will somehow automatically add muscle and make them bigger. This is just not accurate—or gaining muscle would be much easier.

- When people start a diet or purposefully eat less food, one of the major risks is losing muscle mass. You'll lose body weight, but you might also lose a lot of muscle. And that, of course, is a problem because having muscle helps you burn calories, stay active, and be healthy.

- The research to date says that you can preserve muscle mass and decrease fat mass even with severe caloric restriction.

- The ability to maintain muscle while losing fat is one way to rescue our resting metabolism so that it doesn't drop too drastically. This means that you just increased your ability to fight weight regain, or putting all of the weight back on, as is typical after the diet stops or changes.

When lowering your calorie intake in an attempt to lose body fat, you increase your chances of success by increasing, not decreasing, protein in your diet.

During calorie restriction, a shift to increase the number of calories you get from protein—which would replace many of the calories you get from carbohydrates and fats—will improve body composition. Even supplementing with milk has been shown to improve body composition when trying to lose weight.

In terms of recommended amounts, it looks like about two times the recommended dietary allowances can cover most of your bases. That would be about 1.6 grams per kilogram of body weight, or 0.72 grams of protein per pound.

Aging and Anabolic Resistance

Research shows that people who add more protein to their diets tend to improve their body composition, particularly when exercise is also included. But what about the massive amounts of muscle that we risk losing as we age?

If you don't work to keep your muscle mass, you will lose muscle mass every decade after about 30 years old. The health implications and your ability to just move around depend on keeping some of your muscle mass.

When we talk about muscle protein balance, it is important to talk about both the synthesis part, which is known as anabolism (or muscle growth), and the degradation part, known as catabolism (or muscle breakdown). If synthesis matches degradation, you would not gain or lose any muscle. If, however, degradation is greater than synthesis, you would be losing muscle.

Additionally, certain changes occur that make it more difficult for an older adult to use protein to build or maintain muscle mass. The body

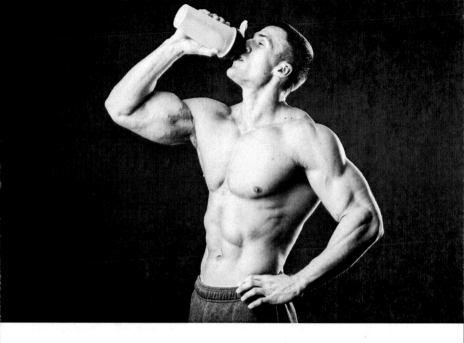

actually starts to resist anabolism, or growth, with age. This process has been coined "anabolic resistance."

Interestingly, even after consuming an amount of protein that is known to increase muscle protein synthesis, the synthesis response is lower in older adults compared to younger adults. So, even though you hear about a specific protein intake—such as 0.8 grams per kilogram of body mass per day—that is recommended to avoid disease states or muscle wasting, it is much too low to actually optimally improve body composition, especially as you age.

If you are 20 years old and you eat or drink about 20 to 25 grams of protein following a workout, you will likely maximize your immediate ability to make new muscle proteins. But you need almost twice this amount (that is, about 40 grams) after exercise when you are older to have the same result as seen in younger people. It is probably quite variable at what age this occurs, but you might consider increasing your after-exercise protein intake after about age 40.

A recent scientific review paper pointed out a number of reasons for why this anabolic resistance might occur as we age, including decreased digestion and absorption of protein, decreased ability for your muscles to absorb amino acids, and decreased anabolic signaling once the protein is eaten.

This anabolic resistance in older, healthy adults can be overcome with a higher intake of dietary protein. The entire process for muscle repair, maintenance, and growth is blunted as we age. You might just need an extra push—such as more protein—to have the response you want.

How much protein should you be consuming to keep your muscle protein synthesis high? One study gave healthy older men 10, 20, or 35 grams of whey protein and found that absorption and muscle protein synthesis was greater with 35 grams compared to 10 and 20 grams.

It looks like there is some sort of anabolic threshold when we talk about protein intake that simply rises as we get older, and that threshold needs to be met to stimulate a response.

An increased protein intake seems to have a long-term effect, as well. Research has shown that more protein in older people help them maintain their muscle mass better than lower protein intake. Overall, if you are an older adult, every time you eat, think about including a lean protein source of food.

Recommendations for Protein Consumption

Unfortunately, the recommendations for daily protein consumption vary across organizations. The American College of Sports Medicine recommends 10 to 35 percent of your total calorie intake to come from protein—which equates to about 200 to 700 calories in a standard 2,000-calorie diet. They also recommend increasing protein intake to 1 gram per kilogram of body weight around age 50 and increasing even further in active older individuals.

But if you are very active, then how much do you need? The International Society of Sports Nutrition recommends 1.4 to 2 grams of protein per kilogram of body weight for active individuals to improve training adaptations to exercise. This is strongly endorsed by the most current research.

Other leading international organizations, such as the Academy of Nutrition and Dietetics and the European Society for Clinical Nutrition and Metabolism, recommend somewhere between 1 and 1.7 grams of protein per kilogram of body weight, depending on your activity level and health status. Overall, recommendations are beginning to increase.

Frequency of Eating and Nighttime Eating

The concept of when we eat and at what frequency we should eat is called nutrient timing.

When do you want to eat? If you like breakfast or a late-night snack, then eating at those times will probably help you stick to the plan. However, the food you pick to eat at those times will make the difference in how your body ultimately stores the energy.

MYTH
Too Much Protein Is Harmful

A myth about eating too much protein is that it will cause your kidneys to shut down, but this is incorrect. There is a lot of research support for a higher-protein diet; studies show no evidence of kidney disease resulting from eating more protein.

On a high-protein diet, your kidneys do perform more work to handle the protein. However, increased action does not equal damage. This is because—like all of our other bodily functions—the kidneys are very good at adapting.

Overall, there is no overwhelming evidence that says that protein harms the body, but anything in excess can potentially be damaging.

How should your daily protein needs be split up over a day for the best results? Eating about 20 grams of protein per meal, spaced evenly throughout the day, is commonly recommended. The research here is mixed, though.

Unfortunately, research shows that older individuals typically consume 8 grams of protein at breakfast, 12 grams of protein at lunch, and a maximum of 40 grams of protein at dinner. This type of spread of protein is considered protein back-loading. It is very common, but for optimal results, it seems that the dose of protein should be spaced a bit more evenly throughout the day, to stimulate muscle protein synthesis.

In overweight and obese older individuals, evenly spaced protein stimulates muscle protein synthesis significantly more effectively than this back-loaded practice. Interestingly, when resistance training is added, muscle protein synthesis normalizes no matter how the protein is eaten. Back-loaded or not, resistance training improves how we respond to eating.

If you simply don't like eating frequently, you can also have great results by eating less frequently. You just need to be sure that when you do eat, you're eating nutrient-dense foods and getting high-quality protein in those foods.

Another time of day that people often want to eat is before bed. It might actually be good for you to eat a small protein snack or drink a protein shake before bed.

When young and older men were given 40 grams of casein protein before bed, their muscle protein synthesis was significantly higher overnight than when they drank a no-calorie drink, regardless of their age.

How do other macronutrients and other forms of protein—besides casein—eaten or consumed before bed affect metabolism and health? In one study, the effect of a nighttime snack on next-day resting metabolic rate was influenced by the sex, age, and fitness level of the person.

What about the effect of nighttime eating on body composition? The first study to look at 12 weeks of nighttime eating before sleep and exercise training found that by simply drinking a protein shake before sleep, muscle size was improved, and so was strength.

It looks like very small, 150-calorie protein drinks before bed might actually be advisable, rather than something to avoid, but much more research is needed in this area.

Protein Powders

It can be difficult to eat a lot of high-protein meals. It just makes you feel very full. So, an easy way to add extra protein is in the form of protein powders. There are many types of protein powders on the market.

There are many forms of protein. Whey protein isolate is considered the purest form of protein. Hydrolyzed whey protein isolate is the most expensive because of the purity and the processes involved to make it. Whey protein concentrate has less filtering and therefore more natural carbohydrates and fats from milk, making the protein content lower in most cases—about 35 to 80 percent protein.

Two other very common sources and types of protein powders are casein, also from milk, and soy protein. Although these proteins also increase muscle protein synthesis, whey is usually considered best for improving muscle protein synthesis, especially post-workout. This is because of whey's higher leucine content—the essential branched-chain amino acid that contributes the most to muscle protein synthesis.

Casein and soy are good options, though, for people who just don't like whey, for those who want something that is slower digesting (casein), or for vegetarians (soy).

Many other sources also exist, such as hemp, pea, and even bug proteins, but less research exists on those.

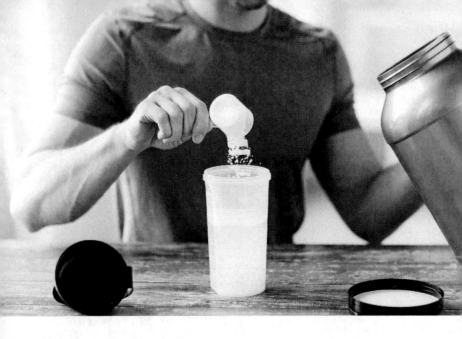

Milk is also an acceptable source of protein and has been found to increase lean body mass more than soy protein after 12 weeks of a resistance-training program. But milk also has both carbohydrates and fat in it.

What do you look for on the label of a supplement? You want the highest percent of protein per scoop. You ideally want a powder with more than 80 percent protein in each scoop.

Take caution, though, when reading the labels on protein powders. Many powders have added proteins that our body cannot use toward building muscle—even if they contribute to the total nitrogen content. Some examples of protein fillers are l-glycine and l-taurine. Supplement companies cleverly market these fillers to make them look like they will help you, but they probably won't.

Overall, protein powders can be a great, convenient way to increase protein intake, and most of them taste great. You can't beat the great effects on body composition with the addition of this supplement to your diet.

Try This

Experiment with protein powders to find one that makes it convenient for you to take in enough protein to optimize your body composition.

Questions to Consider

1. What myths were busted in this lecture?

2. What foods do you eat that contribute to your daily protein needs?

High-Protein Diets and Anabolic Resistance

H ave you heard that a high protein diet will destroy your kidneys? Well this sort of statement has been brought to our attention over the years from many media outlets. However, you'd be hard-pressed to find any research to support this notion, with one major exception: people who have preexisting kidney disease. It is amazing how people are frightened of eating or drinking protein because of how the media have blown this issue so far out of proportion. But, because of this major caveat, it's important to always meet with your physician before drastically changing anything in your diet.

Everybody is unique, and you don't want to rely on the statistics—you want to be sure that you know what's right for you. However, with this caveat, higher than typically recommended protein diets are safe and are effective for improving body composition. I've seen this first-hand in a number of the research studies that I've either directed or helped with. And adding more protein to your diet is really a good idea. But, this leads me to another common myth surrounding protein. Have you heard that most people eat a high protein diet already—particularly in America?

Because Americans are known as meat-eaters and generally eat a lot of food it is common to think that Americans do, indeed, eat more protein than needed. While this may be true for some individuals, we need to consider that recommendations are based on your body weight and not a one size fits all recommendation. So, yes, some Americans may eat more protein than they need. But many don't. A much larger person, for example, needs to eat more protein than a smaller person just to meet the very lowest recommended protein intake.

For example, I just collaborated on a research project where we studied middle-aged people with class 3 obesity, which is the highest level of obesity.

This means that each person in the study had a body mass index, or a weight-to-height ratio that was greater than 40. And some of the people in the study actually did eat normal amounts of protein, but because of their large body weights they were only eating about a quarter of the recommended daily allowance for protein, which, as you know, is 0.8 g of protein per kg—0.36 g per lb—of body your weight. So, in this scenario, despite these obese people eating protein regularly—and likely in an amount that is normal for an average-sized person—it was far too low when body weight was taken into account. It didn't even meet the lowest recommended dose to avoid diseases. And, when you consider that many studies tell us to eat more protein than is currently recommended, especially if you are active, then you may want to change a few things.

So, if you're sitting there questioning how much protein to eat, then you're in luck because, in this lecture, we will talk about the amount, an the timing, and the type of protein that you might need to consume to lose body fat while maintaining muscle mass—even with a low calorie diet. We will also be talking about muscle growth and breakdown, and how, as you grow older, you will need even more protein to support what is happening to your body. So, let's get started.

Let's say that you want to get in shape and you've decided to become fit. You're told by your health professional that you should add more protein to your diet because you're working out now. You may say, "Won't adding protein just make me big and bulky?" Absolutely not. After the myth about protein and the kidneys, this is the next major protein myth that I hear all the time. Many people still think that eating protein will somehow automatically add muscle and make them bigger. This is just not accurate—or gaining muscle would be much, much easier. When people start a diet or purposefully eat less food, one of the major risks is losing muscle mass. Sure, you'll lose body weight, but you may also lose a lot of muscle. And that, of course, is a problem because having muscle mass helps you to burn calories, stay active, and be healthy. So, the question becomes can you preserve muscle mass and decrease fat mass even with severe caloric restriction? Well, the research to date says yes.

Remember the class 3 obese people in the research study I just told you about? Well, they were all put on a very low-calorie diet—I mean absurdly low—lower than I would ever recommend. But, this was a medically mandated low-calorie diet due to the severity of their obesity. Well, when we added 12 weeks of resistance training and much more protein to their very low calorie diets they still lost a lot of weight, but they were able to maintain a greater amount of muscle mass compared to the people who did not incorporate resistance exercise. The cool part is that this was the case even though they were restricted to 800 calories per day. That means even when we are in a severe calorie deficit eating more protein and lifting weights can help prevent significant losses in muscle mass that would otherwise be seen.

Consider how important that is. The ability to maintain muscle while losing fat is one way to rescue our resting metabolism so that it doesn't drop too drastically. This means that you just increased your ability to fight weight regain, or putting all of the weight back on, as is typical after the diet stops or changes. But, this doesn't only apply to those on medically directed extreme weight loss plans and people who are severely obese, or what's referred to as morbidly obese. It also applies to anyone trying to lose body fat. When lowering your calorie intake in an attempt to lose body fat you increase your chances of success by increasing not decreasing the protein in your diet.

So, how much protein, and in turn calories, can you actually add without increasing your body fat? Well, in the most extreme example that I've seen, one study gave young, healthy men 4.4 g of protein per kg of body weight per day for eight weeks. This is nearly 4 times the recommended amount. This turns out to be about an additional 1200 calories for the average 150 lb, or 68 kg, person. With simple calorie counting, you'd expect these guys to have gained a lot of weight, right? But, even with this increase in calories, the men in this study did not gain any body fat or muscle mass.

Now, this huge dose of protein is pretty outrageous and most of the time completely unnecessary, but what about more reasonable increases in protein? Another study did just that. First, they put 39 physically active men and women who were about 21-years-old, and with a normal body mass index of BMI of 22–29, on a low calorie diet. It was about a 40% reduction from what they normally ate. Then, they supplemented the participants with 3 different levels of protein. One group got the recommended dietary allowance, or RDA, for protein, which was 0.8 g per kg of body weight, the second group got 2×RDA at 1.6 g per kg, and the third group got 3×RDA at 2.4 g of protein per kg of body weight.

So, what happened? Turns out that both the 2× and the 3× the recommended protein intake preserved muscle mass and reduced the body fat to the greatest extent while on a low calorie diet. And the group that supplemented with 2× the RDA of protein had the greatest effects. This means that during calorie restriction, a shift to increase the number of calories you get from protein, which would replace many of the calories you get from carbohydrates and fats, will improve body composition. Even supplementing with milk has been shown to improve body composition when trying to lose weight.

Researchers put overweight and obese women on an exercise and low calorie diet for 16 weeks with varying amounts of protein and dairy. They found that all of the women they lost a significant amounts of weigh, but the high-protein and high-dairy group—which was about 30% protein and 15% dairy—lost the most fat from their stomach area and from their visceral fat—that's the fat surrounding your organs and is linked to so many health problems. But, another cool benefit also occurred while these women were on the low calorie diet and exercising—only the high-protein, high-dairy group was able to actually add muscle mass. Not to mention, protein intake from milk and other sources may help decrease your waist circumference and maximize your strength. Sounds pretty good, right?

So simply putting yourself on a low calorie diet isn't enough. Yes, you need to know something about the quantity of food you eat and drink because a deficit in calories does create weight loss, but the type, and quality of your calories matters too. If you want to lose fat but also preserve your muscles, or even add muscle to help with your performance, mobility, and metabolism then you should seriously consider increasing the amount of protein you eat.

So, research pretty clearly shows that people who add more protein to their diets tend to improve their body composition, particularly when exercise is also included. But, what about massive amounts of muscle that we risk losing as we age? As you know, if you don't work to keep your muscle mass, you will lose muscle mass every decade after about 30 years old or so. The health implications and your ability to just move around depend on keeping some of your muscle mass. Have you seen the older people you know losing lots of muscle?

So, what can you do? Particularly as an older adult, is there anything you can do about the amount of protein you consume, to preserve, or even prevent the muscle loss, or even increase muscle protein synthesis? Yes. But first, a little physiology lesson. When we talk about muscle protein balance, it is important to talk about both the synthesis part, which is known as anabolism or muscle growth, and the degradation part, which is known as catabolism or muscle breakdown. If synthesis matches degradation, you would not gain or lose any muscle. If; however, degradation is greater than synthesis, you would be losing muscle.

Additionally, one really interesting thing about aging is that certain changes occur that actually make it harder for an older adult to use protein to build or maintain muscle mass. The body actually starts to resist anabolism or growth with age. This process has cleverly been coined anabolic resistance. Interestingly, even after consuming an amount of protein that is known to increase muscle protein synthesis, the synthesis response is lower in older adults compared to younger adults. So even though you hear about a specific protein intakes like 0.8 g per kg of body mass per day that is recommended to avoid disease states or muscle wasting, and it is far too low to actually optimally improve body composition, especially as you age.

But, what is the effect on muscle protein synthesis if you get your protein dose after exercising? For example, we know that the ideal dose of protein after exercise to stimulate muscle protein synthesis or muscle growth, as well as a host of other benefits, is about 20–25 g of protein. The research was done only with young men; however, most experts use this same range for young women. But, what about in older women and older men? One study gave elderly men 1, 10, 20, or 40 g of protein immediately after resistance training, and found that with 20 g of protein, muscle protein synthesis remained elevated compared to baseline levels of muscle protein synthesis, and that's good. But, here's the kicker, muscle protein synthesis was even higher with a 40 g dose. So, it seems like older muscles respond better to higher protein amounts.

Recently, it has also been shown that even more protein above the RDA, even in young people, may further contribute to the muscle protein balance equation by reducing muscle protein breakdown. So if you're 20 years old and you eat or drink about 25 g of protein following a workout; you will likely maximize your ability to make new muscle proteins. But, you need almost twice this amount—that is, about 40 g—postexercise when you are older in order to have the same result as seen in the younger people. And what age does this occur?

Well, it's probably quite variable. But, I would like to take this into account and consider upping my after-exercise protein intake after about age 40. A recent scientific review paper pointed out a number of reasons why this anabolic resistance might occur as we age. Some of these include: decreased digestion and absorption of protein, decreased ability for your muscles to absorb amino acids, and decreased anabolic signaling once the protein is eaten. Sounds challenging, right? Well, this anabolic resistance in older, healthy adults can be overcome with a higher intake of dietary protein. The entire process for muscle repair, maintenance, and growth is just blunted as we age. You may just need an extra push—like more protein—to have the response that you want.

OK, so you're probably thinking, "just how much protein should I be consuming to keep my muscle protein synthesis high?" One study gave healthy, older men 10, 20, or 35 g of whey protein and found that absorption and muscle protein synthesis was greater with 35 g compared to 10 and 20 g. And it looks like we have some sort of anabolic threshold when we talk about protein intake that simply rises, as we get older. And that threshold needs to be met in order to stimulate a response. An increased protein intake seems to have a long-term effect as well.

One study looked at the level of protein intake in older men and women over 3 years. After a complete dietary analysis, the participants were grouped into 5 groups based on their levels of protein intake. It turns out that the group that consumed the highest average amount of protein—about 19% of their typical diet over the 3-year-period—had the smallest loss in muscle mass over the same time. In fact, they had 40% less muscle loss than the group with the lowest protein intake that only ate about 11% protein in their diets. In other words, more protein in the older people helped them to maintain their muscle mass much better than lower protein intake. Overall, if you are an older adult, do not fear protein. In fact, I would make sure that every time you eat, you include a lean source of protein.

All right, so we've pretty clearly established that you should consume a good amount of protein, and hopefully the case for a protein intake that is greater than 0.8 g of protein per kg of body weight is a no-brainer now. But, what are the actual recommendations for daily protein consumption from different organizations? Unfortunately, the answer varies across organizations. The American College of Sports Medicine recommends 10–35% of your total calorie intake to come from protein, which equates to about 200–700 calories in a standard 2000-calorie diet. They also recommend increasing protein intake to 1.0 g per kg of body weight around age 50, and increasing even further in active, older individuals.

This is not bad considering all of the research supporting more protein for improved body composition, health, and performance, but if you are very active, then what? How much do you need? The International Society of Sports Nutrition recommends 1.4–2.0 g of protein per kg of body weight for active individuals to improve training adaptations to exercise—this is strongly endorsed by the most current research. Other leading international organizations like the Academy of Nutrition and Dietetics and the European Society for Clinical Nutrition and Metabolism recommend somewhere between 1.0 and 1.7 g of protein per kg of body weight depending on your activity level and health status.

So, recommendations are beginning to increase and the research tells the story. And just to recap, some food sources that are great for protein are eggs, lean chicken, beef, and fish, and things like Greek yogurt, nuts, peas, tofu, seeds and quinoa also pack a protein punch. And even though I mentioned this at the beginning of the lecture, it is worth repeating because one question that I continue to get asked regarding the amount of protein we eat is this "Is too much protein harmful? And, Won't my kidneys shut down?"

I want to tell you again—absolutely not. This is wrong. But, the myth persists. We already talked about the research support for a higher protein diet—these studies show no evidence of kidney disease resulting from eating more protein. Here's the deal, on a high protein diet, your kidneys do perform more work to handle the protein. However, increased action does not equal damage. This is because, like all our other bodily functions, the kidneys are very good at adapting. One study found that markers of kidney function are not affected in strength athletes with multiple years of high protein intake. However, there is likely a time when you don't need any more protein.

More than 1.5 g per lb—or 3.3 g per kg—of body weight is not needed or recommended, as 1 g per lb—2.2 g per kg—of body weight is enough and far exceeds the 0.36 g per lb—0.8 g per kg—that is traditionally recommended. Overall, there is no overwhelming evidence that says that protein harms the body, but anything in excess can potentially be damaging. That's just common sense. But; unfortunately, common sense sometimes goes out the window when people talk about new diets and eating fads.

And of course, always double check, and change your diet with your healthcare provider to make sure it's a healthy choice for you. Now, let's go beyond just how much protein we should eat and move on to topics like when we need to eat it, and at what frequency we should eat protein. This is a concept called nutrient timing. The first thing to talk about is when do you want to eat? For example, if you like breakfast, or a late-night snack then eating at those times will probably help you stick to your plan. However, the food you pick and eat at those times will make the difference in how your body ultimately stores the energy.

So, how should your daily protein needs be split up over a day for the best results? Eating about 20 g of protein per meal spaced evenly throughout the day is commonly recommended. The research here is mixed though. Unfortunately, research shows us that older individuals typically consume about 8 g of protein at breakfast, 12 g of protein at lunch, and a maximum of 40 g of protein at dinner. This type of spread of protein is considered protein back-loading. It is very common. But for optimal results, it seems that the dose of protein should be spaced a bit more evenly throughout the day, in order to stimulate muscle protein synthesis. In overweight and obese older individuals, evenly spaced protein stimulates muscle protein synthesis significantly more effectively than this back-loaded practice. Interestingly, when resistance training is added, muscle protein synthesis normalized no matter how they ate their protein. Back-loaded or not, resistance training improves how we respond to eating.

A study that I worked on showed that a higher protein diet—35% of total calorie intake—spaced across 6 meals per day significantly reduced body fat and abdominal fat. And lean mass remained higher compared to the same amount of protein eaten over 3 meals per day. When compared to a more common and lower protein intake—like 15%—the high protein, eaten more frequently approach was also better for body composition and metabolism. Think about it like this, if you can spike your protein synthesis on more than one occasion in a day, you will probably have a better net effect at the end of the day than only spiking your muscle protein synthesis at one meal where you happen to eat all of your daily protein.

But, I also know people who simply don't like eating frequently. It can be a hassle and take too much time. Well, you can also have great results eating less frequently. You just need to be sure that when you do eat, you're eating nutrient dense foods and that you're getting high quality protein in those foods. Another time of day that people often want to eat is before bed. Do you find yourself hungry before bed, maybe wanting a snack but believe that it's not a healthy habit? It's not only not unhealthy it may actually be good for you to eat a small protein snack or drink a protein shake right before bed. When young and older men were given 40 g of casein protein before bed, their muscle protein synthesis was significantly higher overnight than when they drank a no calorie drink. And this was regardless of their age. It worked for young and old alike.

Now, this was not done in women, but I think similar results would occur. This study shows us a couple of things. One, you may be able to improve your body composition by having a nighttime protein snack. And two, although older men have lower rates of muscle protein synthesis than young men, both age groups have an increase in muscle protein synthesis when taking a protein shake before bed. But, how do other macronutrients and other forms of protein eaten before bed—besides casein—affect metabolism and health?

Interestingly, a study from our lab showed in young, active men—whether eating a carbohydrate, whey protein, or casein protein snack before bed that had about 140–150 calories in total—resting energy expenditure the next day was increased compared to eating nothing at night before bed. But, when we did a very similar study in obese women their next morning resting metabolic rate had a more favorable increase if protein was consumed before sleep, but interestingly, not with carbohydrates. The difference was very small, but the pattern that we noticed was pretty interesting. Essentially, the effect of a nighttime snack on next day resting metabolic rate was influenced by the sex, age, and fitness level of the person in the study.

What about the effect of nighttime eating on body composition? Well, we looked at this over a 4-week period where overweight and obese young women had a carbohydrate, whey, or casein snack before bed every night, and they also exercised 3 days per week. Although nobody lost weight, all 3 groups increased their muscle mass in the study. What's more is that the whey and casein groups—they had protein—tended to decrease fat mass, whereas the carbohydrate group had no change. Now, these differences were very small and not statistically significant, but it has pushed us to look further into new research to see exactly what is going on.

The first study to look at 12 weeks of nighttime eating before sleep and exercise training recently found that by simply drinking a protein shake before sleep, muscle size was improved and so was strength. Now, it looks like very small 150-calorie protein drinks before bed may actually be advisable, rather than something to avoid. But, I'll be the first to tell you that much more research is needed in this area and I'll talk much more about nighttime eating later in this course.

In sum, protein consumption should be on the top of your mind and probably timed to multiple feedings in a day to achieve your optimal body composition results. But, it can be difficult to eat a lot of protein meals. It just makes that you feel very full. So, an easy way to add extra protein is in the form of protein powders. There are many types of protein powders on the market so let's just talk about a few things to look for before you purchase one. First, there are many forms of protein. Whey protein isolate is considered the most pure form of protein. Hydrolyzed whey protein isolate is the most expensive because of the purity, and the process involved to make it. But, whey protein concentrate has less filtering and therefore more natural carbohydrates and fats from milk, making the protein content lower in most cases—about 35 to 80% protein depending on what you buy. The other 2 very common sources and types of protein powders are from casein—which is also from milk—and soy protein. Although these proteins also increase muscle protein synthesis, whey is usually considered best for improving muscle protein synthesis, especially post-workout. This is because of whey's higher leucine content—the essential branched-chain amino acid that contributes the most to muscle protein synthesis.

Casein and soy are good options, though, for people who just don't like whey, want something that is slower digesting—that would be casein—or for vegetarians who might choose soy. Many other sources also exist like hemp, pea, and even bug proteins, but less research exists on those. Milk, as you probably guessed, is also an acceptable source of protein and been found to increase lean body mass greater than soy protein after 12 weeks of a resistance-training program. But keep in mind that milk also has both carbohydrates and fat in it.

So what do you look for on the label of a supplement? You want the highest percent of protein per scoop. You ideally want a powder with more than 80% protein in each scoop. For example, 25 g of protein in a 28 g serving scoop equates to 90% protein—the perfect amount. Take caution, though, when reading labels on protein powders. Many powders have added proteins that our body cannot use toward building muscle even if they contribute to the total nitrogen content of the product. Some examples of protein fillers are l-glycine and l-taurine. And supplement companies cleverly market these fillers to make them out to look like they will help you out, but they probably won't. Overall, protein powders can be a great; convenient way to increase protein intake and most of them taste great. You can't beat the great effects on body composition with the addition of this supplement.

So we can see that a protein intake above recommended levels will be beneficial for body composition. And don't worry; if your kidneys are healthy, increasing your protein is completely safe. Using protein supplements is not required, but it can be a very convenient way to get in the required protein amounts no matter what your age and activity level. When it comes to weight loss, the addition of protein to the diet will aid in fat loss and muscle gain or preservation when combined with exercise training even if you are in a severe calorie restriction.

You also know that as you age, maintaining and improving your muscle mass can be a challenge—this is called anabolic resistance. However, when adding a larger than recommended amount of protein to the diet, it has been found that not only is muscle protein synthesis maximized, muscle protein degradation slows down too. In older individuals, it seems as though the higher the protein, the better. In terms of recommended amounts, it looks like about 2× RDA can cover most of your bases. That would be about 1.6 g per kg of body weight or 0.72 g of protein per lb of body weight. If you weigh 150 lb, or 68kg, you would aim for about 110 g of protein per day. This could be 2 eggs for breakfast, a Greek yogurt for a morning snack, a palm sized portion of chicken for lunch, a scoop of protein powder for an afternoon snack, followed by another palm sized portion of lean meat for dinner.

I really hope that you consider analyzing your diet, and maybe increasing your protein intake. It can certainly help combat anabolic resistance and improve body composition. Try this experiment with protein powders to find one that makes it convenient for you to take in enough protein to optimize your body composition.

Critical Micronutrients and Water

I n this lecture, you will learn about what vitamins and minerals are, some specific roles that vitamins and minerals have in your body, what foods make up good sources of some of the major micronutrients, and how to recognize both deficiencies and overloading toxicities that can occur with specific micronutrients. To achieve balance, you should aim to add more nutrient-dense foods like vegetables, fruits, and whole grains to your diet; stay active; and take a multivitamin.

Vitamins

■ Micronutrients include both vitamins and minerals. They do not directly provide energy but play a big role in energy production. Micronutrients are needed only in small quantities, so even small fluctuations of higher or lower intake can have a large impact on body composition, health, and performance.

■ Vitamins serve many important functions in our bodies and are involved in digestion, absorption, energy production, antioxidant purposes, and growth. They are regulators in numerous metabolic reactions that release energy from food or help with energy transfer to produce ATP, the energy currency of our bodies.

■ Vitamins are termed "organic compounds" because they contain carbon, just like all three of the macronutrients: carbohydrates, fats, and proteins. Vitamins also act as cofactors and coenzymes, which are required for various interactions in our metabolic pathways.

For a compound to be considered a vitamin, almost all textbooks will define them as follows.

- Vitamins are natural components of foods, usually present in very small amounts.
- Vitamins are essential for normal physiological function.
- Vitamins, when absent from the diet, will cause a specific deficiency in that particular vitamin.

This means that you must get vitamins from the food you eat.

Vitamins are classified as either fat-soluble or water-soluble, depending on whether they dissolve in fat or water. Fat-soluble vitamins include vitamins A, D, E, and K. The body absorbs them from the gastrointestinal tract and stores them in the liver, fatty tissues, and parts of your cells that contain fat, such as the cell membrane.

Fat-soluble vitamins move in your blood bound to dietary fat. This means that if fat is not part of your diet, you will likely have suboptimal fat absorption and might be set up for a fat-soluble vitamin deficiency. Fat-soluble vitamins are not readily excreted and are stored in your fat cells and liver.

Water-soluble vitamins include the B vitamins and vitamin C. These vitamins are also absorbed from the gastrointestinal tract and must be transported in the blood with what are called carrier proteins.

Water-soluble vitamins are not stored in large amounts in the body because body water turnover is so constant. They are also easily excreted through urine and a little bit through your sweat. Because they are so easily excreted and not stored, a daily intake of less than 50 percent of any of the water-soluble vitamins can lead to deficiency in about four weeks.

This means that if you are missing an entire food group, such as carbohydrates or fats (which can easily happen if you follow a fad diet), it would be fairly easy to be deficient in some vitamins.

- Both deficiencies and toxicities are possible with vitamins. A deficiency is not enough; a toxicity is too much.

- Toxicity is not likely to occur from food alone; it's more common when people are taking supplements. So, don't take more than the recommended dose of whatever supplements you choose to take, and talk to a professional about what you are taking and how much.

- Both deficiencies and toxicities are more likely with certain vitamins and minerals than others. Fat-soluble vitamins are stored more efficiently in the body (there is less fat turnover compared to water turnover). Vitamin A toxicity is the most common form of fat-soluble vitamin toxicity, because it can occur when intake exceeds just two times the needed recommendations.

- When vitamin A accumulates in the liver, you can have both acute and more chronic outcomes. Headache, rashes, visual changes, bone pain, skin cracking, mouth ulcers, yellowing of the skin, nausea, and vomiting are acute outcomes that may occur. Chronic toxicity can even lead to liver damage.

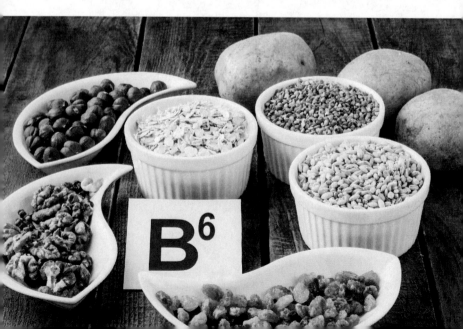

Although there is a word of caution about foods containing vitamin A, you should not be afraid to consume them. Just be aware of how much vitamin A you are consuming.

Water-soluble vitamins, on the other hand, are much less likely to lead to toxicity, but it could occur from overconsumption of niacin, B_6, and vitamin C. Toxicities are far less common from whole-food choices than from supplements, such as multivitamins.

A number of things can impact our overall vitamin needs, such as exercise, stress, aging, sex, and medications. Micronutrient needs will vary from person to person, and a one-size-fits-all approach is not possible.

Another interesting note about vitamins is that their status in foods can change just by how you store food and cook food. Poor storage and preparation of food can result in a decreased vitamin content in your food.

Things like excessive cooking and exposure to light, heat, air, and water can all lower the vitamin content of foods. Generally, it is best to consume food soon after harvest or buy foods that have been frozen quickly after harvest. The sooner that a fresh fruit or vegetable is frozen, the more vitamin content that will be preserved.

Minerals

Minerals are inorganic molecules (meaning molecules without carbon). Like vitamins, they are essential—in very small amounts—and they must be included in our diets because we don't make them naturally.

Similar to vitamins, minerals also serve many different regulatory functions in our bodies. They work as cofactors, meaning that they assist enzymes in energy transformation, contribute to production of other cells and enzymes, and help form red blood cells and bones. Minerals are involved in nerve impulses, body growth and development, water balance, muscle movement, and metabolism.

Electrolytes are minerals that keep our nervous system firing properly. They are electrically charged particles that most commonly include calcium, sodium, potassium, magnesium, and chloride. They help with establishing the electrochemical gradient across cells, which is necessary for proper nerve communication.

Electrolytes also assist with muscle contraction and modulate fluid exchange within the body's fluid compartments. That means that the electrolyte minerals play a big role in how we store water and where we store water. In this way, they influence our body composition and our body's water content quite a bit.

Because we need minerals in very small amounts, it is even more critical not to underestimate the value they have for our bodies.

The two types of minerals are major minerals (also called macrominerals) and trace minerals (also called microminerals). The major minerals include calcium, phosphorus, sodium, and magnesium, and they are required in amounts greater than 100 milligrams per day.

Trace minerals, on the other hand, include minerals like selenium, iron, and zinc. These are required in amounts less than 100 milligrams per day, and typically even less than 15 milligrams per day.

Ingestion of a mineral-containing food does not necessarily translate to 100 percent absorption of the mineral. This concept is called mineral bioavailability. In other words, even though you consume food with minerals, there are several factors that can affect how much of this mineral is actually absorbed from the gut to the blood stream.

In general, there are four factors involved in mineral bioavailability.
1. *The type of food that contains the minerals.* Typically, animal sources have a better bioavailability of minerals than plant sources.
2. *Mineral-to-mineral interactions.* Because minerals tend to move through similar receptors in the gastrointestinal tract, high amounts of one mineral may inhibit, or slow down, absorption of another mineral.

3. *Vitamin-mineral interactions.* A positive interaction example is that vitamin C intake improves iron absorption. A dietician will have additional information about foods you can pair to optimize your supplementation strategies for minerals.

4. *Fiber-mineral interaction.* Fiber can bind to minerals and block or slow their absorption. Typically, our dietary fiber comes from plant sources (this is another reason that animal sources might often be superior in terms of mineral bioavailability).

Consider the food's nutrient density, or how many nutrients it has, compared to its calorie content when you purchase food to eat.

Phytochemicals

Another component of nutrition that is often considered along with micronutrients is phytochemicals, which are biologically active compounds found in plants that provide zero calories or direct energy but can influence your overall health. Currently, only a few of an extensive list of known phytochemicals have been studied.

Phytochemicals have numerous roles but are most often linked to disease prevention. They can function as antioxidants that reduce damage caused by reactive oxygen species, can have hormonelike actions, and can even be considered metabolic boosters.

Food Sources versus Dietary Supplements

Most experts will recommend getting most of your micronutrients from food sources instead of dietary supplements. Research shows that vitamins and minerals from whole foods might have more health benefits than getting the same micronutrients from a supplement.

Although the reason why is not entirely understood, it is thought that the different types of nutrients in whole foods might interact in a synergistic manner that results in the greater absorption of combined micronutrients than when those micronutrients are taken as a separate

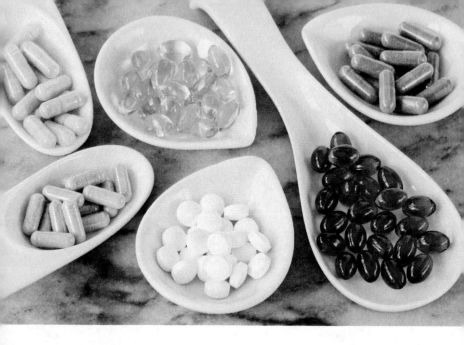

supplement or with a combined multivitamin. Also, there seem to be nutrients that just can't be reproduced in dietary supplements.

Some research also shows that single-nutrient supplements can have adverse effects—such as a higher risk of toxicity or possibly just a nutrient-nutrient interaction that might unfavorably impact nutrient absorption—even though intentions were good.

So, a diet that includes all the macronutrients from whole foods is most likely the best option, and the best place to start, to get the best micronutrient content out of your food. In addition, you'll likely get other active compounds, such as phytonutrients, by eating a diet consisting mostly of whole foods.

The problem is that many people don't eat enough variety of nutrient-dense whole foods in their day-to-day eating. Instead, whole foods get replaced by heavily processed foods for a majority of meals and snacks.

Over time, nutrient deficiencies can come about by relying solely or mostly on these processed and easily accessed foods. Although many processed foods are appealing and convenient, it is probably a good idea to limit them as much as we can.

A low-quality diet can lead to nutrient deficiencies, and deficiencies can lead not only to more than just poor health, but they have also been linked to a greater risk of becoming obese. In addition, if you throw deficiency issues on top of hard exercise training, which can also lead to a greater need for certain nutrients, you could be at a huge risk for deficiency.

The Importance of Water

Water is essential for optimal health and body composition, but many people walk around with less-than-adequate hydration levels. In addition to keeping you hydrated, water helps transport all of the nutrients in your body and helps move metabolic waste products out of your body. Water also plays a huge part in the regulation of body temperature, particularly with exercise.

Aim for about 8 to 10 cups, or about 2 liters, of water per day in addition to eating plenty of fruits and vegetables, which are loaded with water.

Given the prevalence of these vitamin and mineral deficiencies, should you take a vitamin and mineral supplement? It depends. Quite a few people would benefit from taking a multivitamin/multimineral supplement. However, supplementation will not fix a broken diet. Work for a highly nutritious diet first, and then simply use supplements to supplement that diet.

Also, the recommended intakes for vitamins and minerals were established to only prevent against any deficiencies. They don't consider the achievement of optimal health or body composition.

To determine if supplementation might help you, think about how many times you eat per day, what quality of food you generally eat, what medications you take, and how much exercise you do on a daily basis. Then, discuss these factors and concerns with your doctor to decide what is right for you.

Try This

Practice drinking 8 to 10 cups of water per day and monitor your urine color.

Questions to Consider

1. What are the main reasons for vitamins and minerals in the body?

2. What does the research say about micronutrient deficiencies in the United States?

Critical Micronutrients and Water

When we think about the food we eat, we think about the way it looks or the way it tastes. And when I talk to research participants or clients about the particular food choices they make, I always focus more on the macronutrient content of their meals—you know, the amount of carbohydrate, fat and protein that they eat. But, there are other things hiding in what we eat. What I'm talking about is the micronutrient content of our food choices, or the amount of smaller nutrients like vitamins and minerals that our food contains.

The reason we often overlook these micronutrients is because they are required in relatively small amounts compared to the macronutrients. The micronutrients, although needed in small amounts, are absolutely critical to regulating many different cell process, metabolic pathways, and other physiological needs in our bodies. It is also interesting to know that it is not as rare as you might think to be deficient in one or more of them. After I analyze the dietary intakes of my clients, I often see deficiencies in at least one of the micronutrients. If a micronutrient deficiency is present for any prolonged period of time physical symptoms may emerge. Depending on which micronutrient is low in your diet, things like stomach upset, hunger, and appetite changes, fatigue, or even changes in your physical appearance may show up.

Now, you may be saying to yourself, "Well, I don't really see or hear of anyone walking around with vitamin problems." Well you're partially correct—we don't usually see many clinical syndromes in Western culture. However, some experts are quick to point out that despite this fact, cases of suboptimal vitamin status are likely very high. Research has shown that a micronutrient deficiency is associated with becoming overweight or obese, and also it's linked to various cancers, cardiovascular disease, and things like osteoporosis. What's more, many of the most popular diets on the market today are linked to micronutrient deficiencies. So, is it now advised for adults to take at least one multivitamin pill each day?

One of the authors of the 2002 study that led to this recommendation said even people who eat 5 daily servings of fruits and vegetables may not get enough of certain vitamins for optimum health. Most people, for instance, cannot get the healthiest levels of folate and vitamin D and E from recommended diets. Even more evidence shows that just about 80% of Americans do not eat at least 5 servings of fruits and vegetables per day, which is the recommended minimum amount believed to provide sufficient essential nutrients. And, with the exception of Vitamin D, humans cannot synthesize their own vitamins, meaning that we must rely entirely on our food intake to get them. There is no doubt about it; we need to make sure we get adequate amounts of the micronutrients from our foods and supplements. If we don't get them, our performance and our health can go downhill. But, adding extra vitamins on top of what we need won't make you healthier or perform better. So how you exercise and live your life can influence your micronutrient status too.

The relationship is complex, but by the end of this lecture you'll have a better grasp on just how many factors affect our micronutrient levels. Another consideration for optimal health and body composition is the amount of water that you consume. You may be amazed at how many important roles water plays in your body, and how influential proper water intake can be to improving your body composition, health, and performance. In fact, water is needed for optimal digestion and absorption of the macro and micronutrients and makes up a significant portion of our bodies—over 60%. Even though most people know that they should drink water, it has been reported that nearly 3/4 of Americans don't meet the current recommendations set by the Institute of Medicine. And I'll go into those recommendations in a few minutes.

Research also demonstrates that just a 1–2% decrease in your total body water, which is very easy to lose, is associated with impaired mental processing, coordination, and a drop in performance. For example, if you weigh 150 lb, or 68 kg, then a reduction of body water by just 1.5 to 3 lb, or 0.7 to 1.4 kg, measured by body weight could lead to any of these issues especially if this continues over a long time. A weight change this small could come from simply not drinking enough fluid or not eating foods that have a high water content. It could also occur during exercise depending on how much you sweat and how hot and humid it is where you exercise.

This flux in weight might happen in just one day, especially in women, as fluctuations in body water are often affected by the menstrual cycle. If you learn that you have a micronutrient deficiency from an analysis of your blood and nutrient intake, it's important to look further into the overall quality of your diet. And because of the link between micronutrients and metabolism, it's important to know as much as you can about the micronutrients in order to optimize your own body composition. Likewise, having too little water intake—which is more common that you'd think—can lead to changes in food intake, cell structure, blood volume, and even body composition changes. However, drinking too much water can also be a problem—we'll discuss this more soon.

In this lecture, we'll talk about what vitamins and minerals are, some of the more specific roles that vitamins and minerals have in your body, and what foods make up good sources of some of the major micronutrients, and how to recognize both deficiencies and overloading toxicities that can occur with specific micronutrients. You will also learn about the various roles that water plays for the physiological function and how to use water as a tool for feeling and looking your best. So to begin, micronutrients include both vitamins and minerals. They do not directly provide energy, but they do play a big role in energy production. Micronutrients, as the name implies, are needed only in small quantities. So, as you might imagine, even small fluctuations of higher or lower intake can have a large impact on body composition, health and performance. Lets start with Vitamins.

Vitamins serve many important functions in our bodies and are involved in digestion, absorption, and energy production, antioxidant purposes, and growth. They are regulators of numerous metabolic reactions that release energy from food, or help with energy transfer to produce ATP, the energy currency of our bodies. Vitamins are termed organic compounds because they contain carbon just like all 3 of the macronutrients—carbohydrates, fats, and proteins.

Vitamins also act as cofactors and coenzymes, which are required for various interactions in our metabolic pathways. For example, aerobic metabolism requires the shuttling of electrons into the electron transport chain, which is how ATP is made. This shuttling mechanism requires riboflavin and niacin—2 water-soluble vitamins—to function properly. For a compound to be considered a vitamin almost all textbooks will define them like this: Vitamins are natural components of foods usually present in small amounts, vitamins are essential for normal physiological function, and vitamins, when absent from the diet, will cause a specific deficiency in that particular vitamin. What this means is that you must get vitamins from the food you eat.

Even if vitamins are a foreign concept to you, you probably have heard of fat-soluble and water-soluble versions of vitamins. Vitamins are classified as either fat-soluble or water-soluble, depending on if they dissolve in fat or water. Fat-soluble vitamins include A, D, E, and K. The body absorbs them from the gastrointestinal tract and stores them in the liver, fatty tissues, and parts of your cells that contain fat such as the cell membrane. Fat-soluble vitamins move in your blood bound to dietary fat. This means that if fat is not part of your diet, you will likely have suboptimal fat absorption and may be set up for a fat-soluble vitamin deficiency. Fat-soluble vitamins are not readily excreted and are stored in your fat cells and liver.

Water-soluble vitamins include B vitamins, and vitamin C. These vitamins are also absorbed from the gastrointestinal tract and must be transported in the blood with what are called carrier proteins. Water-soluble vitamins are not stored in large amounts in the body because body water turnover is so constant. They are also easily excreted through urine and a little bit through your sweat, and because they are so easily excreted and not stored, a daily intake of less than 50% of any of the water-soluble vitamins can lead to deficiency in about 4 weeks. That means that if you are missing an entire food group like carbohydrates or fats—which can easily happen if you follow a fad diet—it could be fairly easy to be deficient in some vitamins.

You might have noticed that I said B vitamins earlier, note that B vitamins are often called The B complex of vitamins because they comprise many vitamins. You have probably heard of B_6 and B_{12} because they tend to get more press. But, actually, the B vitamins include B_1, which is thiamine, B_2 riboflavin, B_3 Niacin, B_5 pantothenic acid, B_6 pyridoxine, B_7 biotin, B_9 folic acid, and B_{12} or cobalamin. Together, these make up the B complex but each serves a specific role in our overall functioning.

And by now you probably have already figured out that anything that affects your metabolism of food is likely to have a big impact on your body composition. As I mentioned, deficiencies and toxicities are possible with vitamins. A deficiency is not enough; a toxicity is too much. Toxicity is not likely to occur from food alone. It's more common when people are taking supplements. So don't take more than the recommended doses of whatever supplements you choose to take, and talk to a professional about what you are taking and how much.

Both deficiencies and toxicities are more likely with certain vitamins and minerals than others. Fat-soluble vitamins are stored more efficiently in the body—there is less fat turnover compared to water turnover. Vitamin A toxicity is the most common form of a fat-soluble vitamin toxicity because it can occur when intake exceeds just 2 times the needed recommendations. When Vitamin A accumulates in the liver, you can have both acute and more chronic outcomes. Headache, rashes, visual changes, bone pain, skin cracking, mouth ulcers, yellowing of the skin, nausea, and vomiting are acute outcomes that can occur. But, chronic toxicity can even lead to liver damage.

Vitamin A also goes by some other names like retinol or retinoic acid. In fact, vitamin A can come in 2 different forms. There's a preformed vitamin A, which includes retinol and is found in many animal sources like dairy, fish, and meat. The other form, provitamin A, is often referred to as carotenoid and the primary source is from beta-carotene, which is converted to vitamin A in your body. You get provitamin A from things like leafy green vegetables, orange and yellow vegetables, and tomato products. Though, there is a word of caution about foods containing vitamin A, you should not be afraid to consume them. Just beware if you are eating a lot of these foods, combined with daily supplementation through a multi vitamin capsule, and possibly taking in even more for therapeutic use as prescribed by your doctor. But, I can't say it often enough—particularly with medications, multivitamin supplements, and herbal extracts—make sure to talk to your doctor about what you're doing.

Water-soluble vitamins on the other hand are much less likely to lead to toxicity, but it could occur from overconsumption of niacin, B_6, and vitamin C. Again, toxicities are far less common for whole-food choices than from supplements such as multivitamins. But, a number of things can impact our overall vitamin needs such as exercise, stress levels, aging, sex, and medications. Micronutrient needs will vary from person to person so a one-size-fits-all approach is not possible.

Another interesting note about vitamins is that their status in foods can change just by how you store and cook food. Poor storage and preparation of food can result in a decreased vitamin content of your food. This would include things like excessive cooking; exposure to light, heat, air, and water can all lower the vitamin content of foods. Generally, it is best to consume food soon after harvest, or to buy foods that have been frozen quickly after harvest. The sooner that a fresh fruit or vegetable is frozen, the more vitamin content that will be preserved.

The next micronutrient category to discuss is minerals. Minerals are inorganic molecules—meaning molecules without carbon. And like vitamins, they are essential—in very small amounts—and they must be included in our diets because we don't make them naturally. Similar to vitamins, minerals also serve many different regulatory functions in our bodies. They work as cofactors, meaning they assist enzymes in energy transformation, contribute to the production of other cells and enzymes, and help form red blood cells and bones. Minerals are involved in nerve impulses, body growth and development, water balance, muscle movement, and metabolism.

If you have heard of electrolytes, then you may know one function of minerals. When you or your child is ill with the flu, or losing fluids because of vomiting or diarrhea, you may have bought a drink that had electrolytes in it to help protect against dehydration. Electrolytes are minerals that keep our nervous system firing properly. They are electrically charged particles that most commonly include, sodium, potassium, magnesium, and chloride. They help with establishing the electrochemical gradient across cells, which is necessary for proper nerve communication. They also assist with muscle contraction, and modulate fluid exchange within the body's fluids compartments. That means that the electrolyte minerals play a big role in how we store water, and where we store water. So, in this way, they influence our body composition and body water content quite a bit. And because we need minerals in very small amounts, it is even more critical not to underestimate the value that they have in our bodies. Think small, but mighty.

The 2 types of minerals are major minerals, also called macrominerals, and trace minerals, also called microminerals. The major minerals include calcium, phosphorus, sodium, and magnesium among others, and they are required in amounts greater than 100 mg per day. Just a quarter teaspoon provides about 600 mg of sodium. Trace minerals on the other hand include minerals like selenium, iron, and zinc, and these are required in amounts less than 100 mg per day and typically even less than 15 mg per day. One note with minerals is that ingestion of a mineral containing food does not necessarily translate to 100% absorption of the mineral. This concept is called Mineral Bioavailability. In other words, even though you consume food with minerals, there are several factors that can affect how much of this mineral is actually absorbed from the gut to the blood stream.

Let me explain how this works. In our foods there are molecules like oxalates and phytates that can alter mineral absorption, and these are often called binders. They may bind up minerals in the food and change the way you can access or use them—that is, they can change the bioavailability of the minerals. In general, there are 4 factors involved in mineral bioavailability.

First, is the type of food that contains the minerals. Typically, animal sources have better bioavailability of minerals than plant sources. This is because meat has a high mineral content, but no binders—like I mentioned earlier—that can inhibit absorption of minerals. Plants, on the other hand, have a relatively high concentration of binders, making it more difficult to absorb the nutrients within. The second factor in mineral bioavailability is mineral-to-mineral interaction. Because minerals tend to move through similar receptors in the gastrointestinal tract, high amounts of one mineral may inhibit or slow down absorption of another mineral. For example, calcium will inhibit iron absorption. So, if you are targeting foods to increase your iron, as with an iron deficiency, it's best to avoid eating foods high in calcium, like dairy, at the same meal.

Third, there are some vitamin-mineral interactions that will affect mineral bioavailability. One positive interaction example is that vitamin C intake actually improves iron absorption. So, in this case, it might make sense to consume orange juice and a supplement with iron at the same time if you are trying to fix an iron deficiency. A dietician will have additional information about foods that you can pair to optimize your supplementation strategies for minerals. Finally, the fourth factor in mineral bioavailability is a fiber-mineral interaction in which fiber can bind to minerals, and block or slow their absorption. Typically our dietary fiber comes from plant sources—this is another reason that animal sources may often be superior in terms of mineral bioavailability.

So, what does this mean in terms of real food? How can we relate the micronutrients to our food choices? And, how can the presence of micronutrients turn an OK food choice into a great food choice? Well, one very common example is the toss up between whole wheat bread and white bread. This is a question I get from my clients all the time. The argument for whole wheat bread is loosely termed the Whole Grain Advantage, and the basis for this argument comes from whole wheat bread's micronutrient content. For example, when comparing the vitamin E, vitamin B_6, potassium, magnesium, and fiber content of whole wheat versus white bread, there is undeniably a higher amount of these vitamins and minerals in whole wheat. Therefore, all else being equal—that is the total calorie content, the carbohydrate content, etc. of a food—micronutrients could make the difference in making a food more nutrient dense, and should not be overlooked.

But, consider this; too, whole wheat bread is different than simply wheat bread. Wheat bread is at times even more processed than white bread and can even contain fewer nutrients. So, don't be fooled by marketing and packaging and be sure to check food labels when buying products for the words whole grain or whole wheat. We'll talk much more about food labeling later in the course. I need to say, too, that there are other reasons to eat or avoid whole wheat bread, but for now, just consider the nutrient density, or how many nutrients the food has compared to its calorie content, when you purchase foods to eat. This is a great starting point.

Another component of nutrition that is often considered along with micronutrients is Phytochemicals. Phytochemicals are biologically active compounds found in plants that provide zero calories or direct energy, but can influence your overall health. Even now, in 2015, only a few of an extensive list of known phytochemicals have been studied. Some phytochemicals that you may be familiar with are isoflavones from soy and resveratrol from grapes. If you haven't heard of resveratrol from grapes, you've probably have heard about it found in red wine. But keep in mind that it's not yet known for sure which method—grapes or wine—is better for your resveratrol content or your health. And phytochemicals have numerous roles, but are most often linked to disease prevention. They can function as antioxidants that reduce damage caused by reactive oxygen species, they can have hormone-like actions, and they can even be considered metabolic boosters. I hope you're getting the point that our food is very powerful. It has a big influence on almost every function of our bodies.

Most experts will recommend getting most of your micronutrients from food sources instead of dietary supplements. There's actually good research to show that vitamins and minerals from whole foods may have more health benefits than getting the same micronutrients from a supplement. Although the reason why is not entirely understood, it is thought that the different types of nutrients in whole foods may interact in a synergistic manner that results in a greater absorption of the combined micronutrients than when those micronutrients if they're taken as a supplement or as a multivitamin. Also, there seem to be nutrients that just can't be reproduced in dietary supplements.

Some research also shows that single nutrient supplements can have adverse effects—like a higher risk of toxicity, or possibly just a nutrient-nutrient interaction that may unfavorably impact nutrient absorption—even though intentions were good. So, a diet that includes all the macronutrients from whole foods is most likely to be the best option, and the best place to start, in order to get your best micronutrient content out of your food. In addition, you'll likely get other active compounds like phytonutrients by eating a diet consisting mostly of whole foods. The trouble is, a lot of people don't eat enough variety of nutrient dense whole foods in their day-to-day eating. Instead, whole foods get replaced by heavily processed foods for a majority of meals and snacks.

Over time, nutrient deficiencies can come about by relying solely or mostly on these processed and easily accessed foods. Some even call these frankenfoods because of how much they have been processed. Now don't get me wrong, many processed foods are appealing and convenient, but it is probably a good idea to limit them as much as we can. A low quality diet—that many people have—can lead to nutrient deficiencies. And deficiencies can lead not only to more than just poor health; they've also been linked to a greater risk of becoming obese. Recently, it was reported that in the US more than 40% of people are Vitamin A, C, D, E, and calcium or magnesium deficient and greater than 90% don't get enough choline, fiber, or potassium.

Now the EAR, or Estimated Average Requirement—which is the amount needed to meet the needs of 50% of the population—for vitamin A, D, E, calcium, and magnesium compared to normal weight adults. Obese adults also had significantly lower intake of both fiber and potassium, which are linked to your metabolism and your heart health. Even scarier is that over 90% of people, both normal weight and obese, were deficient in fiber, potassium, and choline. With fiber alone, it is thought that for every 10 g you eat, you can reduce your overall risk of mortality risk by up to 34%. And because the nutrients that are low in the US on average are commonly found in foods like fruits, vegetables, whole grains, and dairy, this study may mean that many Americans, and particularly obese Americans, are not eating enough of these foods. In addition, if you throw these deficiency issues on top of hard exercise training, which can also lead to a greater need for certain nutrients, you can easily see how many people could be at a huge risk for deficiency.

So, even with the gold standard option of eating a diet of more nutritious, colorful, and varied whole food sources—we need to be realistic. Given the prevalence of these vitamin and mineral deficiencies, the question becomes "Should I take a vitamin or mineral supplement?" Well, like most good questions in nutrition or sport nutrition, the answer is it depends. The authors of a study on this question looked into supplement use within normal and obese individuals. Not surprisingly, they report that people who take multivitamin and multimineral supplements had lower prevalence of inadequate vitamin and mineral intake.

They go on to write that supplement users were actually more likely to have a healthy diet compared to non-users. It may be that the habit of using a multivitamin is more likely to be done by people who have other healthy habits. But based on this information, and my own personal experience with clients, I would say that quite a few people would benefit from taking a multivitamin, or a multimineral supplement. Many clients that I work with who believe they're eating very well, show up with deficiencies once I analyze their diets and look over their blood work.

However, supplementation will not fix a broken diet. Remember, work for a highly nutritious diet first, and then simply use supplements to supplement that diet. Also, remember, the recommended intakes for vitamins and minerals were established to only prevent against deficiencies. They don't consider the achievement of optimal health or body composition. Do you want to be simply not deficient? Or do you want to be optimal in your micronutrient intake? These are the questions to consider when the "should I supplement" question comes out. You may want to think about how many times you eat per day, what quality of food you generally eat, what medications you take, and how much exercise do you normally have on a daily basis to determine if supplementation will help you. And then, discuss these factors and concerns with your doctor to decide what is right for you.

So, in the end, vitamins and minerals play a huge role in your overall health, how you feel, and what your body composition is or will become. And remember that water's also essential for optimal health and body composition. I'm sure you know that you need it to hydrate, but the fact is that many people walk around with less than adequate hydration levels. In fact, one study even reported that over half of professional basketball players were under-hydrated before the game, and that's in professional athletes. Water helps to transport of all of the nutrients that we just discussed, and helps move metabolic waste products out of your body. Water also plays a huge part in the regulation of body temperature, particularly with exercise. The list goes on and on for water, so be sure you drink up and aim for about 8–10 cups, or 2 liters of water per day in addition to eating plenty of fruits and vegetables which are loaded with water. It may make you get up more to use the bathroom, but that's actually a really healthy side effect to drinking water regularly—more physical activity.

Remember that you can actually drink too much water. This is called hyponatremia, which means low sodium—this can occur when you drink so much water that it actually dilutes, or literally waters down the sodium in your body. This can cause nausea, vomiting, fatigue, and neuromuscular issues like cramps and muscle spasms and even sometimes events like coma or death. Another note is that if you exercise a lot the fluid recommendations get much more detailed, so be sure to ask a professional if you feel like you need more specific information. Simply, monitoring your urine color can help. Aim for a light yellow color—too clear or too dark a urine color should be avoided.

Overall, you should aim to add in more nutrient-dense foods like vegetables, fruits, and whole grains, stay active, and take a multivitamin supplement. It is a balance that we are all striving for—optimal health, optimal nutrition, and optimal body composition. Try this: practice drinking 8–10 cups of water per day, and monitor your urine color.

Food Labeling and Nutritional Choices

What are the rules that we should follow in the grocery store? How can we decipher a food label and know what we're looking for? What can we identify as important for improving body composition, recovery, or optimal aging? There is no perfect formula, magic food group, or even cursed aisle in the supermarket. Rather, there are bad options, better options, and the best options. In this lecture, you will learn how much food to consume each day, what your dietary intake should look like, and how to interpret each section of the Nutrition Facts label.

How Much Food Should You Eat?

▪ How much food should you eat? It depends on who you are, how old you are, how big or small you are, how much muscle you have, what your sex is, and what goals you have. These basic indicators will dictate the energy requirements of your body in general.

▪ At different stages in our lives, we have different energy demands— that is, different amounts of calories that we need to live optimally. For example, a child is constantly growing and developing until the onset of puberty. In comparison to their size, a child will likely require more calories than an adult while they are growing so fast.

▪ A larger person—in terms of body size, not fat mass—is going to require more absolute energy each day than a smaller person, assuming equal activity levels.

▪ Men tend to be larger than women. Therefore, based on the previous principle of body size alone, men will often require greater calorie intake than women. However, a second factor is that, on average, men will have

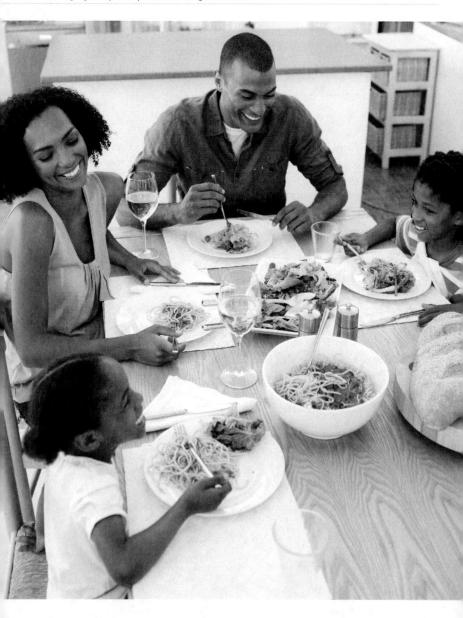

more muscle mass than women. Muscle tissue is highly metabolically active and demands a high energy intake—to keep us moving.

Your relative activity level also determines how much food you need to eat every day. If you exercise a lot, you will probably need more food to refuel and recover. But there are also times when you would not want to replenish your energy stores completely.

The food you require depends on your goals. Are you trying to lose weight? Or are you trying to put on 5 pounds (2.27 kilograms) of muscle mass? In both of these cases, total caloric intake will be different, and so will the components of that caloric intake.

Another area we cannot ignore is genetics. For example, do you have a tendency to gain weight or lose weight easily, and what does your family look like? Answers to these questions are important. However, even a lousy or a fantastic genetic predisposition must be massaged by the other factors that we can control.

On nutrition labels, certain nutrients are "based on a 2,000-calorie diet." Not everyone eats a 2,000-calorie diet; this just reflects the caloric intake of an average-sized person to maintain weight and serves as a basic starting point for most people. The percentages listed on the Nutrition Facts label must be adjusted case by case.

Are All Calories Created Equal?

Is a calorie just a calorie, regardless of if it's 200 calories of pizza or 200 calories of broccoli? If you consumed primarily calories from simple sugars each day, you might not gain any weight overall, but you would be missing a ton of the nutrients that your body requires to function well, and over time, this would alter your body composition and health for the worse.

Importantly, the readout on your scale probably won't change—and you might go on thinking that all is well—but internally the story could be much different. Chances are good that you would develop compromised metabolic, immune, and inflammatory function that, at best, would not allow you to function optimally and, at worst, could lead to serious conditions, such as blood glucose and lipid abnormalities and possibly chronic disease.

While we need to be aware of the number of calories we eat, it is probably more important to worry about the quality of those calories. Essentially, eating nutrient-dense foods provides much more bang for your buck. In fact, you often have to eat quite a bit of the quality foods to meet your calorie needs—so you really can eat more and weigh less.

Nutritional Information Labels

The first thing to look for on a nutritional label is the serving size, located in the top-left corner of the label. The serving size is important because this is the portion that all the nutritional information is based on. If you choose to eat more or less than the serving size listed, your nutritional intake will also be higher or lower for all nutrients.

Next, examine the total number of calories for the given serving size, located at the top of the label. This gives you an idea of how much this product is going to contribute to your entire day's intake. Even though the quantity of calories is less important than the quality of calories, at some point you need to be aware of calories and make sure that you're not eating too many or too few to support your goals.

Just below where the total calories are listed is the list of nutrients provided per serving, including total fat and types of fat, cholesterol, sodium, carbohydrates and sugars, and protein. All the values are given in grams and also as a percent daily value, which provides consumers with a general estimate of how much this serving of this particular food will contribute to overall recommendations for each nutrient each day based on a 2,000-calorie diet.

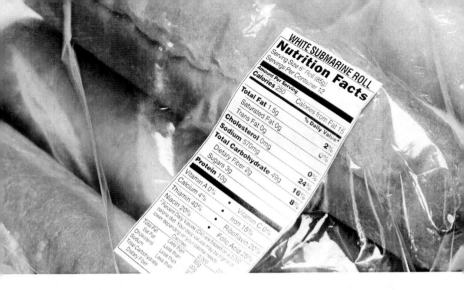

At the bottom of the food label are the amounts of certain vitamins and minerals, such as vitamin A and C, calcium, and iron. This gives you a better idea of the nutrient density of the food you choose to eat. You should choose higher values of these nutrients paired with a lower-calorie amount on the label.

The food label is typically paired with a list of ingredients contained in the product. The higher up on the list, the greater relative amount of the ingredient in the food. The first item listed has the greatest relative amount in the food. You want to see more "natural" or unprocessed ingredients toward the beginning of the list.

It's a good idea to choose foods with as few ingredients as possible to have a better idea of how processed the food is. Today, almost everything is processed to some degree—this is usually for food safety—so choose foods that are as minimally processed as you can.

The food label—specifically, the ingredients list—is also great if you need to identify anything that could trigger a known allergy. If you are unsure about a food or a name on the label, it's better to stick with the motto of "when in doubt, leave it out."

The U.S. Food and Drug Administration proposed a change to the label. The new label was proposed to identify a few things.

- Serving sizes are listed bigger and bolder; they are also updated to reflect more realistic serving sizes.
- The calories will be listed in a larger font.
- Added sugars must be listed on the label.
- There will be other small changes to reflect current nutrition and food science.

Food Labels: Making Good Decisions

Knowing the food label language will only help you make more consistently good decisions for what to buy and eat if you take a little time to look at the label and interpret whether the food has the nutritional makeup and quality to meet your goals.

You should also have an idea of what the recommended ranges are for you to try and eat of each nutrient based on things like your age, weight, and sex. But keep in mind that current science continues to update the recommendations that you should follow.

Let's go through a food label and consider some very general rules of thumb.

- Make sure to get the right amount of protein in your diet. Determine your protein needs based on factors like age, sex, and your goals. Most people will fall somewhere between 1 and 1.5 grams of protein per kilogram of body mass for protein needs. Then, read the Nutrition Facts label to see how much protein you are eating with each meal. Add up the grams of protein and multiply by 4— the conversion factor for protein grams to protein calories.
- Use the Nutrition Facts label to look at your carbohydrate intake. Try to limit the amount of simple sugars you eat or drink, and choose more complex starches instead—foods like vegetables and whole grains, which usually have more fiber, too.

- On the food label, compare the total carbohydrate value to the amount of sugar and fiber in the product. Is there a high amount of sugar compared to the total carbohydrate value? If so, this is probably a simple carbohydrate that should be limited. A food that has a high amount of fiber and low amount of sugar compared to the total carbohydrate in the product is probably the better day-to-day option.

- Some recent research shows that we might be able to better choose our carbohydrates based on the ratio of carbohydrates to fiber (in grams per serving) that are listed on the Nutrition Facts label. If the ratio is greater than 10:1 for carbohydrates to fiber, the recommendation is to avoid this food. If the ratio is less than 10:1, it is likely a good choice, and if the ratio is less than 5:1, it is a great choice.

- Try to identify the whole grains or oats as the first ingredient on the ingredients list at the bottom of the label for carbohydrate foods. A range of 45 to 65 percent of carbohydrate intake in your total diet is typically recommended. For body composition purposes, much of the current research indicates that the lower end of this spectrum is likely a good thing. This means smart carbohydrate choices (as with all the nutrients) at each meal.

- Although there's no gram-per-day recommendation for fat, the U.S. Department of Agriculture provides a general range based on percentage of your total dietary intake, including about 20 to 35 percent of your total calories coming from fats. But new research shows that many people successfully eat more fat than this and still improve body composition and health.

- A better way to consider fats is by types of fats. Choosing a good mix of polyunsaturated, monounsaturated, and saturated fats is a good idea. Also, limiting omega-6 fatty acids from excessive intake of vegetable oils and premade dressings and increasing intake of omega-3 fatty acids (from fish, nuts, and seeds) is another good idea overall.

- As of January 2006, trans fats have been required to be on the Nutrition Facts label. These rarely occur naturally and are considered the *really* bad guys. They're known as lethal because not only do they increase bad cholesterol, but they also decrease good cholesterol and are directly related to heart disease risk. Try to avoid foods high in trans fats.

For fat calories, you need to multiply fat grams by 9, not 4, as you do for both protein and carbohydrates. This means that fat has the highest calorie count per gram of the macronutrients.

Besides the protein, carbohydrates, and fat, also consider the sodium and cholesterol content of foods if you know that you have a negative family or personal disease history with these nutrients. Otherwise, new research indicates far less concern than originally thought.

Also, look at the amount of micronutrients in your food, including vitamins and minerals. A few will be listed on your food label. It is best to aim for 100 percent of the micronutrients in your daily diet from all meals and supplements.

Try This

Read Nutrition Facts labels for sugar content and aim to reduce the amount of added sugars in your overall diet.

Questions to Consider

1. What sources of fat are dominant in your diet?

2. How much added sugar do you get in your typical daily diet?

Food Labeling and Nutritional Choices

With a buffet of different dieting options available, sometimes we forget to look at the basics—like how to read a food label. You see, often times knowing what exactly to look for on a food label can help us make good decisions about our food choices. While this probably sounds easy enough, it can get confusing when you think about serving sizes, carbohydrate, fat, and protein numbers, and vitamin and mineral content. Just trying to sort out the small print of ingredients listed at the bottom of the label can take an advanced degree.

To complicate things further is the fad-based side of nutrition, and overabundance of pseudo-experts that market very well in order to sell their products. The food industry is like any other industry, and it's designed to make money. It's among the top advertisers in the United States. In 2012, $116 million was spent on marketing for fresh fruits and vegetables. You might think, wow, that's a lot of money on advertising. Well, I did too until I saw that the marketing for fast food topped out at over $4.6 billion, the same year. And think about how many labels are on a box of food that try to convince you to buy and eat. The labeling claims are designed to make you think the products are better for you. You are bombarded with slogans like Healthy Choice and Certified Organic.

But do you really need labels to convince you that a food is a healthy choice? I hope not. But here's an interesting fact, the Food and Drug Administration actually has data to show that when the package has labels on the front, you are less likely to read the Nutrition Facts panel where the more reliable information can be found. It's also difficult to stay away from foods with enticing descriptions. You've probably noticed this too when you eat out at a restaurant. You don't often see menu items listed as simply fish or beef; instead you see descriptive words like Chilean Seafood Filet or Omaha Tender Beef. Which one would you be more likely to buy? These evocative descriptions, and these names, are rated as more appealing and tasty.

Without a doubt, big politics are involved in foods that are backed with serious money and marketed to you. The way to approach food, and particularly food labeling, is to be as educated as possible, and then to keep a healthy skepticism when reading labels and advertisements. It's not hard to see that health-related food labeling will likely influence how you feel about certain foods and ultimately what you buy and eat. But it's probably best to limit your purchases of packaged foods and ones with excessive health claims.

So, how do you know what to do? Where are the rules that we should follow in the grocery store? How can we decipher a food label and know what we are really looking for? What can we really identify as important for improving body composition, recovery, or for optimal aging? There is no perfect formula, magic food group, or even a cursed aisle of the supermarket. Rather, there are poor options, better options, and the best options. In this lecture, we will go over how food you consume each day, what your dietary intake should look like, and how to interpret each section of the Nutrition Facts label.

The first question is often "How much food should I eat?" Again, like most difficult questions, the answer is it depends. It depends on who you are, how old you are, how big or small you are, how much muscle you have, what your sex is, and what goals you specifically have. These basic indicators will dictate the energy requirements of your body in general. Let's visit them one by one.

First is Age. At different stages in our lives, we have different energy demands—that is, different amounts of calories that we need to live optimally. Think of a child who is constantly growing and developing until the onset of puberty. In comparison to their size, a child will likely require more calories than an adult while they are growing so fast. And during certain events, like pregnancy and breast-feeding, or recovery from injury or disease, we have increased energy demands, requiring a higher number of calories per day. If you become more sedentary as you age, you will also require fewer calories. But, if you choose to maintain or increase activity as you age, your calorie intake will stay up. However, be careful here. Older adults often don't eat enough calories due to a variety of factors including a loss of appetite. So, based on which stage of life you are in; you will likely require varying amounts of calories.

Next is Body size. A larger person—we're talking actual body size and not fat mass—is going to require more absolute energy each day than a smaller person, assuming equal activity levels. Think of it as a smaller engine versus a larger engine. The small engine just requires less fuel to continue revving compared to the large engine. A reasonable example is, again, an adult and a child. The child is growing and requires specific nutritional needs, but in absolute terms the adult needs more calories because they have a greater body area to support metabolically.

The third component to how much food we need is sex. Men tend to be larger than women. Therefore, based on the previous principle of body size alone, men will often require greater calorie intake than women. However, a second factor is the amount of muscle mass that men carry compared to women on average. And, yes, many examples exist where this is not the case, but on average men will have more muscle mass than women. Think of muscle mass as hungry tissue. Muscle tissue is highly metabolically active, and demands a high-energy intake to keep us moving. With simple math, more muscle mass on your body frame equals more hungry tissue, equals more food needed.

OK, with these factors in mind, you have an idea of what your basic energy demands are compared to your spouse, or your best friend, or your neighbor. But, there's more to the equation. What does your typical day look like? Are you sitting at a desk all day or are you training for a marathon? Or, like most people, are you somewhere in between? Your relative activity level also determines how much food you need to eat every day. If you exercise a lot, you will probably need more food to refuel and recover. But, there are also times when you would not want to replenish your energy stores completely. And the food you require depends on your specific goals.

Are you trying to lose weight? Are you trying to put on 5 lb, or 2.25 kg, of muscle mass? In both of these cases—losing or gaining—total caloric intake will be different, and so will the components of that calorie intake, which I will go later in this lecture. Another area we cannot ignore is your genetics. For example, do you have a tendency to gain weight, or to lose weight easily? And what does your family look like? Answers to these questions are important. However, a lousy or a fantastic genetic predisposition must be massaged by the other factors that we can control. So you can see that your individual characteristics, your goals, and training status, and even your genetics can influence your daily energy needs. In the research lab, using specialized equipment, and calculations, we can also determine your calorie needs.

You might have noticed that on nutrition labels, certain nutrients are based on a 2000-calorie diet, and by now, you know that not everyone eats a 2000-calorie diet. Well, this just reflects the average intake of an average sized person to maintain weight, and serves as the most basic starting point for most people. But, because some people might require 1500 calories and others well over 4000 calories per day, the percentages listed on the nutrition facts label must be adjusted case by case. Also, keep in mind that to convert calories to kilojoules, you multiply by 4.2. So, based on all of these factors, you know roughly how much food you should eat per day, and we'll go into more detail about this in an upcoming lecture. But, how do you apply this information to what you see on a food label?

Let's say that you're 40 years old, 5'10" tall, and weigh about 160 lb and are generally active. Using a metabolic calculator, you see that you should eat roughly 2300 calories per day to maintain your body weight. Now what? Should your only goal be to go out and consume 2300 calories regardless of where those calories come from? Well, this brings up the classic argument of is a calorie is a calorie, regardless of if it's 200 calories of pizza or 200 calories of cake or 200 calories of broccoli.

Based on this logic and your 2300-calorie per day goal, you could consume any of the following to hit your needs, 575 jellybeans, 4 Big Macs, 385 stalks of celery, or a variety of nutrient dense foods all chosen to promote energy, lean mass accumulation, fat loss, and disease prevention. Do you think of these food choices that they have the same effect on your body composition and overall health? Well, they all add up to 2300 calories, right?

I bet that your common sense tells you that this is not the case. While these examples are extreme, they make an important point. If you consumed primarily calories from simple sugars each day—the 575 jellybean example— you might not gain any weight overall, but you could be sure you are missing a ton of nutrients that your body requires to function well, and over time this would alter your body composition and health for the worse. Importantly, the readout on your scale probably won't change—and you may go on thinking that all is well—but, internally, the story could be much different.

Chances are good that you would develop compromised metabolic, immune, and inflammatory function that at best would not allow you to function optimally, and at worst could lead to serious conditions like blood glucose and lipid abnormalities and possibly chronic disease. OK, so the answer is pretty obvious here. While we need to be aware of the amount of calories we eat, it is probably more important to worry about the quality of those calories. For example, let's compare 100 Calories from jellybeans to 100 Calories from spinach—which is about 14 cups of raw spinach.

The jellybeans have about 28 g of carbohydrate, all coming from simple sugars. The spinach, however, has about 14 g of carbohydrate. The spinach also contains about 10–14 grams of protein, exceptional daily values for vitamin A and C, as well as small to moderate amounts of iron and calcium. You can see that even though these 2 foods have the same calorie density, at 100 calories each, the spinach offers a much higher nutrient density— meaning a lot of nutrients with few calories. The spinach has dietary fiber, protein, and a number of vitamins and minerals, and you'd have to eat a lot of it just to get those 100 calories.

Essentially, eating nutrient dense foods provides a way more bang for your buck. In fact, many participants in my studies or clients I've worked with begin eating these foods and find that they have to eat quite a bit of the quality foods to meet their calorie needs. Essentially, you really can eat more and weigh less. In fact, entire books have been written on the topic of is a calorie, really a calorie. But, how do you know what the nutrient density is of your foods? Well, it's simple; check the food label. Here, I will teach exactly you how to do it.

Does this sound daunting? Don't let it be. I've worked with many people who just need a little direction on what to look for. And, once you know, it's simple. Here is an example of a nutritional label for macaroni and cheese. The first thing to look for is the serving size, located in the top left corner of the label. The serving size is important because this is the portion that all of the nutritional information is based on. So, if you choose to eat more or less of the serving size listed, your nutritional intake will also be higher or lower for all of the nutrients. For example, if the label shows that a serving is only 1 cup, and you eat 2 cups of the food, then you need to multiply everything on the label by 2. Make sure you are aware of your serving size when reading the label.

And the next thing to do is examine the total number of calories for the given serving size, located on the top of the label. This gives you an idea as to how much this product is going to contribute to your entire day's intake. You now know that the quantity of calories is less important than the quality of calories, but at some point you need to be aware of it and just make sure you're not eating too much or too little to support your goals. I'm not a big fan of counting calories. But, when just starting out on the journey to improve your body composition, it can be an effective tool until you get the hang of what foods make you feel good, perform well, and improve your body composition.

Now, just below where the total calories are listed, you'll start to see a list of all the nutrients provided per serving including total fat and the types of fat, cholesterol, sodium, carbohydrates, and sugars, and lastly protein. All these values are given in grams and also in a percent daily value. So, what does this mean? Remember when I mentioned the common phrase based on a 2000-calorie diet? Well, this is precisely what the percent daily value relates to.

Here, the label provides consumers with a general estimate of how much this serving of this particular food will contribute to the overall recommendations for each nutrient each day based on a 2000-calorie diet. So if you eat more or fewer than 2000 calories per day these percentages will also change. For example, if you eat more than 2000 calories, the percent of your daily diet listed on the label will decrease, and if you eat less than 2000 calories, then the percent listed on the label will increase. The percent daily values might be useful for some people, but are really most valuable in pointing out red flags—when certain nutrients are extremely high or when certain nutrients are extremely low, or non-existent.

At the bottom of the food label we will see the amounts of certain vitamins and minerals like Vitamin A, Vitamin C, calcium, and iron. This gives you a better idea of the nutrient density of the food you choose to eat. You should choose higher values of these nutrients compared with a lower calorie amount on the label. The food is typically paired with a list of ingredients contained in the product, the higher up on the list, the greater relative amount of the ingredient in the food. So if see an ingredient list with wheat flour, oat flour, corn starch, salt, guar gum, and cane juice, you would know that the wheat flour, the first item listed, has the greatest relative amount in that food.

You want to see more natural or unprocessed ingredients towards the beginning of the list. Some people say this should be names you can read and pronounce. I agree to an extent, but sometimes, there are just long names in a perfectly fine food to eat. I think it's a good idea though to choose foods with as few ingredients as possible in order to have a better idea of how processed the food is that you're eating. But, today almost everything is processed to some degree—this is usually for food safety—so choose foods that are minimally processed as you can.

A food label's also great if you need to identify anything that could trigger an allergy. It is in the ingredients list of the label that you would identify any particular ingredient to avoid. Just be careful, because the front label advertising needs to be compared to the small print on the Nutrition Facts label about where the particular product was processed. In our research, we always tell potential subjects if the food or supplements we are asking them to consume were produced in a factory that co-processed any potential allergenic foods like wheat or shellfish. Just keep in mind that if you are unsure about a food or a name on the label, it's better to stick with the motto of "when in doubt, leave it out."

It seems easy enough; however, the U.S. Food and Drug Administration, or FDA, proposed a change to the label. And that new label was proposed in order to identify a few specific things. Serving sizes are now going to be listed as bigger and bolder; they are also updated to reflect more realistic serving sizes. For example, right now ice cream has a serving size of just 1/2 cup. The changes would increase the serving size to a more realistic size of one cup. Likewise, for soda instead of an 8 oz. serving, it will be 12 or 20 oz. The amount people typically eat or drink. The calories will be listed in a larger font and added sugars must be listed on the label. There will be other small changes to reflect current nutrition and food science. It should be an improvement to help you quickly read and understand more about exactly what you're eating. So, there you have it, the very complex nature of the food label simplified for your use. Your ability to translate the food label will aid tremendously in your quest to know more about what you are eating and help with any body composition changes that you may want to make in the future.

Now, you know the food label language, how does this help you to make more consistent good decisions for what to buy and eat? It will only help if you take just a little bit of time to look at the label and interpret it if the food has the nutritional makeup and quality to meet your goals. For example, take into account the fact that carbohydrates and proteins each provide about 4 calories per gram, but fats provide more at 9 calories per gram.

You should also have an idea of what the recommended ranges are for you to try and eat of each nutrient based on the things like your age, your weight, and your sex. But, keep in mind that current science continues to update the recommendations that you should follow. It may take some getting used to— reading nutrition labels takes time and makes grocery shopping take a lot longer when you first do this. So let's go through a food label and consider some very general rules of thumb. The first thing I would do is make sure to get the right amount of protein in your diet.

It's clear that protein is vital to normal body function and improved body composition. It keeps you full and less likely to gorge at other meals. But, how do you know the correct amount to consume? I'm a fan of using hand sizes to estimate your needs, but it can be good to count calories for a short period of time, until you get into a good routine. So, simply determine your protein needs based upon the numerous factors that we discussed like age, sex, and your goals. Most people will fall somewhere between 1 and 1.5 g of protein per kilogram of body mass for your protein needs. Again, for a 150 lb, or 68 kg, person, this would be between 70 and 100 g of protein per day. Then, read the label to see how much protein you are eating with each meal. And then just add up the grams of protein and multiply by 4—the conversion factor for protein grams to protein calories. Now, you have your calorie intake from protein.

In my research showing improvements in body composition with higher protein, I ask participants to include a good protein source at each meal. It could be eggs in the morning, a protein shake, lean meats, or combinations of vegetables, seeds, beans, and nuts. Once your protein is dialed in, use the Nutrition Facts label to look at your carbohydrate intake. You may be surprised at just how many carbohydrates and sugars are in common foods that you eat. They may be simple sugars like fruits and juices or complex starches like whole grains and vegetables. Also, many empty calories are typically high in carbohydrates—things like candies, sodas, many juices, and white bread.

One good approach is to try and limit the amount of simple sugars you eat or drink and choose more complex starches instead. These foods like vegetables and whole grains usually have more fiber too. On the food label, compare the total carbohydrate value to the amount of sugar and fiber in the product. Is there a high amount of sugar compared to the total carbohydrate value? If so, this is probably a simple carbohydrate that should be limited the only exceptions being certain disease conditions and maybe for some very active people during exercise.

But, is there a high amount of fiber and a low amount of sugar compared to the total carbohydrate in the product? Well, this is probably the better day-to-day option. Keep in mind though that at some level sugar is sugar—whether it is from added sugars, natural sugars, or refined sugars, it all counts towards your sugar or carbohydrate intake. Some recent research even shows that we may be better able to choose our carbohydrates based upon the ratio of carbohydrates to fiber in grams per serving that are listed on the Nutrition Label.

If the ratio is greater than 10:1 for carbohydrates to fiber, the recommendation is to avoid this food. If the ratio is less than 10:1, it is likely a good choice, and if the ratio is less than 5:1, this is a great choice. For example, if your drink has 25 g of sugar and only 1 g of fiber, this is a 25:1 ratio and would be classified as a food to avoid by this scale. This is not perfect because it doesn't include the glycemic index, but it may lead you to better carbohydrate choices. Lastly, you should try to identify whole grains or oats as the first ingredient on the list at the bottom of the label for carbohydrate foods.

A range of 45–65% of carbohydrate intake in your total diet is typically recommended. For body composition purposes, much of the current research is indicating that the lower end of this spectrum is likely a good thing. This means smart carbohydrate choices, as with all the nutrients, at each meal. So, the next logical question is what about fats? The first thing is that when you are eating lean meats, you often have both protein and fat in the food. So, sometimes you don't have to actively seek out more fat to eat. But, there are definitely times when a good mix of the types of fat need to be considered, or total fat needs to be increased or decreased.

The good news is you can find all of the fat information on the label too. Consuming certain types of good fats can actually help to improve body composition. How could that be the case? As we've discussed, fats are generally more satiating than either proteins or carbohydrates—meaning that they leave you feeling full longer and stopping from reaching back for a second helping or snack. Fats are absolutely necessary for many body processes and are the main fuel for the body at rest and during low-to-moderate intensity activity.

So, how many calories should come from fat each day? Which fats are better for us and which fats get the bad rap? How can you distinguish this on the food label? Well, there's no gram per day recommendation for fat. Instead, the U.S. Department of Agriculture—USDA—provides a general range based on the percentage of your total dietary intake, including about 20–

35% of your total calories coming from fat. But, new research shows that many people are successful with more fat than this and still improve body composition and health.

A better way to consider fats is by the types of fats. Choosing a good mix of poly, mono, and saturated fats is a good idea. Also, limiting omega-6 fatty acids from excessive intake of vegetable oils and premade dressings and increasing intake of omega-3 fatty acids from fish, nuts, and seeds is another good idea overall. Also, as of January 2006, trans fats have been required to be on the Nutrition Facts Label. These rarely occur naturally and are considered the really bad guys of nutrition. They are formed when liquid oils are made to be solid—a simple way to increase the shelf-life of products. Essentially, they are man-made by hydrogenation where hydrogen ions are forced into the fat to change is chemical makeup.

The reason they're known as lethal is because not only do they increase bad cholesterol, but they also decrease good cholesterol and are directly related to heart disease risk. In fact, in November 2013, the FDA concluded that partially hydrogenated oils could no longer be considered as GRAS or Generally Recognized As Safe. After lots of bad publicity, manufacturers have decreased the amount of trans fats found in our foods significantly. But, trans fats are still found in many snack-type foods, cookies, crackers, and food fried in partially hydrogenated oils.

Refer to the ingredients list to avoid being tricked. Some products will report zero trans fats on the nutrition label, but hydrogenated oil in the ingredients list. Well, partially hydrogenated oils are the alter ego of trans fats. The 2 are equivalent. So, it's best to try and avoid foods high in trans fats by reading the labels carefully. But give yourself a break because they are hidden in many of your favorites I bet. A great place to start your fat intake—one of the quality kind—is to make it about 20–35% of your total daily calorie intake.

Remember that for fat calories, you need to multiply the fat grams by 9, not 4 as you did for both protein and carbohydrates. This means that fat has the highest calorie count per gram of the macronutrients. So if, by chance, you aim for 60–100 g of fat per day, this equals 540–900 calories from fat alone.

One interesting side note is that alcohol provides about 7 calories per gram, making it more energy dense than either carbohydrates or protein.

Besides, the big 3—protein, carbohydrates, and fat—also consider the sodium and cholesterol content of foods if you know you have a poor family or personal disease history with these nutrients. Otherwise, new research indicates far less concern than originally thought. Also, look at the amount of micronutrients in your food—including vitamins and minerals—a few will be listed on your food label. It is best to aim for about 100% of the micronutrients in your daily diet from all meals and supplements.

So, to summarize, let's reexamine some key points. Your diet quality is the most important aspect to improving body composition because all calories are not created equal. As it is often said, consider eating better rather than just eating less. And know what to look for on the Nutrition Facts Label. This can help you to identify better choices. Look for protein in your food choices, see what types of sugars you are consuming, and aim for quality fats. Take your time on your next visit to the grocery store. Try to use your knowledge of the food label to make the best choices you can.

If your food choices don't pass with flying colors, don't worry. You will gradually become more attuned to what's a poor option, and what's a better option, and what's the best option. There is no perfect diet. Just better combinations of foods than others. Those Nutrition Facts tell us about the quality and the quantity of the calories in our diet. Eventually, you will easily read labels and then enjoy the freedom of not having to count calories. Instead, you will look for nutrient dense foods that nourish your body and improve your health and body composition. It will literally feel like you can eat more and feel better. Try this, read your nutrition facts labels for the sugar content and aim to reduce the amount of added sugars in your overall diet.

Nutrient Timing and Frequency

The purpose of this lecture is to discuss the different components of nutrient timing—specifically, pre-exercise, during-exercise, and postexercise nutrition—and to shed some light on which tactics seem to work best for body composition and performance. Keep in mind that although common recommendations exist, nutrition is very individualized. Overall, make sure that you are getting adequate carbohydrates, fats, protein, and micronutrients throughout the day to fuel your lifestyle, and understand that this might differ drastically from person to person. Then, try some timing strategies to see if they work for you.

Nutrient Timing

- Timing when to eat our meals around exercise is important for many reasons. We need energy to fuel our workouts—perhaps multiple bouts in one day—but at the same time, we don't want to eat too much or too close to a training session or we might experience gastrointestinal issues that could make us feel terrible and ruin our workout.

- Nutrient timing is an overarching idea that encompasses a variety of strategies that might be directed toward performance, recovery from strenuous exercise, improving body composition, or a combination of all three.

Pre-Exercise Nutrition

- You need fuel and energy to exercise. Your body needs at least some fuel in the tank to perform optimally. Glycogen, which is the storage form of carbohydrates in the body, is the main fuel source during moderate to vigorous exercise, so it stands to reason that carbohydrates are an important pre-exercise nutrient.

These energy stores are sometimes the limiting factor in exercise, and running out can be the cause for running out of fuel in many long-distance exercises—essentially, your tank is empty. Thus, it is recommended that consuming carbohydrates prior to exercise (referred to as "carb loading") will fill up the tank. But how much you need depends on what your purpose is and what level of activity you are doing.

Many leading sports nutritionists instruct IRONMAN athletes—who swim 2.4 miles, bike 112 miles, and then run 26.2 miles—to increase their carbohydrate consumption to about 70 percent of their diet 5 to 7 days before a competition by adding things like oatmeal, rice, pasta, and bread to almost every meal.

Frankly, the details of optimal pre-exercise nutritional strategies are less important to the average person. That's not to say that pre-exercise nutrition is not important—it certainly is—but simply getting in some good nutrient sources with carbohydrates and protein, ideally 3 to 4 hours before exercise, is all you should concentrate on.

Be conscious of the total calories that you are taking in and burning during exercise so that you don't end up overeating, adding too much to your total caloric intake, and ultimately hurting your body composition or performance goals.

Many people prefer to work out in the morning before eating breakfast. If that is you, and you like that, go for it. But if you work out for more than 90 minutes, or at a vigorous intensity, you might consider fueling up a little and see how it makes you feel.

During-Exercise Nutrition

A common misconception is that you need sugar-filled sports drinks to rehydrate, no matter what type of exercise you are doing. If you are exercising for less than 60 to 90 minutes, all you really need is about a cup of water to keep you hydrated—no extra calories needed.

If you are participating in long-distance or time-consuming endurance events like marathons, then you certainly need to replenish your body with additional calories during exercise, and sports drinks are a great way to do this.

For endurance exercise of longer than 60 to 90 minutes, general recommendations for athletes are to take in between 30 and 60 grams of carbohydrates per hour during exercise to extend endurance performance.

This is a wide range because everybody is different. It is a trial-and-error process to find which fueling strategy works best for you based on what your goals are. If you can only tolerate the lower end of the 30- to 60-gram range, that doesn't mean that you are a worse athlete. Additionally, your stomach—just like your muscles—can be trained to tolerate more.

This emphasis on eating carbohydrate during exercise becomes even more important if you have not carb loaded, not consumed pre-exercise meals, or have restricted energy intake for weight loss.

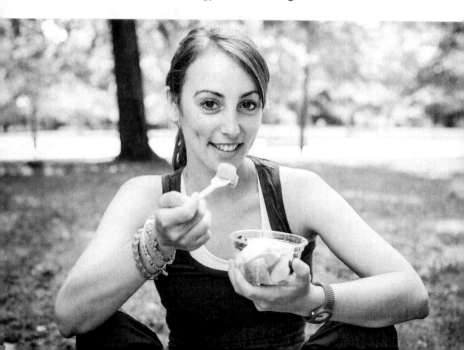

What type of carbohydrates should you eat before and during exercise? The common recommendation is to eat fast-digesting, or high-glycemic-index, carbohydrates during exercise. These include foods and drinks like sports beverages, premade gels, and whole foods like bread, jelly, and fruit.

One note of caution is that high-fructose products (such as some sports drinks) and foods (such as a lot of actual fruit) can lead to upset stomach and diarrhea. Most sports drinks have a combination of fructose and glucose, and you need to experiment with them to see what works for you.

In addition to protein prior to exercise, protein during exercise is important. Decades of research has shown that a carbohydrate-and-protein mix improves performance and lengthens time to exhaustion during endurance exercise when compared to just carbohydrates alone. These studies have all used sports drinks that include carbohydrates and protein.

The general recommendation for resistance training—because you should be doing a combination of both cardio work and resistance training—is that you include both carbohydrates and protein. The media pushes protein and resistance training so much that many people think that you only need protein during resistance training, but carbohydrates are also important.

Consuming carbohydrate in combination with protein will provide the most benefits during resistance exercise, and we've seen this in the research for endurance exercise, too. You'll optimize muscle glycogen, encourage better results, and help repair muscles by using a beverage that contains both carbohydrate and protein.

Postexercise Nutrition

The postexercise period is widely considered the most critical part of nutrient timing. Theoretically, consuming the proper ratio of nutrients immediately following exercise can initiate the rebuilding of damaged muscle tissue and restoration of energy reserves. This might enhance both body composition and exercise performance.

This entire concept of consuming nutrients immediately after exercise for maximal gains is often referred to as the "window of opportunity" or your "anabolic window." Generally, this anabolic window is considered to be within 30 and 60 minutes after your workout.

The following are some general recommendations for replenishing your fuel stores after exercise.

- The first issue is your rate of muscle glycogen resynthesis, or how quickly you can restock your stored glucose in your muscles and liver after you depleted them during exercise. Eating carbohydrates within 30 minutes of finishing your exercise seems to result in a greater rate of muscle glycogen resynthesis than if you delay eating carbohydrates by just 2 hours.

- Some studies have suggested up to 1.5 grams of carbohydrates per kilogram of body weight after a workout. But far less than this amount of carbohydrates will have a beneficial result for glycogen resynthesis.

- Immediately after exercise, you should aim for a higher-glycemic-index carbohydrate source, such as a bagel, a muffin, pasta, or cereal. Some research shows that a beverage with glucose and fructose might take advantage of certain sugar transporters and allow for the best rate of glycogen resynthesis.

- The research also shows that adding protein to your carbohydrates after your workout might help further increase glycogen storage and also increase muscle protein synthesis. The ratio of 3 to 4 grams of carbohydrate per 1 gram of protein in the post-workout meal is the general recommendation for these benefits to occur.

While there is scientific evidence to support the idea of an anabolic window, it appears as if it is not as important as we originally thought.

For athletes who are competing extremely hard and are performing two or more workouts per day, this window is very important to maximize muscle glycogen resynthesis and protein synthesis so that they can begin the recovery process as soon as possible. They need to train or compete within just a few hours.

However, for most individuals, while this window still exists, it is not necessary to change your habits to take advantage of it, but doing so might optimize your results. Unless you exercise again within a few hours, you should probably shift your focus more to the total amount of protein and carbohydrate you eat over the course of the day as opposed to hitting that window. For improvements in body composition, it is key to understand your total daily needs.

Meal Frequency

The information on how often you should eat, called meal frequency, is all over the place. Some suggest three meals per day while others suggest six, and some even suggest below and above these recommendations.

Research suggests that just by increasing protein and eating more frequently, you can improve your body composition, improve satiety, and boost metabolism. But if it's not high in protein, consuming three versus six meals per day doesn't seem to matter.

In other words, you can eat several small meals each day or you can eat the traditional three big meals each day, and there's almost no physiological difference. Just decide what you like and what fits your life.

Eating frequently might help with optimizing some aspects of performance, body composition, and health, but it is likely overemphasized in many people. Eating frequently might keep you from being over-hungry and gorging at the next meal, but you have to get to know your eating patterns and habits to see if it will work for your lifestyle.

Try eating six smaller but protein-rich meals per day to see if it works for your lifestyle and goals.

1. What will you change with regard to your nutrient timing based on the information from this lecture?

2. Is there a specific food type and timing that is right for you?

Nutrient Timing and Frequency

With an overwhelming amount of nutrition information available, from peer-reviewed journals to magazine covers to website forums and blogs, it can seem almost impossible to choose what foods are the best to eat—let alone when you should be eating them. One really fit friend—someone who you assume knows what they're talking about—tells you to cut out carbohydrates and eat protein 6 times per day, while you just read some science in a magazine saying that carbohydrates are essential, too much protein may hurt you, and maybe you should only eat 3 meals a day. So where do you even start?

Well, in the field of performance nutrition, new science comes out daily, which is a good thing because it shows that the subject is progressive, and dynamic, and it is not defiant to change, but it can also be overwhelming because what you thought was best for you yesterday is probably contradicted today. Too often media outlets leave out many of the details that are absolutely critical to the outcome from the research study. For example, I just read a research article where the average caloric intake of the participants in the study was right around 6,000 calories per day and they all lost weight. So what if the magazine headline read, "Eat 6,000 calories per day and lose weight!" Sounds pretty good right?

Well, what I didn't tell you was that the study was done on cyclists during just one day of the Tour de France where they expended that many calories or more. And that's a big difference, right? This shows that the details of the research matter. For this lecture we will tackle the questions of when and how many times you should eat throughout the day and in-and-around exercise, especially to improve body composition. Without even considering what you should be eating, the concept of nutrient timing—or quite simply when you should be eating—can seem pretty complex, but let's start at the most basic level right now.

If I asked you if you should drink water during a long hot jog in the heat, or wait until after your jog to drink water, you'd probably already know that nutrient timing is important. In this case, timing your water to take during your run would be most helpful. Well, nutrient timing can be applied to all sorts of aspects of eating and drinking to achieve optimal body composition. You know that the RDA for protein is 0.8g/kg of body weight to stave off disease. For sake of making this easy, let's round that 0.8g/kg to 1.0g/kg. Let's say you have a 75 kg man—or roughly 165 lb—and he consumes all of the recommended 75 g of protein on a daily basis. Fantastic, sounds spot on, right? Now, what if I told you he consumed all 75 g of that protein during his 6:00 AM breakfast? Does your opinion change? Does it still sound great to you? Probably not. The whole point here is that we all intuitively know that when you eat—your nutrient timing—is an important factor.

The purpose of this lecture is to discuss the different components of nutrient timing and to shed some light on which tactics seem to work best for body composition and performance. Now, before we get started, a key note to keep in mind throughout this lecture is that although there are common recommendations that exist, nutrition itself is very individualized. What works for one person may not work for another person as well, and a person's goals—like weight loss, an endurance race, or a bodybuilding competition—will alter optimal nutrient intake.

If you're like most people, then you probably wonder what to eat before or after your workout. Or, if a sports drink is something you should be sipping on at the gym. Well, timing when to eat our meals around exercise is important for many reasons. We need energy to fuel our workouts, perhaps even multiple bouts in one day, but at the same time we don't want to eat too much or too close to a training session or you may experience gastrointestinal issues that could make you feel terrible and ruin your workout. We are all aware that exercise can be tough enough as it is, so you don't want any additional issues.

Now before we really dive into the details of pre, during, and post-exercise nutrition, you should know that nutrient timing is an overarching idea that encompasses a variety of strategies that may be directed towards performance, recovery from strenuous exercise, improving body composition, or a combination of all 3. So, what should you do before exercise? Let's start with the obvious—you need the fuel and energy to exercise. Simple enough?

Your body needs at least some fuel in the tank to perform optimally. Glycogen, which is the storage form of carbohydrates in the body, is the main fuel source during moderate to vigorous exercise, so it stands to reason that carbohydrates are an important pre-exercise nutrient, right? These energy stores are sometimes the limiting factor in exercise, and running out can be the cause for "bonking" or "hitting the wall" as many long-distance exercisers can tell you about. Essentially, you run out of fuel and your tank is empty. Thus, it is recommended that consuming carbohydrates prior to exercise will fill up the tank. This is usually talked about as carbohydrate loading. But how much? Well, it depends on your purpose, and what level of activity you are doing.

Recently, I was in Tennessee to watch the Ironman Chattanooga, an event where athletes swim 2.4 miles, bike 112 miles, and then run 26.2 miles—an amazing feat. Is carbohydrate loading important to these athletes? You bet it is. Most of these athletes compete at a high intensity for anywhere between 8–14 hours continuously. So not only is pre-exercise an important nutrition component, but so is during and post-exercise nutrition. During these races, athletes depend upon sports drinks and gels, pre-made sandwiches, and all sorts of foods that the athlete can eat without getting an upset stomach, and that they can carry with them while riding a bike or running. No wonder nutrition is considered the 4th event along with swimming, biking, and running for triathletes.

Many leading Sports Nutritionists instruct these athletes to take up their carbohydrate consumption to about 70% of their diet 5–7 days before a competition by adding things like oatmeal, rice, pasta, and bread to almost every meal. However, does this really apply to the average person? To answer that, ask yourself if you exercise that much? Chances are that you don't, and there's certainly nothing wrong with that. These people are exercising anywhere from 10–20 or more hours per week. But, how should you change your pre-exercise nutrition if this carbohydrate loading isn't necessary for your average 30-minute jog or spin class at the gym every Tuesday?

Frankly, the details of optimal pre-exercise nutritional strategies are less important to the average person. That's not to say that pre-exercise nutrition is not important—it most certainly is—however, simply getting in some good nutrition sources with carbohydrates and protein is all I would suggest concentrating on. I see time and time again people making the relationship between exercise and nutrition much more difficult that it really needs to be. In my experience with sports nutrition consulting, I have seen the greatest results in performance and body composition changes when things are simplified—and this crosses over all types of clients I've worked with—from age-group triathletes to Olympians.

So just get in some good carbohydrate and protein ideally 3–4 hours before exercise. Be conscious of total calories that you are taking in and burning during exercise so that you don't end up overeating, or adding too much to your total caloric intake, and ultimately hurting your body composition or performance goals. You could simply eat 2 eggs and a banana or have a glass of milk. Also, I know many people who prefer to work out in the morning before they eat breakfast. If that's you, and you like that, then go for it. But, if you work out for more than 90 minutes, or at a vigorous intensity, you might consider fueling up a little and see how it makes you feel.

What about during exercise? Have you ever seen people carry Gatorade with them to a 5k race, or huge jugs of sports drinks at the gym when only running on a treadmill for 20 minutes at a steady, moderate pace? Well, common misconception is that you need these sugar filled drinks to rehydrate no matter what type of exercise you are doing. However, if you are exercising for less than 60–90 minutes, all you really need to worry about is water. No extra calories needed.

Remember the muscle glycogen we talked about earlier and how it is the primary fuel for your body with hard exercise? Well one hour of high intensity exercise will only burn through about half of those glycogen stores. So, while your favorite sports drink might taste delicious, for exercise of these shorter durations, consumption of sports drinks during the exercise itself will not really be beneficial to you. And if you're trying to lose weight or improve body composition, then these are really just added calories in the form of sugar that you don't really need.

In my time doing sports nutrition research and working with sports nutritionists and collegiate athletes, it is amazing how improvements in body composition occur even in college level athletes by monitoring nothing else but their sports drink consumption. The problem is that it tastes great and most people think that they need it to replenish. Don't get me wrong, it can help, but consuming these throughout the day and in excessive amounts is not only impractical, but it may also hurt your performance and body composition. That being said, sports drinks aren't evil—in certain situations they are needed. But, the details matter too—who is it, what exercise, how long, and how intense?

If you are participating in long-distance or time-consuming endurance events like marathons, then you certainly need to replenish your body with additional calories during exercise, and sports drinks are a great way to do this. For endurance exercise that's longer than 60–90 minutes, general recommendations for athletes are to take in between 30–60 g of carbohydrates per hour during exercise to extend performance. For example, you'll get about 50 g of carbohydrates from 2 medium-sized bananas or 2 cups of most cereals or sports drinks.

Now, I want to note that 30–60 g of carbohydrates per hour is a pretty wide range. The reason this is such a wide range is that everybody is different. Some stomachs can't handle the higher end of this range and will have GI issues or feel bloated. That definitely won't help their performance. For example, one of my colleagues is working with a former collegiate athlete who had a very sensitive stomach when racing in college—to the point of not being able to consume any nutrition within 2 hours of racing—but now, at the age of 30, he can handle the upper end of this 30–60 gram range while exercising.

I bring this up to illustrate a few points about during exercise nutrition. Everybody is different. It truly is a trial and error process to what fueling strategy works best for you based on your goals. To further that point, if you can only tolerate the lower end of 30–60 g range that doesn't mean that you are a worse athlete, and your stomach—just like your muscles—can be trained. In fact, this is a very hot topic of conversation with elite endurance athletes globally right now as some people are suggesting that select individuals may be able to train their body to take in north of 80 g per hour with extensive training. This would be well more than 2 large bananas and a large sports drink per hour, while exercising. This emphasis on eating carbohydrate during exercise becomes even more important if you have not carbohydrate loaded, not consumed pre-exercise meals, or have restricted energy intake for a weight and fat loss purpose.

Along these same lines, do you know what type of carbohydrate you should eat before and during exercise? The common recommendation is to eat a fast digesting or high glycemic index carbohydrate during activity. These include foods and drinks like sports beverages, pre-made gels, and whole foods like bread, jelly, and fruit. One note of caution is that high-fructose products, like some sports drinks, and foods like actual fruit, can lead to an upset stomach and even diarrhea. Most sports drinks have a combination of fructose and glucose, and you just need to experiment with them to see what works for you. My lab is actively researching this area, and we are testing all types of carbohydrates and modified carbohydrates for their effectiveness. Again, I wouldn't even consider these carbohydrate drinks if you're not exercising for more than 60–90 minutes. They simply aren't needed in that scenario.

Now, we've talked about protein prior to exercise, but protein during exercise is important as well. Decades of research have shown a carbohydrate and protein mix improves performance and lengthens time to exhaustion during endurance exercise when compared to just carbohydrate alone. These studies have all used sports drink products that include carbohydrates and protein. Just check you're the Nutrition Facts label to see if your favorite drink has both carbohydrates and protein. One complaint that I often hear from both clients and students is that sports nutrition and exercise physiology concentrate too much on endurance sports.

Well, let's talk about resistance training since most of you will likely be doing a combination of both cardio work and resistance training—at least I hope so. That is the general recommendation that you are to include both. The fact is that the media pushes protein and resistance training so much that many people think you only need protein during resistance training, but carbohydrates are important too.

A natural response to any stressful situation, including exercise, is to produce a hormone called cortisol. Cortisol has many actions in your body and it is necessary for optimal functioning. However, too much cortisol and particularly, chronically elevated cortisol can break down your lean muscle mass. But, eating carbohydrates can help to minimize the production of cortisol during exercise.

I'll explain this. One research study had participants complete 60 minutes of resistance training while consuming one of 3 beverages. A 6% carbohydrate solution—like most sports drinks on the shelves these days, a 6% carbohydrate + 6 g of essential amino acid solution, or a placebo beverage. They found that serum levels of cortisol—a stress hormone that contributes to the breakdown of your lean muscle—increased 105% in the placebo group, while the carbohydrate group increased only 11%, and the carbohydrate + essential amino acid group had only a 7% increase in cortisol.

These results suggest that consuming carbohydrates in combination with protein will provide the most benefits during resistance exercise, and we've seen this in the research for endurance exercise too. You'll optimize muscle glycogen, encourage better results, and help repair muscles by using a carbohydrate and protein beverage. It's funny how far apart the resistance and endurance exercise seem, but how similar the nutritional requirement are for them. Even though there are small differences in the details of what to eat and how much to eat before and during endurance and resistance training, both carbohydrates and proteins are important for optimal performance and body composition.

Now, that we have discussed pre and during exercise nutrition, let's take a look at post-exercise nutrition. The post-exercise period is widely considered the most critical part of nutrient timing. Theoretically, consuming the proper ratio of nutrients immediately following exercise can initiate the rebuilding of damaged muscle tissue and restoration of energy reserves. This may enhance both body composition and exercise performance.

This entire concept of consuming nutrients immediately post-exercise for maximal gains is often referred to as the window of opportunity, or your anabolic window. Generally, this anabolic window is considered to be within 30–60 minutes after your workout. But, is this anabolic window as small as we think? Do we need to rush to the protein powder or smoothie station as soon as we drop a weight or get off the treadmill in order to maximize muscle protein synthesis and recover fully?

Or for that matter, does it even matter at all? Is it really a window of opportunity? Let's start by looking at general recommendations for replenishing your fuel stores post-exercise. The first issue is that your rate of muscle glycogen re-synthesis or how quickly can you restock your stored glucose in your muscles and liver after you depleted them during exercise. Eating carbohydrates within 30 minutes of finishing your exercise seems to result in a greater rate of muscle glycogen re-synthesis than if you delay eating carbohydrates by just 2 hours. The benefit to eating quickly after a workout is thought to be due to your muscles being more insulin sensitive at this time. This means that your muscles make more efficient use of insulin immediately after exercise. Some studies have suggested up to 1.5 g of carbohydrates per kilogram body weight or 225 g of carbohydrates for a 150 lb, or 68 kg, person after a workout, but far less than this is actually needed or beneficial for glycogen re-synthesis.

Immediately post-exercise, you should aim for a higher glycemic index carbohydrate source like a bagel, a muffin, pasta, or cereal. Some research shows that a beverage with glucose and fructose might take advantage of certain sugar transporters and allow for the best rate of glycogen re-synthesis. The research also shows that adding protein to your carbohydrates after your workout may help to further the increase in glycogen storage and also increase muscle protein synthesis. And it's the ratio of 3–4 g of carbohydrate per 1 g of protein in the post-workout meal is the general recommendation for these benefits to occur.

So now let's go back to this question of the anabolic window. This concept suggests that in order to maximize muscle protein synthesis and prevent protein breakdown, you should consume nutrients as soon as possible after working out. That seems like common sense, right? The quicker you get your fuel back into your cells; the quicker you can build muscle. Well, it's not that easy. While there is plenty of research regarding this window of opportunity, there is beginning to be a new school of thought on this. Don't get me wrong—if you were to ask me, "Does the anabolic window exist?" My answer would be an unwavering yes.

But, if you were to ask me, "Is it really a window of opportunity?" In other words, is this something you need to take advantage of? My answer would be it depends. There is scientific evidence to support the idea of an anabolic window, but it appears that it is not as important as we originally thought. For athletes who are competing extremely hard, or performing 2 or more workouts per day, then the window of opportunity is very important to maximize muscle glycogen re-synthesis and protein synthesis so they can begin the recovery process as soon as possible. They need to train or compete within just a few hours.

However, for most individuals, while this window of opportunity still exists, it is not necessary to change your habits to take advantage of it, but doing so may optimize your results. For example, if you work out on Monday morning, and then eat normally all day long, by the time you get to your workout on Tuesday morning, you'll have no issues with glycogen storage or protein synthesis.

But, can you restore or repair faster by consuming the proper nutrients immediately post-workout? Maybe, but if you don't, it's not really a big deal. Unless you exercise again within a few hours, I would suggest you shift your focus more to the total amount of protein and carbohydrate you eat over the course of the day as opposed to hitting the window of opportunity. For improvements in body composition, it is likely a key to understand your total daily needs. I personally aim for a post-workout nutrition shake, but this is part of my normal habit and in line with my current exercise goals.

A mistake I see a lot is when people who are interested in fat loss, worry too much about pre-, during, and post-workout foods. I'll often see a big pre-workout fuel-up, a sports drink during exercise, and then rushing home after the workout to eat again even though they're still stuffed from all that food, and they only worked out for 45 minutes. This is simply too much. The food doesn't match the goal. It is a clear case of a little bit of information getting way out of control. For this person, some light food to fuel an intense workout would be great. Sipping water during the workout is good too. And then, just simply getting into the next appropriate meal, filled with lean proteins, healthy vegetables, and fruit, and some whole grains would be just fine. Super easy, super simple.

Another area that get's a bit confusing is how often you should eat. This is called Meal Frequency. How many meals should you eat per day? The information out there is all over the place. Some suggest 3 meals; some suggest 6, some even below or above these recommendations. What about calorie distribution? Should you eat more calories in the morning or at night? Or does it even matter?

A study that I helped with a few years back investigated whether a high protein diet, which was 35% protein, consumed in either 3 or 6 meals per day versus a standard diet of 3 meals a day—15% protein—would improve body composition and metabolism in overweight individuals. To determine what improved body composition would look like, we measured total body fat, abdominal fat, lean body mass, post-meal thermogenesis or the increase in metabolism following a meal, and leptin production. And leptin is a hormone that regulates hunger—we'll talk more about it in another lecture.

We found that total body fat and abdominal fat significantly decreased in both high protein groups. And lean body mass, post-meal thermogenesis, and leptin increased when high protein meals were eaten 6 times per day. So that's pretty great. Just by increasing protein and eating more frequently, you can improve your body composition, improve satiety, and boost metabolism. However, keep in mind that the population in this group was overweight. These results may not carry over to other populations, but it was an interesting finding regardless.

The truth of the matter is, if it's not high in protein, consuming 3 versus 6 meals per day doesn't really seem to matter. The *Journal of the International Society of Sports Nutrition* reported that as long as we eat the right foods in the right amounts, meal frequency seems to be a matter of personal preference more than anything else. In other words, you can eat a lot of small meals each day—something like consuming a small meal ever few hours—or you can eat the traditional 3 big meals each day and there's almost no physiological difference. Just decide what you like and what fits your life.

For me, I've always been a 6 meals per day person. I started this just because I was hungry, and I was always running from sport to sport. I know plenty of super fit people who practice this strategy. But, I also know people who have excellent body composition who don't like being bothered by eating so much. Again, you need to ask yourself, "What works for me?" This applies to other topics dealing with nutrient timing too. I could argue to death either side of the eat breakfast or skip breakfast debate, and the same thing goes for should you stack most of your food towards the beginning or end of the day debate. There is evidence, and good research, to support both arguments. So with all this contradicting information, what do you do?

I suggest trying both to see what works best for you; keep an open mind. As I mentioned before, nutrition is very individualized, and we are all unique, so one script for what to eat is not appropriate for everybody. There are a few guidelines, but they can be adapted. So what's the bottom line with meal frequency? Eating frequently may help with optimizing some aspects of performance, body composition, and health. But, it is likely over-emphasized in many people.

The general consensus from the research is that the number of meals you eat per day has no benefit except when high protein is involved and maybe only in specific populations. In the end, eating frequently may keep you from feeling over-hungry and gorging at the next meal. But, you have to know your eating patterns and habits to see if it will work for your lifestyle. I'm often asked this question too, "Can I eat late at night?" Well, stay tuned because in the next lecture I will spend the entire time going through the myths and facts about nighttime eating and discuss a lot of new information on the topic.

At this point, I'd like to help you digest all of this information that really seems to go opposite directions at times. As I've said multiple times what you do depends on your goals. Athletes have different nutritional needs than the average person, for instance, and even with these 2 groups different goals can drastically affect individual approaches to the same problem.

Within reason, there is no right or wrong answer when it comes to the various aspects of nutrient timing and choices, so long as you're making positive steps towards achieving your goals. Choose whichever plan works for you, and your lifestyle, check with your doctor to make sure it's good for you, and then stick to it.

It seems to me that some people are so focused on the nitty gritty of nutrient timing, that they forget about the big picture, which is to improve and optimize your body composition, health, and performance. Focusing too much on meal timing can be stressful. So, don't let it be. The less stressful you can make it; the easier it is to incorporate it into your life. Overall, I suggest that you concentrate more on the overall composition of your diet throughout the day, and the habits that you can easily change, before moving into advanced nutrient timing strategies.

The take-home message is this, make sure that you are getting adequate carbohydrates, fats, and proteins, and micronutrients throughout the day to fuel your lifestyle, and understand that this may differ drastically from person to person. Then, try some of the various timing strategies that we just went over and see if they work well for you. Try this, start by eating 6 smaller but protein-rich meals per day to see if it works for your lifestyle and your goals.

Lecture 13

Nighttime Eating

For a long time, it was believed that eating late in the night before going to sleep was bad for your health and would automatically make you gain fat. But emerging research has shown that small, protein-type beverages consumed before sleep might have a number of advantages—particularly when paired with a dynamic exercise program. After this lecture, you will have a better understanding of nighttime eating and why many people thought it was off-limits. You will also learn how eating protein at night, particularly before bed, can potentially impact body composition and overall health.

Eating before Bed: Research and Physiology

- We all have a circadian clock, or circadian timing system, that is like an internal clock that regulates our physiology with our daily behaviors and surrounding environment. For many of us, our typical circadian clock keeps us awake and active during the daytime hours and less active during the evening and night hours.

- Our circadian clock adjusts our physiology to coincide with these typical periods of activity and rest throughout the day. Because many of us are less active in the evening and late-night hours, our clock is programmed to slow our internal system down at those times, too.

- But does a less active system at night translate to fat gain if you eat at night? It depends. The food we consume essentially has two fates: It's either stored for later use or burned for energy (oxidation). Because our biological clock slows things down at night, it seems obvious that any food we eat at night will more likely be stored rather than burned during this time. So, this might be strike one against eating at night.

When you eat carbohydrates, for example, they are broken down into smaller components, like glucose, that enter your blood. In response to the glucose, insulin is secreted from your pancreas to get the glucose into your cells. This effectively lowers blood glucose back to "normal."

A potential strike two against eating at night is that research shows that for the same amount of glucose, greater amounts of insulin are required to remove it from the blood during the night as compared to the day. More insulin produced means more storage at night.

If nighttime eating is not done often, there is likely no problem. But if repeated over time, chronically high insulin can lead to desensitization of the insulin receptors and possibly to future problems with glucose control.

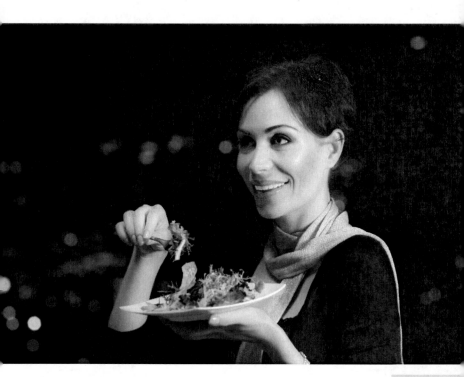

Research has also shown that the energy cost of digesting and processing your food—that is, the thermic effect of food—decreases at night. That means that if you eat the same exact meal for breakfast as you do for dinner, you'll have lower energy expenditure in the evening.

We also know that we do not feel as full when we eat food toward the later part of the day, so there's a chance that we'll eat more. In addition, it takes longer for food eaten later in the day to be emptied from the stomach and into the intestines during this time.

So, our physiology at night favors storage when we eat toward the later part of the day. This might not be ideal for body composition. Based on this information, could nighttime be the wrong time to eat? Is there a wrong time of day for people to eat if they want to maintain or lose fat?

While some of the research done in this area has been focused on specific groups of people—such as night-shift workers and people with night eating syndrome who ate late at night—and there is also controversy with what defines nighttime eating, the takeaway message is not controversial: If you consume the majority of your food in the evening and night hours as opposed to during the daytime hours and in excess of your energy needs, then you will likely have some unfavorable changes in your body composition.

But many of us eat our food at various intervals throughout the day and not primarily at one point of the day or another. Also, most people sleep during the night and work during the day.

So, one way that researchers define nighttime eating, or presleep eating, is simply taking in an additional snack after dinner and before going to bed.

It might just be a matter of knowing what our best food choices are if we want to eat at night. We know that large portions are not ideal, but what about low-calorie, nutrient-dense options? What about protein?

Consuming Protein before Bed: Active People

Many athletes and bodybuilders typically consume protein before bed, but are they reaping any benefits? For very active people, the rationale for consuming protein before bed is the belief that it would keep you anabolic overnight and promote muscle growth or repair.

Remember that "anabolic" means promoting a metabolic environment to stimulate, in this case, muscle building. The idea is that perhaps, over the long term, this continual anabolic state could lead to increases in muscle recovery and performance. Eating protein before bed to keep muscle growth continuing overnight might give you a competitive edge or allow you to recover better.

Whey protein is a very common supplement used by athletes and everyday gym-goers. However, casein protein, which makes up 80 percent of the protein in milk, has been highlighted as the best to be consumed before sleep due to its slow release from the stomach.

Casein is found in higher concentrations in foods like cottage cheese and Greek yogurt. The theory is that this allows for prolonged anabolism or, at least, less muscle breakdown overnight while you are sleeping.

It wasn't until 2012 that research-based evidence on the impact of consuming casein protein before bed was available. Professor Luc Van Loon and his research team in the Netherlands were the first to show us that consuming casein protein before bed increases muscle protein synthesis overnight. The studies demonstrated a few new things: We can digest and absorb protein at night, and we can increase muscle protein synthesis while sleeping.

In a follow-up study, Professor Van Loon's group was able to show true improvements in body composition when protein was consumed at night during a 12-week resistance exercise program. This shows us that specifically eating protein at night before bed can increase muscle mass in the long term.

Furthermore, research has shown that providing casein, whey, or carbohydrates within 30 minutes of going to bed led to greater resting energy expenditure (so burning more calories) in physically active men the next morning—compared to the lower resting energy expenditure when the men were given a placebo at night before bed.

Research has also found that fat burning was better when fit young men drank either a placebo or a casein protein shake compared to when they were given whey protein or carbohydrates.

This shows that the subjects who drank a placebo, which had no calories, and those who drank about 150 calories of casein protein both responded with a nice fat-oxidation or fat-burning response. This was a better response than provided by drinking whey protein or carbohydrates.

Taken together, this information tells us that if you are an active individual or athlete, consuming something before bed is better than going to bed on an empty stomach if you want to maximize your calorie-burning potential. It also suggests that casein may be better than whey, because casein seems to increase muscle growth overnight, and may promote a greater fat utilization.

Consuming Protein before Bed: Overweight and Obese People

Drinking small amounts of protein before bed seems to be beneficial for active people, but what about for overweight and obese people? Remember that the main reason to avoid nighttime eating was because we were told that it would make us store calories rather than burn them—that is, gain fat. But is this the case when you eat specifically after dinner and before sleep *and* you eat only a small portion?

To answer this, researchers provided a small, low-calorie protein-and-carbohydrate snack (in the form of cereal and milk) to overweight and obese people 90 minutes after dinner. This was opposed to the typical high-calorie, high-fat meals that they were used to eating at night. They did this every day for four weeks.

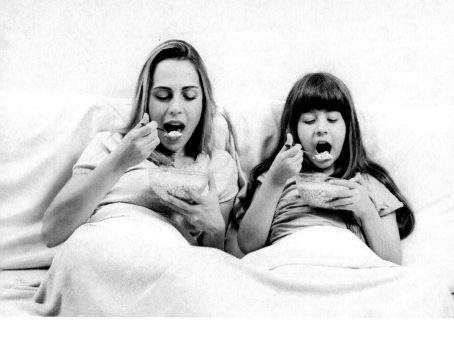

They found that the people who ate the cereal at night before sleep (which was about 130 calories of food) ended up lowering the total number of calories that they ate all day long on average over the four-week study. This led them to lose body weight in this study.

Just knowing that you are "allowed" to eat again later in the evening might stop you from taking bigger servings or going for seconds at your other meals. Still, this was the only study to see nighttime feeding in a positive light for people who were not active or fit.

What would happen if the nighttime snack were a low-calorie protein beverage (of about 150 to 160 calories) instead of the protein plus carb cereal snack?

Researchers gave one of three beverages—casein protein, whey protein, or a carbohydrate drink—to overweight and obese people within 30 minutes of going to bed and found that the participants felt fuller and had less desire to eat the next morning regardless of what they consumed (protein or carbohydrates).

Perhaps this was beneficial in terms of reducing total calorie intake the next day, similar to the cereal study. But because the study was only one night long and researchers didn't measure how much food participants ate for breakfast or if they ate less overall as a result of nighttime eating, they don't really know if the presleep snacks had an impact on total calorie intake.

Unfortunately, researchers also found that all groups, regardless of what they consumed, had higher insulin levels the next morning compared to normal. This was not an ideal finding because obesity is already associated with insulin resistance, or a lowered ability to use the insulin that is produced.

But the obvious solution to this problem is exercise. Exercise training increases insulin sensitivity, so adding daily exercise over a longer period might stop or reverse this acute insulin resistance associated with eating before bed in overweight and obese people.

When researchers carried out nighttime feeding of protein or carbohydrates before bed with the subjects for four weeks and added three days per week of exercise training, insulin levels did not change from baseline.

In addition, the group consuming the casein beverage felt fuller at the end of the four weeks compared to the groups consuming whey and carbohydrates. This study shows a possible advantage to casein protein.

Furthermore, there were slight decreases in body fat and slight increases in lean mass in all groups, while body weight stayed the same. In other words, there was no change in body weight, but body composition was slightly better.

So, it turns out that there might be some real advantages to eating a small protein snack late at night. We also know that increasing protein in your diet is advantageous for body composition over longer studies. This nighttime addition of protein will help increase total protein intake in your day.

Try This

If you are hungry at night before bedtime, try having a small protein beverage or protein food.

Questions to Consider

1. What are some things you tend to eat before bed? What are some alternatives that you can try instead?

2. What are three reasons why you might consider eating a small protein-centric snack before bed?

Nighttime Eating

If you're like me, then you get hungry again before you head to bed at night. I know we've already discussed topics like when to eat and how much to eat, but nobody ever specifically talks about one of the most common questions that I get which is, "What can I eat at night before sleep?" Usually, this question is crammed between a few other questions like, "Won't eating at night make me fat?" Or "Can I really eat before bed?" For a long time, it was believed that eating late at night before going to sleep was bad for your health and would automatically make you gain fat.

Eat past eight equals gain weight, right? Well, not quite. You see, there are several things we need to consider when the topic of nighttime eating is brought up, and a few questions come to my mind for me. I wanted to know where these recommendations were coming from? Where's the scientific evidence? And how is nighttime eating defined? Does this mean I should be monitoring what time I eat dinner? How does the nighttime meal size and composition influence my health? And, of course, are carbohydrates evil?

Lucky for me, I had a way to find these answers. And just like that, nighttime feeding has been a major research focus in my lab at Florida State University. The original premise for starting this line of research stemmed from my glory day as a collegiate ice hockey player. I remember reading about the need to stop eating late at night to avoid gaining fat or feeling lousy. Then, various TV shows and media experts began to speak up about it too. I mean everybody just knew that if you want to have a great body composition, you should avoid eating late at night—after dinner—at all costs. The trouble was, that I always ate before going to bed. I thought it would be good to help my body recover from practice and workouts so that I could become a better player. And just about everybody I knew who had low body fat and good muscle mass would not only eat at all times of the day, but would purposefully eat before bed and drink a protein shake or have some kind of protein before going to sleep.

So, how could this huge gap exists between the people I knew who ate before bed and still felt great, and had excellent body composition, and performed well, and the opposite message that many in the media were telling us? Well, the short answer is that many things influenced this public health message. And I'll go over them in this lecture. After this lecture, you'll have a better understanding of nighttime eating and why many people thought it was off-limits. You will also learn about eating protein at night, particularly before bed, can potentially impact body composition and overall health.

I'm sure you've come across something or someone telling you that nighttime eating is bad and that you should have a set stop time each night for the eating. To understand why most people think that eating at night is bad, we need to dive into some research and physiology. An easy place to start would be with your circadian clock or circadian timing system. You see we all have an internal clock that regulates our physiology with our daily behaviors and surrounding environment. So for many of us, our typical circadian clock keeps us awake and active during the daytime hours and less active during the evening and night hours. Our circadian clock adjusts our physiology to coincide with these typical periods of activity and rest throughout the day. Because many of us are less active in the evening and late night hours, our clock is programmed to slow our internal system down at those times, too. But, does a less active system at night translate to fat gain if you eat at night? As any good scientist might say, the answer is it depends.

Recall that the food consumed essentially has 2 fates, it is either stored for later use or burned for energy. Since our biological clock slows things down at night, it seems obvious that food we eat at night will more likely be stored rather than burned during this time. So this may be strike one against eating at night. Now, remember we learned that when you eat carbohydrates; for example, the carbohydrates are broken down into smaller components like glucose that enter your blood. In response to the glucose, insulin is secreted from your pancreas to get the glucose into the cells. This effectively lowers blood glucose back to normal.

Here's a potential strike 2 against eating at night. Research shows that for the same amount of glucose, greater amounts of insulin are required to remove it from the blood during the night as compared to the day. More insulin produced equals more storage at night. If nighttime eating is not done often, there is likely no problem. But, if it's repeated over time, chronically high insulin can lead to a desensitization of the insulin receptors and possibly lead to future problems with your glucose control. Research has also shown that the energy cost of digesting and processing your food—that is, the thermic effect of food—goes down at night. That means that if you eat the same exact meal for breakfast as you do for dinner, you'll have a lower energy expenditure in the evening.

We also know that we do not feel as full when we eat foods toward the later part of the day, so there's a chance we'll eat more food. And one more point about nighttime digestion; it takes longer for food eaten later in the day to be emptied from the stomach and into the intestines during this time. To sum it up, when we eat at night, more insulin is needed, we feel less full so we eat more, and we have a slower digestion, and less energy is used to digest and process food. This tells me that our physiology at night favors storage when we eat towards the later part of the day.

This may not be ideal for body composition. Do you see how the message quickly spread to avoid eating in the evening? I sure do. So, based on the information could nighttime eating be the wrong time to eat? Well, a study with animals surely has us all convinced that this might be the case. If you change the feeding time of mice, so that they are fed a high fat diet during the time when they normally sleep—which, in mice this is during the daylight hours—as opposed to when they are normally awake—which, is during the night for mice—the mice gained more fat.

This looks like there may actually be a wrong time of day to eat—at least for mice. An interesting finding for sure, but I was told to never trust a rat or a mouse. Does this hold true for humans? Is there a wrong time of day for people to eat if they want to maintain or lose fat? If you take the time to do a little research on night eating and humans, you'll see that much of scientific evidence that is cited for why we shouldn't eat at night was based primarily on people who work the night-shift in jobs that provide service 24 hours such as hospitals, and people with Night Eating Syndrome—this is an eating disorder characterized by eating more than half of your daily food intake after dinner, waking up from sleep to eat, and having little appetite for breakfast.

Here, the story was pretty clear too, Night Shift Workers and people with Night Eating Syndrome who ate late at night ended up getting people bigger, fatter, and less healthy. At this point you might think that the story of don't eat at night seems to be logical, but there are some other things to consider. For example, in addition to late night eating these individuals also have disturbed or restricted sleep and we know that the less sleep you get, the greater your chances for overweight and obesity. Now, to mention the obvious response to sleeping less at night—more opportunity to eat—you have more hours in the day when you might eat, and this could obviously lead to trouble if you're trying to achieve your optimal body composition. There is also controversy with what defines nighttime eating. Much of the research on this topic uses different criteria for night eating. Some will say that it's the total calories consumed within a specified time frame. For example, calories consumed between 5pm and midnight. Others will say it is waking up throughout the night to eat. And the typical dinner meal may or may not be included in what is defined as nighttime eating.

What is not controversial is the take away message that if you consume the majority of your food in the evening and night hours as opposed to during the daytime hours and in excess of your energy needs, then yes, you will likely have some unfavorable changes in your body composition. But let's be realistic here. Many of us eat our food at various intervals throughout the day and not primarily at one point in the day or another. Also, most people actually sleep during the night and work during the day. So, the way that my research group defines nighttime eating, or presleep eating, is simply taking in an additional snack after dinner and before going to bed.

It may just be a matter of knowing what our best food choices are if we want to eat at night. We know that large portions are not ideal but what about low-calorie, nutrient-dense options? What about protein? Like I mentioned earlier, many athletes and body builders typically consume protein before bed, but are they reaping any benefits?

In this field of performance nutrition and exercise physiology, we think about feeding our bodies all the time. We basically know how to feed ourselves throughout the day, and in relation to exercise, in order to optimize body composition and health. This is not surprising as much of the available research is tailored towards this optimization. For very active people, the rationale for consuming protein before bed is the belief that it would keep you anabolic overnight or promote muscle growth and repair. Remember that anabolic means promoting a metabolic environment to stimulate, in this case, muscle building. The idea is that perhaps, over the long-term, this continual anabolic state could lead to increased muscle recovery and performance. Simply, eating protein before bed to keep muscle growth continuing overnight could give you a competitive edge against the competition, or simply allow you to recover better.

Before we get into that possibility, let's briefly go over our options for what that before bed protein snack might consist of. We know that whey protein is a very common supplement used every day by athletes and gym-goers. However, casein protein, which makes up 80% of the protein in milk, has been highlighted as the best to consume before sleep due to its slow release from the stomach. Casein is found in higher concentrations in foods like cottage cheese and Greek Yogurt. The theory is that this allows for prolonged anabolism or, at least, less muscle breakdown overnight while you're sleeping.

It wasn't until 2012 that research-based evidence on the impact of consuming casein protein before bed was available. In some very nice studies, Professor Luc Van Loon and his research team in the Netherlands were the first to show us that consuming casein protein before bed increases muscle protein synthesis overnight. Specifically, they compared physically active young men who consumed either 40 g of casein protein equaling 160 calories or a placebo drink 2 1/2 hours after a lower body resistance exercise workout, but within 30 minutes of going to bed. It turned out that the group who drank the casein protein had greater overnight muscle protein synthesis compared to drinking no protein.

They then completed a similar study in elderly men showing that casein protein at night before sleep—but this time via nasogastric tubing, so not exactly drinking it—had the exact same outcome, an increase in muscle protein synthesis. These studies demonstrated a few things. One, we can digest and absorb protein at night, and two, we can actually increase muscle protein synthesis while sleeping. Until this point though, the studies had not been long enough to show that the increase in muscle protein synthesis would actually lead to more muscle mass or better body composition—but it certainly looked like it would.

So in a follow-up study from Professor Van Loon's group, they examined whether acute changes in muscle protein synthesis could translate to changes in muscle size and strength with long-term daily protein intake before bed combined with resistance training. They had all the research subjects complete resistance exercise for 12 weeks. At the same time, they gave one group a protein and carbohydrate drink made of about 28 g of casein and 15 g of carbohydrates every night before sleep. The other group got a no-calorie placebo. During the 12-week training, the group consuming the protein and carbohydrate drink appeared to have greater increases in muscle fiber size and maximal strength than the group getting no-calories, protein, or carbohydrates before bed. This study was able to show true improvements in body composition when protein was consumed at night during a 12-week resistance exercise program. We must consider that protein intake was not matched, though, between groups, but this does show us that specifically eating protein at night before bed can increase muscle mass in the long-term.

Now, that we know casein protein before bed is beneficial for muscle growth, you might be wondering if there are any other benefits from consuming casein at night. If so, how do these benefits compare to whey protein and even carbohydrates? Fortunately, work from my lab answers a few of these questions. We found that providing casein, whey, or carbohydrates within 30 minutes of going to bed led to greater resting energy expenditure—so burning more calories—in physically active men the next morning compared to a lower resting energy expenditure when the men were given a placebo at night before bed. We also found that burning fat was better when fit young men drank either a placebo, or a casein protein shake compared to when they were given whey protein or carbohydrates. This shows me that the subjects who drank a placebo, which had no calories, and drinking about 150 calories of casein protein both responded with a nice fat oxidation or fat-burning response—a better response than drinking whey protein or carbohydrates.

Taken together, this information tells us that if you are an active individual or athlete, consuming something before bed is better than going to bed on an empty stomach if you want to maximize your calorie burning potential. It also suggests that casein may be better than whey, as casein seems to increase muscle growth overnight, and may promote a greater fat utilization. So drinking small amounts of protein before bed seems to be beneficial for active people, but what about for overweight and obese people? Remember that the main reason to avoid nighttime eating was because we were told that it would make us store calories rather than burn them—that is, gain fat. But is this the case when you eat specifically after dinner and before sleep, and you eat only a small portion?

To answer this, researchers provided small, low-calorie, protein, and carbohydrates snack in the form of cereal and milk to overweight and obese people 90 minutes after dinner. This was opposed to the typical high-calorie, high fat meals that these people were used to eating at night. They did this every day for 4 weeks straight. What they found was that the people who were compliant and ate the cereal at night before sleep, which was about 130 calories of food, ended up lowering the total number of calories that they ate all day long on average over the 4-week study. This led them to actually lose body weight in this study.

My guess is that just knowing that you are allowed to eat again later on in the evening might stop you from taking bigger servings or going up for seconds at your other meals. Still, this is the only study to see nighttime feeding in a positive light for people who were not active or fit. We wondered what would happen if the nighttime snack was a low-calorie protein beverage, 150–160 calories, instead of the protein plus carbohydrate cereal snack? Would appetite change? Would body composition improve? Were there any health changes that might come up? What about any cardiometabolic issues or benefits associated with consuming protein or other foods before bed? We looked into this and gave one of 3 beverages—casein protein, whey protein, or a carbohydrate drink—to overweight and obese people within 30 minutes of going to bed.

We found that the research participants ended up feeling fuller and had less desire to eat the next morning regardless of what they consumed. Protein or carbohydrates, it didn't matter; there was no difference between them. Our first thought was that this might be beneficial in terms of reducing total calorie intake the next day—similar to the cereal study I just mentioned. But, because the study was only one night long and we didn't measure how much food they ate for breakfast, or if they ate less overall as a result of nighttime eating, we don't really know if the presleep snacks had an impact on total calorie intake—they simply reported feeling more full and had less desire to eat.

And unfortunately, we also found that all groups, regardless of what they consumed, had higher insulin levels the next morning compared to normal. This was not an ideal finding because we know that obesity is already associated with insulin resistance, or a lowered ability to use the insulin that is produced. So we weren't pleased that their insulin levels were higher. Well, what's the obvious solution to this problem? Exercise.

You are all well aware that exercise training increases insulin sensitivity. So doesn't it make sense that adding daily exercise over a long period may stop or reverse this acute insulin resistance associated with eating before bed in overweight and obese people? Well, that is exactly what we found. When we carried out nighttime feeding of protein or carbohydrates before bed with our subjects for 4 weeks straight and included 3 days per week of exercise training insulin levels did not change from baseline. So that solved the problem. Subjects could have their bedtime snack, could feel fuller— an advantage when you're trying to lower calorie intake—and with added exercise, their insulin levels remained stable. We were also able to show that the group consuming the casein beverage felt fuller at the end of the 4 weeks compared to the groups consuming whey and carbohydrates. Looks like a possible advantage to casein protein from this study. But, you must be wondering if there were any changes in body composition with the addition of exercise? Did the protein groups have a better outcome?

Well, we did show slight decreases in body fat and slight increases in lean mass in all groups, while body weight stayed the same. This should ring some bells, there was no change in body weight, but body composition was ever so slightly better. We also noticed that metabolic rate was increased for the protein groups, but decreased for the carbohydrate group. This was not large enough to be considered statistically significant, but the magnitude of change was interesting to us. Because all the groups improved body composition, regardless of what they ate before bed, we know that it was the exercise that was most important in body composition change, and not necessarily the impact of that before-bed protein on appetite.

But, the greater message might be that despite having about a 150-calorie snack, in this case from protein or a carbohydrate shake, before bed, body composition still improved with exercise training. The women in the study did not gain weight or fat. That's a great thing. What's more? In a different study, we also found improvements in cardiovascular health as a result of exercise and drinking protein before bed in overweight and obese women. So it turns out that there may be some real advantages to these small, protein snacks late at night.

We also know that increasing protein in your diet is advantageous for body composition over the longer studies. This nighttime addition of protein will help to increase total protein intake in your entire day. One of the many questions that still remains is what actually happens to fat during the overnight period in response to protein before bed? Well, my lab just finished up a studying looking at how casein before bed influences overnight lipolysis or fat breakdown and mobilization, in belly fat. The study hasn't been published as of December 2015 when we taped this course, so I can't quite tell you all of the results, but let's just say that we are excited to share the news.

What I want you to understand is that a broad statement like don't eat after 7 pm is outdated and based upon research that may not even apply to people like you. It turns out that large meals that are very high in calories and eaten late at night don't seem to be tolerated as well as the same meal eaten earlier in the day. But, you now know about all the emerging research that is beginning to tell a clearer story. And the story is that small, protein type beverages, consumed before sleep may have a number of advantages—particularly when paired with dynamic exercise training. Things like improved muscle protein synthesis, increased muscle mass, increased strength, increased metabolism, and reduced desire to eat.

There is no need to fear eating at night, but the right choices need to be made to ward off fat gain and weight gain. For now, it looks like casein is the protein of choice for presleep consumption in active individuals—and not that much, only 150 calories. So try this, if you are hungry at night before sleep, try having a small protein beverage or protein food.

Evaluating Dietary Supplements

The field of performance nutrition is extremely dynamic. There is new research coming out almost daily that can change the general consensus on any single topic. While there are many performance supplements that show no real benefit, other supplements could be quite beneficial to health, body composition, and performance, as you will learn in this lecture. In fact, some performance supplements have shown safety and efficacy for a long time and have now made their way into the clinical world to alleviate and prevent diseases.

Supplement Facts Panel

- A dietary supplement has a very long definition. Technically, they are defined as a product that is intended to supplement the diet and contains one or more of the following ingredients: a vitamin, mineral, an herb or other botanical, an amino acid that is a concentrate, a metabolite, a constituent, an extract, or a combination of any of these.

- Note that these products are not intended to replace food that is already in your diet.

- There are some differences between a conventional food label with the Nutrition Facts panel and the Supplement Facts panel.

- You'll often see a section with a "proprietary blend" listed. This means that rather than giving specific amounts of specific ingredients, they are bunched together under "proprietary blend," and only a single amount of all ingredients in the blend is listed. This is a list of ingredients that are part of a product formula specific to a particular manufacturer. It is their secret ingredient.

The Food and Drug Administration does not require the amount of the ingredients in the proprietary blend formula to be listed, which is where consumers tend to run into trouble with supplements. You don't have to avoid products with a proprietary blend, but be sure to work with a sports nutritionist and your physician to see what will work best for you.

If you do see the dose listed—which many quality companies include on their labels already—it's best to be sure that it matches what the research evidence shows actually works for humans.

Fat-Loss Supplements: Caffeine

Contrary to what you might think, some fat-burning supplements on the market actually work and are safe. Most of these supplements target fat loss in one of three ways: by increasing the fat you burn for energy, by blocking fat storage in your body, or by controlling your calorie intake by suppressing hunger. However, of all the marketed products, only a few have good research-based evidence.

The most common supplement in the fat-burning category is caffeine. In fact, caffeine is the most popularly consumed drug in the world and is found in coffee, tea, soda, and even chocolate.

Caffeine is thought to be a weight-loss supplement because it increases resting energy expenditure by 7 to 15 percent in some studies. The active compound of caffeine, called methylxanthine, acts as a heart muscle, skeletal muscle, and central nervous system stimulant. This is why you might get the jitters when you have an extra cup of coffee in the morning.

Some people need to be careful because the extra stimulation from caffeine can be too much. But this only needs to really be taken as a precaution if you have a preexisting heart condition or are extremely sensitive to caffeine. As always, check with your doctor regarding your individual health status.

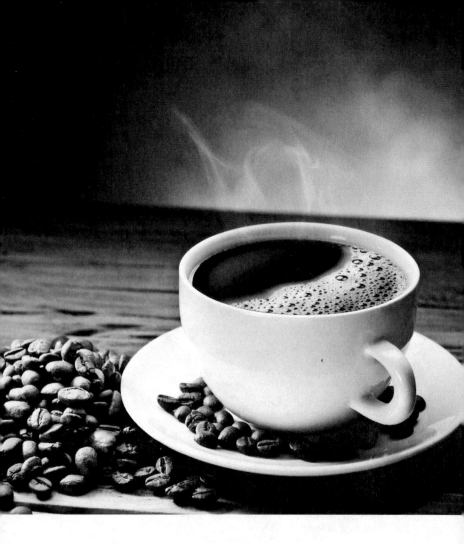

Most of the studies show that to have a noticeable metabolic-increasing effect, roughly 3 to 6 milligrams of caffeine per kilogram of body mass must be consumed at one time. This equates to about 1 to 2 normal-sized servings, such as 16- to 20-ounce cups of coffee, depending on the strength of the brew.

If you don't like drinking that much liquid, there are caffeine tablets available on the market that are pretty inexpensive and contain about 200 milligrams per pill. Just keep in mind that an excess of pretty much anything that you put into your body will likely cause problems and could even be deadly.

You can probably see how this might lead to cost and/or efficacy issues of caffeine. For fat loss, start with many of the other nutrition and exercise factors offered in this course first. Then, if you truly want to try caffeine for fat-loss purposes, it could be useful if done properly.

It is best to have caffeine 30 to 45 minutes before exercise and/or first thing in the morning before breakfast. For best results, caffeine should be taken on an empty stomach. Consuming it with food, especially carbohydrates, diminishes its effects by lowering plasma caffeine concentrations as well as delaying the time to peak caffeine concentration in your blood.

Drinking your coffee with little or no additives, such as cream, sugar, or milk, might be most helpful (not to mention lowering your overall calorie intake).

The downside to caffeine is that the effect of caffeine on weight loss is not the same for everyone. It seems to work best for younger people and for those who are more physically fit.

Also, if you consume lots of caffeine, it is thought that you become less sensitive to its fat-loss and exercise-performance effects.

A common concern that people have with caffeine is that it will cause dehydration. However, numerous studies have shown that this is a myth and that there is no evidence to support it.

Fat-Loss Supplements: Green Tea

Green tea has become increasingly popular in American culture over the past decade, with all kinds of products that contain green tea or green tea extracts. It has been used in Eastern cultures for much longer to increase mental awareness, improve digestion, regulate body temperature, act as an antioxidant, and for its antiobesity and anticancer effects.

The active ingredient in green tea is called epigallocatechin gallate (EGCG). In some studies, EGCG has been shown to increase energy expenditure by about 4 percent and increase fat burning by 10 percent compared to a placebo.

Interestingly, when combined with caffeine, there seems to be a synergistic effect between caffeine and EGCG, which in some studies has been shown to ramp up fat burning more than caffeine or EGCG alone.

But don't run to the supermarket and start buying everything with green tea just yet. To have a beneficial effect, research shows that you need to consume about 750 milligrams, or about 15 cups, per day of EGCG.

But you don't have to drink all of your EGCG. Many EGCG supplements are found in capsulated form, with about 400 milligrams per pill. Check with your doctor to make sure that your choices are healthy ones.

Many teas and supplements contain both EGCG and caffeine. But even drinking decaffeinated green tea might improve body composition.

Fat-Loss Supplements: Capsaicin

Capsaicin is a spice that causes the perceived "hotness" you feel when eating spicy foods. This pungent extract has been shown to increase thermogenesis and energy expenditure.

The issue with this is that many of these studies use rats and not humans as research subjects. So, you have to be cautious about generalizing results to humans.

The data for humans is less impressive, but body fat reductions have been reported. The issue is that there is a high rate of weight regain,

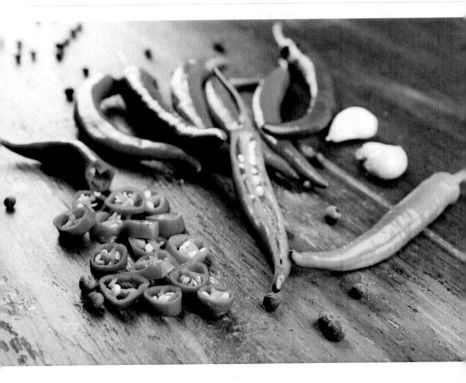

and the participants had trouble sticking to the dosage that is thought to be required for a beneficial effect.

Fat-Loss Supplements: Carnitine

Another debatable supplement for fat loss is called carnitine, which is a fat carrier, or gatekeeper, that helps transfer fat into the mitochondria, where it gets oxidized for fuel. Logically, it makes sense to think that if you increase the amount of carnitine, then you could get more fat into the right place to burn for energy.

Unfortunately, that is not the case in 99 percent of the research on this topic. Until more long-term studies are completed, it doesn't appear to be worth it.

Muscle-Gain Supplements: Creatine

The biggest player in the category of supplements that are thought to increase your muscle mass is creatine, or creatine monohydrate. Creatine is one the most popular supplements ever produced and the most thoroughly researched of any supplement.

We produce creatine naturally in the liver and kidneys. It is stored either as free creatine or bound to a phosphate in skeletal muscle. Naturally, the creatine phosphate energy system is used to provide energy for maximal-intensity, short-duration exercise. Creatine supplies a phosphate to adenosine diphosphate to create adenosine triphosphate, or ATP—the energy we need to do everything.

As a supplement, creatine is often used to help build muscle, improve strength and power, and increase anaerobic, short-duration exercise (i.e., power lifting or sprinting). The standard serving of creatine is 5 grams, which is equal to the amount of creatine in about 2.5 pounds of raw meat. So, it is much easier to take a small scoop of creatine versus eating an entire plate of steak.

There are several forms of creatine on the market, but the one that has the most research support and effectiveness is creatine monohydrate. Several hundred peer-reviewed research studies have evaluated this form, and more than 70 percent of these studies show a significant improvement in exercise capacity and increases in muscle mass.

Most experts attribute the beneficial changes to body composition and performance from creatine to the improved ability to do more quality work during exercise. But research also shows some improvements to actual cellular processes for muscle gain, too.

And due to the repeatable success of creatine use for improving both body composition and performance, creatine is now being studied and used with great interest for use with clinical populations and in disease prevention.

Creatine has now been shown to improve muscle mass and outcomes in people with muscular dystrophy, leukemia, traumatic brain injury, and infants born with errors in normal metabolic function.

A common myth is that creatine is a steroid and will damage your kidneys. Creatine is not a steroid; it is simply the combination of three amino acids. The research shows that creatine is safe and effective among young and old, male and female, and healthy and diseased populations. In the absence of any preexisting conditions, such as kidney disease, creatine is a supplement that has consistently been shown to be beneficial.

The most common side effect reported is weight gain. However, this is probably the type that you want, because creatine increases muscle mass. Also note that some cases of gastrointestinal upset have been noted in the literature. The most common dose is 5 grams per day (about 1 tablespoon).

Muscle-Gain Supplements: Beta-Alanine

Another supplement that might help with muscle mass and performance is called beta-alanine, which has been shown to improve performance and exercise capacity as well as permit greater intensity and volume of exercise training.

Beta-alanine, which is an amino acid made in the liver, combines with another amino acid called histidine to form a new protein molecule called carnosine in the muscle. Carnosine then acts to buffer, or soak up, the acidity, or hydrogen ions, that is created during very difficult exercise.

When accumulated, hydrogen ions cause muscle pain and fatigue, so if the hydrogen ions are controlled, theoretically, you could exercise longer and/or at a higher intensity. And higher-intensity exercise for longer should help improve body composition.

Many studies support the use of beta-alanine to increase performance and body composition in both men and women. About 3 to 6 grams per day for 4 weeks can increase intramuscular carnosine and improve performance. Typically, this dose should be split up throughout the day for best results.

One side effect to note is that beta-alanine is often associated with a tingling feeling or numbness in the extremities called paresthesia. It is temporary but annoying. And not all people have this feeling, but it is reported in many of the research studies. As a result, some companies have made extended-release capsules to allow a slow release of beta-alanine, which can help reduce or diminish any of the paresthesia effects.

Try This

Try adding 5 grams per day of creatine monohydrate to your daily routine.

Questions to Consider

1. What supplements do you already take? Are there any supplements hidden in common foods or beverages that you consume?

2. What myths have been busted based on the new information you've learned from this lecture? What supplements do you think you would be willing to try after learning what you learned in this lecture?

Evaluating Dietary Supplements

Many of you have heard the saying whole foods first when it comes to your diet and the famous Hippocrates quote "Let food be thy medicine and medicine be thy food."

Of course, we know that food is necessary to fuel our daily activities, and the composition of what we eat may affect our body composition and performance. However, is there a point where food may not be enough to work to our optimal level and peak capacity? Is there a need to add supplements into our diet on top of what we eat?

You also know from the micronutrients lecture that many people end up with minor deficiencies in one nutrient or another. But, you may be wondering, what about all the other supplements you hear about? It is no secret that many people are looking to gain an extra edge for fat loss, body transformation, energy levels, and performance.

These supplements or ergogenic aids as they're often categorized as are termed sports and performance nutrition or sports supplements because many athletes also are looking for an edge. But, so are many other people as well. These supplements come in many shapes and sizes, from pills to powders to gels, and the general public eats them up.

It's quite surprising to see how much money is spent on supplements each year. A study by Persistence Market Research released a report recently that stated that the global sports nutrition market, which includes sports foods, and drinks, and supplements, was valued at $20.7 Billion—yes billion—and is projected to reach a whopping $37.7 billion by the year 2019.

With the overwhelming amount of advice and testimonials about consuming supplements, it is difficult to determine which of these products work, which are a waste of your money, and which products could be harmful.

It seems that almost weekly there is a story in the news about contaminated supplements that creates the image that supplements are completely unregulated. Well, this is not true and, like many news stories, often one bad scenario paints the entire industry with the same brush. Admittedly, it can be quite confusing, and even the most experienced consumer has doubts. It's confusing even for people like me, who studies these supplements on a regular basis, to know just what to choose. How do you know that the doctor pushing this new miracle product isn't being paid by the company to promote it?

The field of performance nutrition is extremely dynamic. There is new research coming out almost daily that can change the general consensus on any single topic. While there are many performance supplements that show no real benefit, other supplements could actually be quite beneficial to health, body composition, and performance. In fact, some performance supplements have shown safety and efficacy for a long time, and have now made their way into the clinical world to alleviate and prevent diseases; I'll discuss it all with you in this lecture. A lot of money is being pumped into this niche market, and the purpose of this lecture is to distinguish the performance supplements that actually work, based on reliable and consistent research, versus those that only lighten your wallet.

Let's begin by discussing what dietary supplements are, and how to read their labels, known as the Supplement Facts panel. Well, a dietary supplement has a very long definition. Technically, they are defined as a product that is intended to supplement the diet and contains one or more of the following ingredients: a vitamin, mineral, herb or other botanical, an amino acid that is a concentrate, metabolite, constituent, extract, or a combination of any of these. Notice how these products are not intended to replace food that is already in your diet. You know how to read a conventional food label with the nutrition facts panel, but there are some differences between this label and the Supplement Facts panel that we should highlight before we dive into the specifics.

You'll often see a section with a proprietary blend listed. This means that rather than giving specific amounts of specific ingredients, they are bunched together under proprietary blend, and only one single amount of all the ingredients in the blend is listed. This is a list of ingredients that are part of a product formula specific to a particular manufacturer. It's their secret ingredient. The Food and Drug Administration does not require the amount of the ingredients in the proprietary blend formula to be listed, which is where consumers tend to run into trouble with supplements. It's very important to check the labels on any supplement to make sure you know what you're taking. If you see proprietary blend, you just don't know how much of each ingredient is in your product. You don't have to avoid products with a proprietary blend, just be sure to work with a sports nutritionist and your physician to see what will work best for you.

If you do see the dose listed—which many quality companies include on their labels already—it's best to be sure that it matches what the research evidence shows actually works for humans. I'll discuss specific examples in just a few minutes. But now that we've covered how to interpret the Supplement Facts labels let's talk about supplements for fat loss, muscle gain and even those that are used for disease prevention. Keep in mind that the choice to take any of these should be thought out and be extremely careful in terms of balancing them with your other healthy lifestyle choices you make. As always, it's a good idea to check with your health professional before adding a supplement to your diet.

Let's start with Fat-Loss Supplements. It seems like nowadays, everyone wants to burn fat the easy way. Every time I open up a fitness magazine, there is an advertisement for a new metabolic booster and some products that are even making their way back to the shelves after being banned in the past for having things like ephedrine, a chemical linked to one death and a slew of serious health problems.

The question is, do any fat-burning supplements actually work and are they safe? And the answer is, actually, yes, some do work, and some are safe. Most of these supplements target fat loss in one of three ways: by increasing the fat you burn for energy, by blocking fat storage in your body, or by controlling your calorie intake by suppressing hunger. However, of all the marketed products, only a few have good research-based evidence. The most common supplement in the fat burning category is probably something you've already had today. It is caffeine. In fact, caffeine is the most popularly consumed drug in the world and is also found in many products like coffee, tea, soda, and even chocolate.

Caffeine is thought to be a weight-loss supplement because it increases resting energy expenditure by 7–15% in some studies. The active compound in caffeine is called *methylxanthine* and acts on the heart muscle, skeletal muscle, and central nervous system as a stimulant. This is why you may get the jitters when you've had that extra cup of joe in the morning. Now, some people need to be careful because the extra stimulation from caffeine can be too much. But, this only needs to really be taken as a precaution if you have a preexisting heart condition or are just extremely sensitive to caffeine. Again, always check with your doctor regarding your own individual health status.

So what is the right balance? Most of the studies show that in order to have a noticeable metabolic increasing effect, roughly 3–6 mg of caffeine per kg of body mass must be consumed at one time. So for example, if you are a 155-pound—or 70kg—person, you would take in 210 to 420 mg of caffeine. This equates to about 1–2 normal sized servings, like 16-20 oz, cups of coffee, depending on the strength of the brew. However, if you don't like drinking that much liquid, there are caffeine tablets available on the market that are pretty cheap and contain about 200mg per pill. Just keep in mind that an excess of pretty much anything you put into your body will likely cause problems and could even be deadly.

You can probably see how this might lead to cost and/or efficiency issues of caffeine. I would recommend, for fat loss, to start with many of the other nutrition and exercise factors I'm discussing with you in the course. Then, if you truly want to try caffeine for fat loss purposes, it could be useful if done properly. So, when should you take caffeine? It is best to take it 30-45 minutes before exercise and/or first thing in the morning before breakfast. For best results, caffeine should be taken on an empty stomach because consuming it with food, especially carbohydrates, diminishes its effects by lowering plasma caffeine concentrations as well as delaying the time to peak caffeine concentration in your blood. So, yes, drinking your coffee with little or no additives like cream, sugar, or milk may be most helpful not to mention lowering your overall calorie intake.

So how does caffeine promote fat loss? Out of a number of potential mechanisms for how caffeine works to promote fat loss, there are two that are thought to work most readily in humans. The first is the inhibition of an enzyme known as *phosphodiesterase* or PDE. In a normal scenario, PDE essentially puts the brakes on fat loss. Caffeine is thought to stop PDE or stop the brakes, which allows fatty acids to be released from fat tissue. Then more energy can be burned from fat for weight loss.

The second mechanism involves the inhibition of a molecule called adenosine. Normally, adenosine will slow or stop the neurotransmitter called norepinephrine. Norepinephrine assists in releasing fat from fat cells and increases energy expenditure to promote weight loss. So by taking caffeine you inhibit adenosine's actions, and norepinephrine can do its work on fat loss.

Now, just because caffeine may increase your ability to get fat out of your fat cells and into your blood—a process called lipolysis—does not mean that you can lose fat and not have to exercise. In order to burn or use the fat that is now in your blood, you have to exercise too. Otherwise, you have a good chance of just circulating the fat around your body and then restoring it, or re-esterifying it as fat. The downside to caffeine is that the effect of caffeine on weight loss is not the same for everyone. It seems that it works best for younger people and for those who are more physically fit. Seems unfair, right?

Also, if you consume lots of caffeine, it is thought that you become less sensitive to its effects on fat loss and performance. Yes, caffeine has been shown to improve exercise performance. However, habitual intake does not affect caffeine concentrations in the blood, and people with more fat mass tend to have higher plasma caffeine concentration than lean individuals. This just means that caffeine stays at an elevated concentration, but it's possible that this could lead to some desensitization where it just takes more and more caffeine to have the same response. A common concern that people have with caffeine is that it will cause dehydration. However, numerous studies have shown that this is a myth and that there is no evidence to support it. Well, why then does it make me urinate more is the common question I get? The answer is probably because you are drinking quite a bit of liquid to get your caffeine intake. More liquid equals more urination.

Another supplement with a potential fat loss effect is green tea. This drink has become increasingly popular in American culture over the past decade with all sorts of products now including green tea or green tea extracts. It has been used in Eastern cultures for much longer to increase mental awareness, improve digestion, and regulate body temperature; in addition to acting as an antioxidant and for its anti-obesity and anti-cancer effects. The active ingredient in green tea is called *epigallocatechin gallate*, commonly known as EGCG.

Essentially, EGCG is thought to block an enzyme called catechol-O-methyltransferase, or COMT that prevents norepinephrine from being degraded and prolongs norepinephrine's thermic action in your body. Remember that norepinephrine's thermogenic effect consists of helping to release fat from fat cells, and to increase energy expenditure.

In some studies, EGCG has been shown to increase energy expenditure by about 4% and increase fat burning by roughly 10% compared to a placebo. Interestingly, when combined with caffeine, which also preserves norepinephrine's thermogenic action, there seems to be a synergistic effect between caffeine and EGCG, which in some studies has been shown to ramp up fat burning more than caffeine or EGCG alone.

But, I wouldn't run off to the supermarket and start buying everything with green tea just yet. In order to have a beneficial effect, the research shows that you need to consume about 750mg per day of EGCG. This is a huge dose. One cup of green tea only has about 50mg of EGCG, which means you would need to drink about 15 cups of green tea per day. But you don't have to turn green drinking all your EGCG. Many EGCG supplements are found in capsulated form with about 400 mg per pill. So, taking two per day would achieve the required amount shown to be effective in research studies. I'll remind you again to check with your doctor about all of this—to make sure that your choices are healthy ones.

Many teas and supplements contain both EGCG and caffeine. But, even drinking decaffeinated green tea may improve body composition. A recent study found that consuming a decaffeinated green tea extract of 571 mg of EGCG/day for 4 weeks, resulted in almost a 2% decrease in body fat and a large 25% increase in fat oxidation during moderate-intensity exercise. Interestingly, the decaf green tea also improved exercise performance in these young men.

While caffeine and EGCG in tea are two of the main fat loss supplements on the market, let's take a look at some others that are easily accessible and have some evidence to back them up. Capsaicin is a spice that causes the perceived hotness that you feel when eating spicy foods. This pungent extract has been shown to increase thermogenesis and energy expenditure by enhancing—you guessed it—norepinephrine release.

The issue with this is that many of these studies have used rats and not humans as research subjects. So you have to be cautious about generalizing these results to humans. The data for humans is less impressive. But, body fat reductions have been reported. The issue is that there is a high rate of weight regain, and the participants had trouble sticking to the dosage that is thought to be required for a beneficial effect.

Another debatable supplement for fat loss is called carnitine. Carnitine is a fat carrier or gatekeeper that helps transfer fat into the mitochondria where it gets oxidized for fuel. Logically, it makes sense that if you increase the amount of carnitine, then you could get more fat into the right place to burn it for energy. Well, unfortunately, that is not the case in 99% of the research on this topic. Until more long-term studies are completed, it doesn't appear to be worth it. Numerous other supplements exist like conjugated linoleic acid or CLA, Chitosan, and yohimbine, and others. However, in research trials with humans, there is not enough evidence, in my opinion, to show any fat loss effect from these supplements that is consistent.

So, for fat loss supplements, only a few have real evidence to support their use. Time and time again, the beneficial effect from these supplements comes when combined with exercise training. Even for the products that have demonstrated the ability to increase thermogenesis and overall calorie burn, it is usually quite small. This just means that if you bank on a supplement to help you lose weight or lose fat without considering your overall nutrition and exercise habits, you are in for a long, expensive, and unsuccessful battle with body composition. In fact, many people feel that when they take fat loss supplements, they can loosen up their good eating patterns because the pill will do the work for them. This couldn't be any further from the truth. In fact, we published research on an ineffective weight loss pill that contained caffeine, green tea, CLA and some amino acids. Turns out that after 8 weeks of taking the pill but not exercising, resulted in no changes in body composition at all.

Now that we have talked about weight loss supplements let's talk about some supplements that are thought to increase your muscle mass. The biggest player here is creatine or creatine monohydrate. Creatine is one the most popular supplements ever produced, and the most thoroughly researched of any supplement.

We produce creatine naturally in the liver and the kidneys. It is stored either as free creatine or bound to a phosphate molecule in skeletal muscle. Naturally, the creatine phosphate energy system is used to provide energy for maximal intensity, short duration exercise. Creatine supplies a phosphate to adenosine-di-phosphate to create Adenosine-tri-phosphate the energy we need to do everything.

As a supplement, creatine is often used build muscle, improve strength and power, and increase anaerobic, short-duration exercise—things like powerlifting or sprinting. The standard serving of creatine is 5 g, which is equal to the amount of creatine of about 2.5 lbs of raw meat. So, needless to say, it is a lot easier to take one tiny scoop of creatine versus eating an entire plate of steak.

There are several forms of creatine on the market, but the one that has the most research support and effectiveness is creatine monohydrate. Several hundred peer-reviewed research studies have evaluated this form, and more than 70% of those studies show a significant improvement in exercise capacity and increases in muscle mass. So let's take a look at some of the research that has been done with creatine to build muscle mass.

In my lab, we had 29 healthy resistance-trained young men consume 21 g of a multi-ingredient performance supplement, which contained creatine, for 6 weeks. During this time, they also lifted weights 3 times per week. The results of this study showed a significant 4.7% increase in muscle mass and a 1.6% average decrease in total fat mass.

The good news is that creatine seems to work in both younger and in older people. In fact, men and women over age 65 who took 5 g of creatine monohydrate per day for 2 weeks and lifted weights 3 times per week, had a significant increase in muscle mass and overall strength. There was an average increase of almost 4 lbs, or 1.8 kg, of muscle mass in the creatine group compared to less than a 1lbs, or 0.45 kg, increase in the placebo group.

Creatine has even been studied in children. One study had 16 young teenage male swimmers compete in two all-out 100% effort 100-meter swims. After supplementation with 20 g per day of creatine monohydrate for 5 days, there was a 2-second improvement in time to complete the two sprints. Almost no time change was reported in the placebo group.

How does creatine help? Most experts attribute the beneficial changes to body composition and performance from creatine to the improved ability to do more quality work during exercise. But, research also shows some improvements to actual cellular processes for muscle gain too.

And due to the repeatable success of creatine use for improving both body composition and performance, creatine is now being studied and used with great interest for clinical populations and in disease prevention.

Creatine has now been shown to improve muscle mass and outcomes in people with muscular dystrophy, leukemia, traumatic brain injury, and infants born with errors of normal metabolic function. It is amazing how this traditional sports supplement is now being used for neuromuscular and neurological conditions. Creatine doses that are similar to what we've discussed have been documented to enter your central nervous system and influence brain concentrations of creatine phosphate after both 7 and 28 days of supplementation. Because creatine enters your brain, it has some evidence to support a positive effects in cases of traumatic brain injury and even some evidence for stroke patients to improve brain function.

In addition, patients with muscular dystrophy are now shown to benefit from creatine supplementation improve nerve function, muscle mass, muscle strength, and power. Even in traditional cases of sarcopenia, or the age-related loss in muscle mass, including creatine and resistance training is shown to increase muscle mass and decrease fat mass.

Now, a common myth is that creatine is a steroid and will damage your kidneys. Creatine is not a steroid; it is simply the combination of three amino acids. The research shows creatine is safe and effective among young and old, male and female, and healthy and diseased populations. In the absence of any pre-existing conditions like kidney disease, creatine is a supplement that has consistently shown to be beneficial.

The most common side effect reported is weight gain. However, this is probably the type that you want, because creatine increases muscle mass. Remember, it is more about body composition that body weight. Also, note that some cases of gastrointestinal upset have also been noted in the literature. The most common dose is 5 g per day about 1 tbsp.

Research shows that creatine builds and preserves muscle mass, so it may be an ideal supplement across the lifespan stages, and not just for the young people trying to put on muscle. Because so many people lose muscle as they age, it might also be a good idea to use creatine to try and prevent some of the muscle loss. It is something that I recommend to my parents and my family.

Another supplement that may help with muscle mass and performance is called beta-alanine. It has been shown to improve performance and exercise capacity as well as to permit greater intensity and volume of exercise training. Sounds pretty good, right? So how does it work? Essentially, beta-alanine, which is an amino acid made in the liver, combines with another amino acid called *histidine* to form a new protein molecule called *carnosine* in the muscle. Carnosine then acts to buffer or soak up the acidity or hydrogen ions that are created during very difficult exercise.

When accumulated, hydrogen ions cause muscle pain and fatigue, so if the hydrogen ions are controlled, theoretically, you could exercise longer and at a higher intensity. You see how once again higher intensity exercise for longer should help to improve body composition. For example, one study had men take 3.2 g per day of beta-alanine with 10.5 g per day of creatine, or 10.5 g per day of creatine only, or 10.5 g per day of dextrose—a sugar placebo—for 10 weeks during a resistance training program. It was found that the beta-alanine plus creatine group had the greatest improvement in muscle mass and the largest decrease in fat mass over the course of the study.

Other research has tested 4 g of beta-alanine per day compared to a placebo for 8 weeks during a high-intensity, interval sprinting, and resistance training program in young men. The results showed that despite both groups losing weight, the composition of the weight was different. On average, the group taking beta-alanine gained more muscle mass. Other studies are beginning to pile up too—many that support the use of beta-alanine to increase performance and body composition in both men and women.

So, how much do you need to be effective? About 3–6 g per day for 4 weeks can increase intramuscular carnosine and improve performance. Typically, this dose should be split up throughout the day for best results, for example, taking 1.5 g 3 times per day.

One side effect to note is that beta-alanine is often associated with a tingling feeling or numbness in your extremities that's called paresthesia. This, sometimes, is temporary but annoying. And not all people have this feeling, but it is reported in many of the research studies. As a result, some companies have made extended-release capsules to allow a slow release of beta-alanine. This slow release can help reduce or diminish any of the paresthesia effects.

My lab has completed two small pilot studies with the use of beta-alanine in both Parkinson's and Multiple Sclerosis patients to see if it improved their physical function. That data is still being analyzed but in a short 4-week study, performance was not improved any more than a placebo. So once again, while there is cross-over from sports science to diseased populations, much more work will be needed just to see what products will work for each condition. It is a very exciting time to be in this field for sure. With all this being said, it seems that beta-alanine improves performance by being converted to carnosine, but more work is underway to pinpoint exactly how beta-alanine improves performance.

Other great muscle building or muscle maintenance supplements exist including amino acids like leucine and whole proteins that we discussed earlier. Another supplement called HMB that stands for beta-hydroxy-beta-methylbutyrate also shows some promise to help build muscle strength, and particularly in non-athletes—but more research is needed.

So, some supplements like caffeine, EGCG, creatine, and beta-alanine, have been studied repeatedly over the years in many different populations. They have been shown to be effective in many different types of exercise modalities, too.

What is really cool is that these traditional sports performance supplements are crossing over into the clinical world and being used to assist with improving or preventing chronic diseases. The most prevalent examples to date include creatine for neurological disorders to improve nerve function and muscle strength. In an ideal world, I could put things simply and say, these supplements I've discussed will work for you. But, this area, along with the entire field of sports nutrition, is not so clear cut. There are a lot of gray areas. With supplementation, individual factors such as training status, sex, age, and performance goals, all play a large role in the efficacy of these products. So, my recommendation is that you focus first on high-quality nutrition and exercise quality as a whole as the best strategy for improving your lifestyle and attaining your initial goals.

Remember, most of you take supplements already. They are in most of the common packaged foods that you eat or beverages that you drink. But, sports supplements are a bit different, and it is important to understand that supplements are intended to be added to a nutritious diet and not replace the foods that we eat. So, try this: Try adding 5 g per day of creatine monohydrate to your daily routine and see how you feel.

Energy Balance and Weight Control

This lecture will cover the topic of energy balance and weight control. You will learn about the major components of food and exercise that might shift your energy balance to favor weight loss or weight gain. The point is to expand your understanding of how energy balance contributes to changes in body composition and health. You will also learn what situations impact your calorie burn and the common ways that you might easily fall into a positive energy balance without even knowing it.

Food Intake and Energy Expenditure

- Most people don't track food intake or bother to read labels or weigh food items. This might not be a practical way to live your life, but it can be useful for some people, even if you just periodically check your calorie intake to keep yourself on track.

- Knowing the relationship between your food intake and energy expenditure can be extremely helpful for figuring out if you will lose weight, maintain weight, or gain weight. The quality of your food choices makes a big difference in weight loss and weight gain goals, but at some point, knowing your routine calorie intake and expenditure is a good idea, too, and often a great place to start if you want to be more active in managing your body composition.

- Many of our official dietary recommendations are based on the calorie content of foods. While this intention was good, it puts certain high-calorie but nutrient-dense foods like nuts, seeds, and eggs into a high-caution list, simply because the calorie content is high.

- We know now that these foods are actually beneficial for weight loss and prevention of weight gain when added to the diet. But when considering only the calorie content, they mistakenly seem like a bad choice.

Even more interesting is that foods like whole eggs are often considered in the same category of "eat sparingly" as cookies and cakes. But eggs and cookies/cake have very different impacts physiologically.

Nevertheless, even if certain foods might be associated with weight loss or gain, calories ultimately do matter, to some extent, in your weight-management success.

The energy balance equation is used with regard to body weight control. Energy balance simply means that the energy that you expend from normal daily energy needs (such as breathing, staying awake, digestion and absorption, and physical activity) or extra activity (such as exercise) is matched or balanced by the energy that you take in from foods and beverages.

There are three basic conditions to be aware of with the energy balance equation: energy balance, where the food calories that you take in match the calories that you expend or burn; positive energy balance, where you eat more calories than expended (or more in than out); and negative energy balance, where more energy is expended than consumed (or more out than in).

Theoretically, if you are in energy balance, you will not lose or gain any weight. In a positive energy balance, you will gain weight. In a negative energy balance, you will lose weight.

Regardless of whether you're in a positive or negative energy balance, there are numerous changes that occur to your body—cellularly, metabolically, and hormonally—to facilitate weight gain or loss.

When we think about energy balance, we need to pay attention to how many calories we need to eat and drink to begin losing weight (or perhaps gaining weight). This is not considering the quality of calories, though.

Energy In

How many calories do you need to cut from your diet, or what deficit do you need to create, to lose weight? How many calories will it take to lose just one pound?

For years, textbooks and experts have asserted that one pound of fat is equivalent to 3,500 calories. So, if you aim for a reduction in one pound of fat per week by modifying your diet alone (not considering exercise), then you would simply eat 500 fewer calories per day for one week.

If you eat 500 fewer calories per day and lose one pound per week, why not up this to a reduction of 1,000 calories per day or more from your typical diet and lose 2 or 3 pounds per week? The "more is better" mantra does not always suit us well with diet or exercise.

If your energy deficit is more than about 1,000 calories per day, it is generally not well tolerated. This is due to many factors, but primarily when you drop your calories by too much, you will also lose muscle—which you do not want.

Too great a calorie deficit also runs a greater risk of missing out on key nutrients, such as vitamins and minerals, and you would likely see your energy levels drop and your fatigue increase—not to mention, you'll probably feel hungry.

One myth that has come about from this 3,500-calorie rule is that weight will simply continue to drop at the same rate—otherwise known as a linear model of weight loss. But it turns out that this rule actually greatly overestimates weight loss, meaning that 3,500 calories might translate to less than one pound of weight loss.

So, an update was made, and the new model for weight loss is called the thermodynamic model, or simply the dynamic model, of weight loss and takes into consideration your baseline body composition, age, height, sex, and degree of calorie restriction. This results in a curvilinear pattern of weight loss over time rather than the traditional linear model of weight loss and is much more accurate in actual trends for weight loss.

Counting Calories

Food contains energy that has the potential to be converted into useful work once metabolized, or broken down, by your body. That energy is measured in units called calories. So, what is a calorie, and how do we know how many calories are in each food we choose to eat?

Technically, a calorie is a unit of heat measurement defined as the amount of energy required to raise the temperature of one kilogram of water by one degree Celsius. By using this definition, you are actually describing a kilocalorie, which is the type of calorie that you see on nutrient labels.

In reality, calories are sort of made up. You don't really eat calories; you eat different kinds of food with different amounts of nutrients in them. However, we give foods a calorie count by burning them in a bomb calorimeter and measuring how much heat is given off.

Each gram of carbohydrate equals 4 calories. A gram of protein also equals 4 calories, and a gram of fat equals 9 calories. When you burn 1 gram of carbohydrate, 4.18 calories are released. When you burn 1 gram of protein, 5.65 calories are released, and when you burn 1 gram of fat, 9.44 calories are released.

These numbers can vary by the type of carbohydrate, protein, and fat that you burn, as well. And these numbers are slightly different than the 4, 4, 9 that are commonly taught in nutrition and exercise science classes.

This is because the digestion and absorption rates of nutrients are less than 100 percent in most foods. This results in a reduced energy intake than when measured by direct calorimetry in a bomb calorimeter.

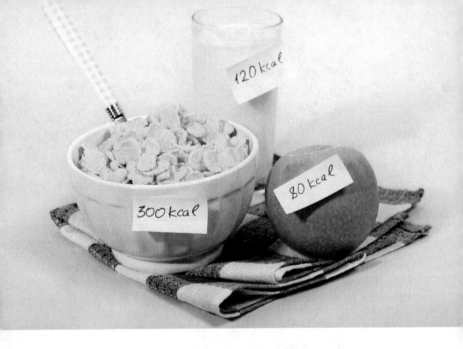

Many factors impact how many calories you actually can use in your body. Some of these might be how the food is grown, such as the soil conditions, what the animal's diet contained, and how ripe the food was when harvested. Even how you cook or prepare the meal makes a difference.

In general, the macronutrient with the highest coefficient of digestibility is carbohydrates at 97 percent, followed by fats at 95 percent and proteins at 92 percent. There can also be variation within a food category.

So, the process of determining the calories in foods is probably more extensive than you imagined. It might also be a shock to see how inexact the process is. In fact, the calories listed on food labels are really just approximations because the data from the bomb calorimeter has a degree of variability.

Energy Out

Just as we can measure the calories contained in certain foods, we have ways to scientifically measure the energy that you expend each day. Direct calorimetry is the most accurate way to measure your energy expenditure, but it is very expensive and highly impractical. You don't actually go into a bomb calorimeter and ignite, but the process is similar in many ways.

Indirect calorimetry, which measures within ± 1 percent of the direct method, is more often used in lab settings. Indirect calorimetry measures your breath—specifically the oxygen that you use and the carbon dioxide that you exhale.

On average, about 5 calories are burned for every 1 liter of oxygen that you consume. Using this fact as well as indirect calorimetry, we can calculate how many calories you are burning and from which macronutrient.

This is done by determining the respiratory exchange ratio, which is calculated by dividing the amount of carbon dioxide produced or exhaled by the amount of oxygen that you consume or inhale. Values range between 0.7 and 1. Even though things like hyperventilation or excessive acid buffering in the cells can skew this ratio a bit, it does give an excellent estimation of fuel use.

By understanding how much of what type of fuel you are burning for energy, you have a good idea of energy expenditure, which you need with your calorie intake to calculate your overall energy balance and primary nutrient needs for your lifestyle. Even better, you will also have a huge advantage from knowing how the foods you eat impact this balance and, ultimately, why and how eating and exercising contribute to your body composition.

There are also many very good metabolic equations—such as Harris-Benedict equation and the Cunningham equation—that have been developed to estimate energy expenditure. These equations are based on many things, such as age, gender, height, weight, and daily activity levels. These formulas are an excellent place to start and give a practical estimate when used properly.

It is important to remember that these equations are only estimations. Metabolism is constantly changing based on the needs of the individual, so it is important to reevaluate a person's nutrition plan based on performance, body weight, and body composition over time.

Total Daily Energy Expenditure

Four components contribute to your total daily energy expenditure, or all of the calories that you burn in a day.

- Resting metabolic rate, which is the energy required to maintain the systems of your body at rest.
- Thermic effect of food, which is the amount of energy required to digest the food you eat.
- Thermic effect of activity, which is the energy expended doing active things, such as working around the house or doing structured exercise.
- Non-exercise activity thermogenesis, which includes unplanned activity, such as tapping your feet or bouncing your knees.

Of the components of our total daily energy expenditure, by far the largest is your resting metabolic rate. About 60 to 80 percent of the oxygen you consume and calories you burn goes to just keeping you alive at rest.

Many factors influence resting metabolic rate, including age, sex, genetics, energy intake (whether fasting or fed), body size, lean body mass, body temperature or climate, caffeine or nicotine consumption, and exercise. Obviously, there are some uncontrollable characteristics that play a part in determining it.

Huge meals with high calorie counts have a larger thermic effect of food. Protein-rich foods also have the greatest effect on increasing calorie burn, because they are the most difficult to digest and absorb— which is one reason that added protein in the diet can be helpful for body composition.

The amount of exercise and activity you do will determine how much of a role the thermic effect of activity and non-exercise activity thermogenesis play into your overall energy expenditure.

Try This

Calculate your resting metabolic rate to have an idea about your daily caloric needs.

Questions to Consider

1. What sources of carbohydrate in your diet would be best for optimizing your body composition?

2. How much added sugar do you think you consume in your typical daily diet?

Energy Balance and Weight Control

We need to eat. For a whole ton of reasons, we need to eat food. Carbohydrates, fats, and proteins all end up supplying us with ATP we need to drive metabolic reactions, physical movement, and everything in between. In this lecture, we will cover the topic of energy balance and weight control. Ultimately, these concepts are often tangled up and made much more complicated than they really need to be.

We've already touched upon the energy balance equation with regard to body weight control. Energy balance is simply meaning that the energy that you expend from normal daily energy needs like breathing, staying awake, digestion and absorption, and physical activity or extra activity like exercise is matched or balanced to the energy that you take in from foods and beverages. If you are really in energy balance, you will not lose or gain any body weight. Well this equation is currently being challenged by research— for example, is it just the number of calories that matter? Or is it really the type or quality of those calories that matters most?

Well, calorie quality does matter a lot—you know that eating 500 calories from Potato Chips is different from eating 500 calories from Spinach. But we need to consider energy balance too. Constantly under-eating will lead to weight loss, and constantly overeating will lead to weight gain. So it's absolutely critical to understand the impact of both the quality of the calories and the quantity of calories on your body's body composition and health. This is why the calories count is often highlighted in large font on new food labels. Think about how many companies clearly label their products as low calorie or zero calorie foods.

In this lecture, we will cover the major components of food and exercise that may shift your energy balance to favor weight loss or weight gain. The point is to expand your understanding of how energy balance contributes to changes in body composition and health.

Most people don't track food intake or bother to read labels or weigh food items. And I'm not suggesting that this is a practical way to live your life. But it can be useful for some people even if you just periodically check your calorie intake to keep yourself honest.

Knowing the relationship between your food intake and your energy expenditure can be extremely helpful for figuring out if you will lose weight, maintain weight, or gain weight. We know that quality of your food choices makes a big difference in weight loss and weight gain goals, but at some point, knowing your routine calorie intake and energy expenditure is simply a good idea too, and often a great place to start if you want to be more active in managing your body composition.

It is important to recognize that many of our official dietary recommendations are based upon the calorie content of foods. While this intention was good, it puts certain high-calorie foods but nutrient dense foods like nuts, seeds, and eggs into a high-caution list simply because the calorie content is high. We know now that these foods are actually beneficial for weight loss and prevention of weight gain when added to the diet. But when considering only the calorie content, they mistakenly seem like a bad choice. Even more interesting is that foods like whole eggs are in often considered in the same category of eat sparingly as cookies and cakes. But as we've discussed, eggs on the one hand and cookies and cake on the other have very different impacts physiologically.

Nevertheless, even if certain foods may be associated with weight loss or gain, calories ultimately do matter, to some extent, in your weight management success. And the energy balance equation is a great place to start this lecture.

There are three basic conditions to be aware of with the energy balance equation. They are energy balance, where the food calories that you take in match the calories that you expend or burn. Positive energy balance, where you eat more calories than expended or more coming in than going out, and lastly, negative energy balance where more energy is expended than you take in. Theoretically, if you are in energy balance, you will not lose or gain any weight. In a positive energy balance, you will gain weight. In a negative energy balance, you will lose weight.

Either way, be it positive or negative energy balance, there are numerous changes that occur to your body—cellularly, metabolically, and hormonally—to facilitate weight gain or loss. Take, for example, extreme weight loss where morbidly obese people defined as those with a body mass index, or weight to height ratio above 40, or having over 100 excess lbs of fat are placed on medically supervised diets as an alternative to gastric bypass surgery. This could be a woman who is 5 feet tall and weighs 205 lbs or more.

When put on very-low-calorie, medically-monitored diets of 800 calories per day—which believe it or not is the common medical treatment at bariatric centers in the U.S.—these people lost a massive amount of weight. On average, about 40 lbs, or 18 kg, or more is lost in about a 12-week treatment period. But here is the problem. That weight loss is not only coming from fat. In this example, the 40-lbs, or 18 kg, weight loss is usually about 75% fat and about 25% muscle. That 25% loss of muscle mass is not desirable, and for this reason, new research, including my own, seeks ways to modify these medically supervised, very low-calorie diets to get the most weight loss from fat while keeping as much muscle as possible.

Now, keep in mind that an 800-calorie diet is not for the typical person and is not recommended. This is a drastically low dietary intake that is only recommended under medical supervision. For our purposes, keep in mind that there are likely several effective dietary strategies to improve weight loss without sacrificing muscle. For example, regular exercise and some specific dietary habits like increase protein intake are usually necessary. Regardless, when we think about energy balance we need to pay attention to how many calories we need to eat and drink to begin losing weight or perhaps gaining weight and the patterns may surprise you. This is not considering the quality of calories, though. We also will take a deeper look at what other situations impact your calorie burn and the common ways that we may easily fall into a positive energy balance without even knowing it.

Let's start with a very simple question and probably one of the first when you feel you've got a positive energy balance, or more energy coming in that is being expended. How many calories do I need to cut from my diet or what deficit do I need to create in order to lose weight? And, let's take it one more step, how many calories will it take to lose just one lbs?

For years, textbooks and experts have asserted that one lbs of fat is equivalent to 3,500 calories. So, if you aim for a reduction in one lbs of fat per week by modifying your diet alone and not considering exercise, then you would simply eat 500 less calories per day for one week. Now, that's actually pretty easy to wrap your mind around, just skip a daily dessert or an extra serving at dinner.

You might say, well if I eat 500 calories less per day and lose 1 lbs per week, why not up this to a reduction of 1000 calories per day or more from my typical diet and lose 2–3 lbs per week? Well, the more is better mantra does not always suit us well with diet and with exercise. Just recall the example about weight loss coming from both fat and muscle. It turns out that if your energy deficit is over about 1000 calories per day, it is generally not well tolerated. This is due to many factors, but primarily when you drop your calories by too much, you will also lose muscle—which you do not want.

Too great a calorie deficit also runs a greater risk of missing out on key nutrients, like your vitamins and minerals, and you would likely see your energy levels drop and your fatigue increase. Not to mention, you'll probably feel hungry. One myth that has come about from this 3500 calorie rule is that weight will simply continue to drop at the same rate, otherwise known as the linear model of weight loss.

Well, in a very nice article in the *International Journal of Obesity*, the authors studied the 3500-calorie rule to see how it lined up with actual weight loss. It turns out that the 3500 calorie rule actually way overestimates weight loss, meaning, that 3500 calories may translate to less than 1 lbs of weight loss.

So an update was made. And the new model for weight loss is called the thermodynamic model or simply the dynamic model of weight loss, and it takes into consideration your baseline body composition, age, height, sex, and degree of calorie restriction. This results in a curvilinear pattern of weight loss over time rather than the traditional linear model of weight loss and is much more accurate in actual trends for weight loss. In simple terms, the 3500 calorie rule over-predicts weight loss, and the new dynamic model gives a more realistic number for any weight loss expectations. Luckily, the authors of this research paper have also provided a nice downloadable weight change predictor that is found online. At this point, it is clear that you first want to figure out how much energy, or how many calories, you should take in to maintain or manipulate your own energy balance equation.

You know that food contains energy that has the potential to be converted into useful work once metabolized or broken down by your body. That energy is measured in units called calories. So, what is a calorie and how do we know how many calories are in each food that we choose to eat? Well, the calorie discussion can be confusing. Technically, a calorie is a unit of heat measurement defined like this: The amount of energy required to raise the temperature of one kg of water by 1°C.

Something that many people don't know is that by using this definition, you are actually describing what is also called a kilocalorie or kcal. This is the typical calorie that that you see on Nutrient Fact labels. And, in reality, calories are sort of made up. You don't really eat calories; you eat different kinds of food with different amounts of nutrients in them. But, we give foods a calorie count by burning them in something called a bomb calorimeter and measuring how much heat is given off. Scientists put food into this machine, and then they ignite the food. As heat is given off, it heats up the chamber that the food is in. The air leaves the chamber and flows through water that surrounds the chamber. Scientists then measure the change in water temperature, and from that change in temperature, calculate how many calories were in the food.

You have learned that each g of carbohydrate equals 4 calories; a g of protein also equals 4 calories, and a g of fat is 9 calories. You may be wondering how the 4, 4, 9 calorie count for each g of carbohydrate, protein, and fat that you eat is calculated. Well, actually, when you burn 1 g of carbohydrate

4.18 calories are released. When you burn 1 g of protein, 5.65 calories are released, and when you burn 1 g of fat, 9.44 calories are released. And we can't forget alcohol, which releases 7.09 calories when combusted.

These numbers can vary by the type of carbohydrate, protein, and fat that you burn as well. And, what is interesting is that these numbers are slightly different than the 4, 4, 9 that are commonly taught in nutrition and exercise science classes. This is because the digestion and absorption rates of nutrients are less than 100% in most foods. This results in a reduced energy intake than when measured it directly in a bomb calorimeter.

Another way of looking at this is as gross energy versus net energy. The gross energy value is assigned to a food after being burned in a bomb calorimeter. The net energy value takes into account something called the coefficient of digestibility, or the percent of the ingested food that actually makes it through the gut and into your bloodstream.

For example, dietary fiber reduces the percent of the food that is useable by the body for energy production. Which makes sense, because we often hear of fiber as a nutrient that promotes regularity or regular bowel movements.

It turns out that many factors impact how many calories you actually can use in your body. Some of these might be how the food is grown—like the soil conditions, what the animal's diet contained, how ripe the food was when harvested—even how you cook and prepare the meal makes a difference. In general, the macronutrient with the highest coefficient of digestibility is carbohydrates at 97%, followed by fats at 95%, and finally proteins at 92%. An interesting note is that there can also be variation even within a food category.

So, as you can see, the process of determining the calories in foods is probably more extensive than you imagined. It may also be a shock to see how inexact the process is. In fact, the calories listed on food labels are really just approximations because you can be sure that the data from the bomb calorimeter has a degree of variability—I mean getting accurate combustion numbers on all the different foods and food combinations available is never going to happen. So, we take the best estimate. So, after accounting for the absorption of the nutrients, 1 g of carbohydrate and protein provide 4 calories each; 1 g of fat provides 9 calories, and 1 g of alcohol provides 7 calories.

But, you have to still keep in mind that research has estimated an error of up to 25% may be seen in the typical nutrition databases that you might use to calculate your calorie intake. We just don't know how each individual will respond to the food and how much energy it will take to digest, absorb, transport, and ultimately excrete these foods. So, now you can probably see how calculating calories might give you a snapshot of the 'Energy In' part of the energy balance equation, but there are still some kinks in the system. It does give you an idea of how things change over time, and I think it is useful to check in with your total calorie intake to keep those things honest. But again, consider the quality of the foods you eat and not simply the quantity. In many cases, you can eat a lot more quality food and still maintain or lose weight by focusing on the quality instead of simply the quantity of food that you eat.

All right—we've discussed the energy in, the calorie counting part of the energy balance equation. Now, what about the energy out or energy expenditure portion of the energy balance equation? I'm sure you are aware of the main things that you do each day that require you to use energy and burn calories. But, do you know how to actually measure or quantify how much energy you expend in a typical day? Well, just like you saw with measuring the calories contained in certain foods, we have ways to scientifically measure the energy that you expend each day.

Direct calorimetry is the most accurate way to measure your energy expenditure, but it is very expensive and highly impractical. This method is usually reserved for people who volunteer as research participants in large-scale clinical exercise and nutrition research studies. For the sake of clarity, you don't actually go into a bomb calorimeter and ignite. I'll describe how this method works for humans. It is actually quite similar in many ways, though.

For direct calorimetry, you are housed in a well-insulated chamber called a metabolic chamber that is surrounded by a known amount of water for a set amount of time. Let's choose 24 hours for this example. Once you enter the chamber, you would not leave it for the entire 24 hours. As you know, you are always producing heat to some extent. The heat that you give off in the metabolic chamber—from your basic metabolic requirements—will dissipate into the room and heat up the environment of the chamber you are in.

Just think about a time when you've been in a small room with lots of people. The room gets warm quickly and if there is no airflow especially. Well, the change in the temperature of the insulated chamber will ultimately change the temperature of the known volume of water that surrounds that chamber. Then, the change in temperature of the water is used to calculate energy expenditure or the calories that are burned. However, due to the impracticality and expensiveness of direct calorimetry, indirect calorimetry is more often used in lab settings.

Indirect calorimetry measures within ± 1% of the direct method and does not require a special chamber. Indirect calorimetry measures your breath—specifically the oxygen that you use and the carbon dioxide that you exhale.

How does this work? Recall that during metabolism oxygen is used and carbon dioxide is produced. Oxygen is needed to produce ATP during rest and during slow-to-moderate intensity exercise. At the same time, as you break down stored fuels in your body for energy, you produce a lot of carbon dioxide. And, carbohydrates, fats, and protein all have different amounts of oxygen that is needed to fully break them down for energy, meaning that different amounts of carbon dioxide and oxygen in your breath can indicate the type of fuel that you are burning.

On average, about 5 calories are burned for every 1 liter of oxygen that you consume. So putting this all together, we actually know how many calories you are burning and from which macronutrient. This is done by calculating what is called the respiratory exchange ratio, which is calculated by dividing the amount of carbon dioxide produced or exhaled, by the amount of oxygen that you consume or inhale. Values range between 0.7 and 1.0. Even though things like hyperventilation or excessive acid buffering in the cells can skew this ratio a bit, it does give an excellent estimation of fuel use.

For example, if you are burning mostly carbohydrates, your RER would be 1.0—top of the range. An RER of 1.0 is equivalent to about 5 calories per liter of oxygen that you consume. This would occur while exercising very hard. Now, if you are burning mostly fat, your RER would be lower at 0.7, which is equivalent to about 4.7 calories per liter oxygen consumed. This would occur while resting and while lying around.

But most people tend to eat a mix of fuels from carbohydrates, proteins, and fats—and as a result, people don't usually burn just carbohydrates or just fats. So the RER for this scenario would be right in the middle of 0.7 and 1.0 with a value of about 0.85 or 4.86 calories per liter of Oxygen indicating that you have a mixed use of fuels. Because protein is not used nearly as much as carbohydrates and fats for energy production, it is not pinpointed on the RER scale. We can also calculate exactly how much fat or carbohydrate you oxidize using standard scientific equations.

All right, so, what does this mean for you? Well, by understanding how much of what type of fuel you are burning for energy, you have a good idea of energy expenditure—which you need with your calorie intake in order to calculate your overall energy balance, and primary nutrient needs for your lifestyle. Even better, you will also have a huge advantage from knowing how the foods you eat impact this balance and ultimately, why and how eating and exercising contribute to your body composition.

Knowing that the average woman weighs 156 lbs, or 71 kg, let's use that an example now to calculate her energy expenditure using indirect calorimetry. Well, at rest, about 3.5 ml of oxygen are consumed per minute. So, to learn how much oxygen she uses every hour, we multiply 3.5 ml times 60 minutes. She uses 210 ml of oxygen per hour. Then we multiply her oxygen use by her weight in kg, which is 71kg. So, 210 ml times 71 kg, equals about 15,000 ml or 15 liters of oxygen per hour. Then, multiplying this out over 24 hours, our subject consumes 360 liters of oxygen per day. Knowing this, we can multiply her daily oxygen intake—360 l—by 4.86 calories, the number of calories burned from a typical mixed diet of carbohydrates, proteins, and fats. We come up with an indirect calorimetric energy expenditure of roughly 1,750 calories burned per day just at rest.

Now—this 1750 calories doesn't include the energy this woman would need to digest food, walk around or exercise. So you can see that she would want to eat above 1,750 calories to account for these other daily activities to stay in energy balance. Most Universities will offer this type of service if you're interested in an evaluation for yourself. They can give you some detailed numbers to understand exactly what your resting metabolic rate is.

Luckily for us, there are also many very good predictive equations that have been developed to estimate energy expenditure. These equations are based upon many things like age, sex, height, and weight and daily activity levels. These formulas are an excellent place to start to give a practical estimate when used properly. Some commonly used metabolic equations include the Harris-Benedict equation and the Cunningham equation. The Harris-Benedict Equation differentiates between males and females and uses height, weight, and age to evaluate metabolic rate. What I like about the Cunningham equation is that it also takes into account your lean body mass.

These are just two of many predictive equation possibilities. When these equations are used, the value given indicates the person's resting metabolic rate—when he or she is not doing any exercise, for example. So, the resting value then needs to be multiplied by an activity factor to get the actual daily needs that account for exercise and activity patterns that you normally take part in.

Activity factors range from about 1.2 to 2.0. For example, you would multiply by about 1.3 for sedentary people or those just doing light activity. You would multiply by about 1.7 for people who exercise daily at a moderate to high intensity. And you would multiply by 2.0 or more for very hard exercise training and people who work out more than once per day to estimate actual calorie needs. So the coefficient is larger for those who do more exercise, which makes sense. It is important to remember that these equations are only estimations. Metabolism is constantly changing based upon needs of the individual, so it is important to re-evaluate a person's nutrition plan based on performance, body weight, and body composition over time.

So, now that you know about how we calculate energy expenditure, or the calories used, for rest and activity, we need to consider how this fits into the energy balance equation. Remember that energy balance is where the food calories that you take in match the calories that you expend or burn. So the next step is to consider and evaluate all of the major components of what makes up your total daily energy expenditure or all of the calories that you burn in a day.

Well, earlier I mentioned that total daily energy expenditure is made up of three components. However, in this lecture, we'll talk about four components that contribute to your total energy expenditure. These are your resting metabolic rate; your thermic effect of food, which is the amount of energy required to digest the food you eat; your thermic effect of activity, which is the energy expended doing active things like working around the house or doing structured exercise. And four would be your non-exercise activity thermogenesis or NEAT which includes unplanned activity like tapping your feet or bouncing your knees.

Of the components of our total daily energy expenditure, by far the largest one that I mentioned is your resting metabolic rate. Resting metabolic rate is defined as the energy required to maintain the systems of your body at rest. About 60 to 80% of the oxygen you consume and the calories you burn goes to just keeping you alive at rest. For very active people, resting metabolic rate may make up less of your total energy expenditure as a percentage because physical activity likely makes up a much larger portion of total energy use in your day. Many factors influence resting metabolic rate, including age, sex, genetics, energy intake whether fasted or fed, body size, lean body mass, body temperature, the climate that you're in, caffeine or nicotine consumption, and exercise. Clearly there are some uncontrollable characteristics that play a part in determining it.

The second component of total daily energy expenditure I mentioned is the thermic effect of food, which is defined as the energy required to digest, absorb, transport, metabolize and store you food. Huge meals with high-calorie counts have a larger TEF. We also know that protein-rich foods also have the greatest effect on increasing calorie burn as they are the most difficult to digest and absorb—which is one reason added protein in the diet can be helpful for body composition.

And finally, the last components of your total daily energy expenditure are the thermic effect of activity and non-exercise activity thermogenesis, or NEAT. These include the energy cost of daily activities including planned exercise, walking to work, or taking the stairs and involuntary muscular activities like knee bouncing, toe tapping, or fidgeting. Obviously, the amount of exercise and activity you do will determine how much of a role TEA or NEAT plays into your overall energy expenditure. For most people who do not exercise much at all, then TEA might make up 10–15% of your total daily energy expenditure. But if you are really exercising a lot then this could be upwards of 30%. Seems like reason enough to try and fit exercise into your day, right?

You've probably also heard that exercise will increase your metabolism. Well, it definitely will increase oxygen consumption, and it can do so for a few hours up to a few days after you finish exercising if done properly. Interestingly, if you exercise regularly for a few weeks or years and then stop for some reason for an extended period of time, your resting metabolism can also decrease. We have even shown that after collegiate swimmers stopped swimming for 5 weeks, they had a significant 7% decrease in Resting Metabolic Rate. So, it is important to maintain your great exercise habits for life.

Now that you understand the energy balance equation, I'm sure you can identify one or two habits in your lifestyle that you can modify to improve one of the aspects of your energy balance. In fact, energy imbalances like eating even just slightly more calories than you expend can translate to significant weight gain over time. Usually, this is how weight gain sneaks up on us, and it's just not noticeable when the weight gain is 5 lbs over the course of an entire year. But in 5 years, this is 25 lbs of extra weight—which I'm sure you will notice.

It is also important to understand that your body will typically fight to be in energy balance and will make adjustments without you even knowing it. This is why weight gain and weight loss typically stall or plateau over time.

I want you to understand that that while individual foods definitely impact our metabolism, weight, and body composition, the bigger picture includes an overhaul of the energy balance equation including food quality and food quantity and the exercises that we choose to take part in. The good news is that most often when you choose to eat higher quality foods, the food quantity piece of the energy balance tends to regulate itself.

Try This: Calculate your resting metabolic rate to have an idea of about how many calories you burn daily.

The Caloric Cost of Exercise

This lecture will take a closer look at the ways we can expend energy and how we might use that information in our efforts to strengthen or alter our body composition. There are many different types of exercise that can help you reach your goals—from small adjustments, such as taking the stairs at work, walking around more, and perhaps getting a standup desk if you have a desk job, to full-blown structured exercise plans. As you will learn, the body needs a combination of proper fueling and exercise to optimize its potential.

The Caloric Cost of Exercise

- If you want to manipulate your body composition, it is important to know the quality of your calories, how many calories you are eating and drinking, and how many calories you are expending.

- Various types of exercises demand varying amounts of energy—walking versus running, for example—and these energy demands are measured scientifically through metabolic testing, which measures the amount of oxygen you take in during an activity. The more strenuous or intense the activity is, the greater the oxygen consumption.

- We have all kinds of technology that estimate calories burned, but not long ago, the caloric cost of exercise was traditionally measured in metabolic equivalents (mets). You might have seen the term "mets" on the exercise equipment in your home or at the local gym. It is simply another way to assess or quantify the intensity level of your exercise.

- One metabolic equivalent is equal to the oxygen consumption of your body at rest, or 3.5 milliliters per kilogram of body weight per minute. When measuring mets, everything is compared to the cost of energy at rest. The more strenuous the exercise, the higher the met value will be—that is, the higher the caloric expenditure will be in relation to resting.

Using mets as a measure of your exercise intensity might seem strange, but if you are trying to determine the number of calories you burn when you are exercising—in other words, your caloric cost of exercise—then a great estimate is to simply multiply the met value by your body weight in kilograms.

Calories are essential; don't treat them as the enemy. Food is fuel. Fuel your body properly for optimal body composition and performance in any aspect of your life—mental or physical.

For most of us, our main energy source during exercise comes in the form of muscle glycogen. Your body has plenty of fuel to perform most forms of exercise—generally about two hours of moderate- to high-intensity exercise.

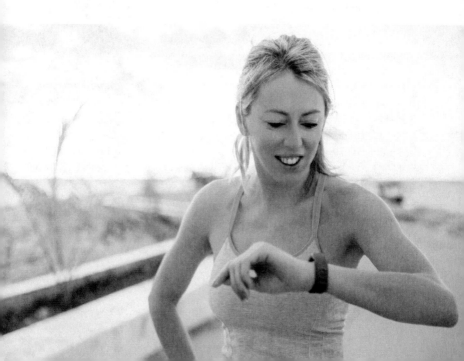

But sometimes we do run out, which is part of the reason you see athletes collapse from time to time. Their bodies have run out of the ability to access and utilize fuel. They might have the mental fortitude to continue, but the body's systems begin to shut down.

The body is remarkable at properly operating all of its intricate systems most of the time—from muscles to enzymes to atoms—in complete unison. But it requires good-quality fuel.

Exercise and Your Metabolism

Exercise increases your caloric expenditure above resting levels, or your resting metabolic rate (RMR), based on how long and intensely you exercise. But does this increase in metabolism last after you finish exercising? In other words, does this increase in caloric expenditure help you burn more calories throughout the day?

Research has shown that your energy expenditure does remain elevated after cessation of exercise. But it is important to note that the amount of elevation in metabolism is dependent primarily on the intensity of the exercise and, to a lesser degree, the duration of your exercise. In other words, what you do during exercise makes a difference in your RMR.

Pretty much the same concept applies to lifting weights. Plenty of research has shown that vigorous weight training can increase your metabolic rate for hours after exercise. However, the average person who takes long breaks between sets will likely not see a large enough elevation to play a significant role on total daily energy expenditure.

You might have heard, too, that exercise increases your RMR all day long—meaning 24 hours or more. There has been quite a bit of research showing that the combination of high exercise energy expenditure and high energy intake in endurance-trained people can elevate RMR for a short period of time (from a few hours all the way up to about 24 hours), but not permanently.

However, there doesn't seem to be substantial evidence that this elevated RMR will occur at all with normal, recreationally active people—although some research has shown benefits in the elderly.

The effect of weight training on RMR is interesting. Weight training might play a large role in total daily energy expenditure—but the caveat is that it's not likely to dramatically increase your RMR, or postexercise energy expenditure, outside of the exercise itself.

How does high-intensity interval training (HIIT) compare to endurance training in burning calories and raising your RMR?

If you are trying to lose weight and improve body composition through exercise, it's likely that you have been told to do aerobic exercise because it is thought to increase both cardiorespiratory fitness and to help lose weight and fat.

Most aerobic exercise interventions consist of moderate-intensity steady-state exercise for about 30 to 40 minutes for 3 to 4 days per week over a 4- to 6-month period. Unfortunately, research on these kinds of exercise programs, more often than not, have shown only a minimal fat loss. In contrast, a lot of the research shows that HIIT exercise results in significant fat loss.

This might sound counterintuitive because you know that higher-intensity exercise burns more carbohydrates, while lower-intensity exercise burns more fat. However, the key to body fat manipulation is all about the total number of calories burned.

Luckily, some research has directly compared traditional aerobic exercise to HIIT. One study showed that young women in a group who did HIIT lost 2.5 kilograms, or about 5.5 pounds, more fat over the course of a 15-week exercise plan than did the aerobic group—in about half of the exercise time. In other words, higher-intensity exercise might be much more time efficient for weight loss and improvement in body composition.

The caloric cost of this type of exercise will benefit us all. In fact, much of the research regarding HIIT shows that individuals can exercise for a shorter duration but still lose more fat, gain more muscle, and thus improve body composition and health to a greater degree than they can with a traditional aerobic program.

Non-Exercise Calorie Burn

What about caloric expenditure when you're not exercising? What you do the rest of your day can also make a big difference in your physical activity levels and body composition.

A common misperception is that only physical activity or exercise—such as running, biking, walking, or lifting weights—is needed to get any sort of health benefit. However, just as snacking on the wrong things throughout the day can make you gain weight, small acts of physical activity throughout the day can make you healthier and even improve body composition.

Very simple things—such as taking the stairs rather than taking the escalator or elevator—can improve your health over the course of time by adding to the total caloric expenditure of the day.

Not only does taking the stairs improve leg strength and cardiovascular fitness, but research has shown that the average person will burn just more than 1 calorie per stair they climb, or about 15 calories for every flight of stairs. This caloric expenditure is based on a 150- to 160-pound person, so a lighter person will burn fewer calories and a heavier person will burn more.

In addition, research has shown that walking down stairs burns about one-third the number of calories as climbing stairs—so about 5 calories per flight descended, making a total of 20 calories per time you go up and down a flight of stairs. Furthermore, more often than not, you will actually save time taking the stairs.

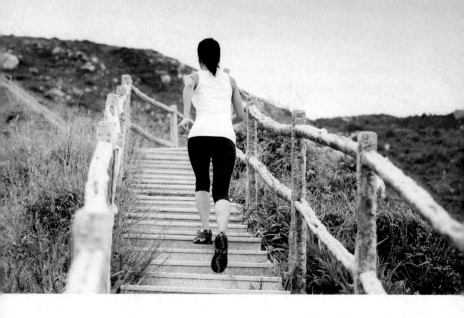

Over the course of a month or a year, these calories add up and can really improve your health and help you improve your body composition, without even working out. Simple daily habits can consciously be altered to improve your health.

You might be pretty sedentary if you are sitting down at work for too long, even if you exercise most days of the week for a certain amount of time. In a typical workweek, people spend on average six hours per day sitting at their desks.

If this is the case for you, consider buying a standup desk for your office. Changing to a standing desk can reduce your risk of obesity, type 2 diabetes, cardiovascular disease, cancer, and overall mortality.

Your heart rate naturally increases as you change from lying down to sitting to standing, and the difference from sitting to standing is approximately 5 to 10 beats per minute, which equates to 0.35 to 0.7 calories per minute.

While this doesn't sound like much, it adds up to somewhere between 25 and 50 calories per hour for a simple change. Given that the average person spends 5 hours and 41 minutes per day sitting at a desk, simply standing instead of sitting could burn almost 285 calories.

If you stand, you'll probably want to start standing for short periods and work up to longer durations. And make sure that you keep shifting around while you stand.

Improved health and body composition do not happen overnight. Changing habits over the long term are what really make the difference, and small changes as well as larger ones matter.

Try This

Pick a new form of activity and include it at least once per week in your weekly routine.

Questions to Consider

1. How can you adapt your daily routine to add simple ways of increasing your energy expenditure? Can you take the stairs? Can you add a short walk or exercise every hour at work?

2. What is the major determining factor for keeping your metabolism high after a workout?

The Caloric Cost of Exercise

We eat and we expend energy. In this lecture, we'll take a closer look at the ways we can expend energy, and how we might use that information in our efforts to strengthen or alter our body composition.

Remember that there are three primary different components to energy expenditure: Resting metabolic rate or RMR, the thermic effect of food, and the thermic effect of activity. These are the three components which should add up to determine the total amount of calories that you expend, or burn, in one day.

Just to recap, resting metabolic rate, or RMR, makes up the majority of your daily energy expenditure—it is estimated to make up somewhere between 60% and 80% of your total energy expenditure output. This is the energy your body needs to stay alive or as the names suggest, simply the energy needed for basic bodily functions at rest.

The thermic effect of food, or TEF, is the energy needed for your body to digest and absorb the food you eat. For example, approximately 30% of the calories in protein are used just to break it down, while only 10% of the calories are used from carbohydrates and nearly 0% from fats. This is the scientific reasoning that explains why one calorie taken in does not mean one calorie is stored.

Last but certainly not least is your thermic effect of activity—this is simply your daily activity. This component includes the calories expended on any kind of deliberate or spontaneous activity throughout the course of the day. This may include your scheduled walk or run in the morning, but it also includes things like standing up and down, taking the stairs or even pacing when your favorite sports team is about to win. The activity part of your total energy expenditure is what I'll focus on for the next few lectures.

So, what is the caloric cost of exercise? Or what are the energy demands of our muscles? If you want to manipulate your body composition, it is important to know the quality of your calories and how many calories you are eating and drinking and how many calories you are expending. Various types of exercises demand varying amounts of energy—walking versus running for example—and these energy demands are measured scientifically through what we call metabolic testing.

Metabolic testing measures the amount of oxygen you take in during activity. The more strenuous or intense the activity is, the greater the oxygen consumption. On average, humans consume 3.5 ml of oxygen per kg of their body weight per minute at rest.

Now we have all kinds of technology that estimate calories burned, but, not long ago, the caloric cost of exercise was traditionally measured in what we call mets or metabolic equivalents. Many of you have even seen the mets term on the exercise equipment in your home or at your local gym—I saw both calories and mets on the treadmill I was using this morning. It is simply another way to assess or quantify the intensity level of your exercise. One metabolic equivalent is equal to the oxygen consumption of your body at rest, or as we just discussed, 3.5 ml/kg/min. When measuring mets, everything is compared to the cost of energy at rest.

So, the more strenuous the exercise, the higher the met value will be—that is, the higher the caloric expenditure will be in relation to resting. For example, running at 10 mph, or a 6:00 min/mile pace, equals 14.5 mets, and that means it requires 14.5 times more energy than resting. Now using mets as a measure of your exercise intensity might seem a bit odd and strange at first, but if you are trying to determine the number of calories you burn when you are exercising—in other words, your caloric cost of exercise—then a great estimate is to simply multiply the met value by your body weight in kg. For example, if you are exercising at an intensity of 10 mets on a stationary cycle in your local gym and you weigh 80 kg or 176 lbs, then you are expending approximately 800 kcal per hour of exercise. Just a side note: I know this is much easier for those of you who use the metric system already, everything in science is based on the metric system, but for those of you who don't, all you have to do to figure out your weight in kg is to divide your weight in lbs by 2.2.

OK, so the science part is great and all, but you might be asking: What about me? How does this apply to my daily life? How long does it take to burn off that bag of chips I just ate or the two extra cookies I ate after dinner last night? Do I have to walk for an hour? Walk for two? Let's tackle these questions with a little case study of our own.

As you probably already know, the type of exercise you participate in dictates how many calories you burn. How many of you have heard someone say, you burn more fat walking than you do running, so why run? Walking hits my fat burning zone.

Because of the way the body's three energy systems work—that is, the creatine phosphate, the glycolytic and the oxidative systems—a lower intensity activity should burn more fat right?

Well, this is partially correct. A higher percentage of fat is burned from the total calories you use during low-intensity exercise. However, the tricky part rests with the actual number of calories burned from the exercise.

Even though during high-intensity exercise a lower percentage of fat is burned, the total number of calories burned is typically far greater than during low-intensity exercise. So, the absolute amount of fat burned is typically greater with high-intensity exercise. So let's say I walk for an hour and burn 300 total calories and 50% of that is from fat. I have burned 150 calories of fat. Now let's say I run for an hour and burn 1000 total calories. Even if only 25% is from fat, I have now burned 250 calories of fat with the higher intensity exercise. So, despite a lower percentage of fat burned when you run hard, you actually burn more fat because the caloric cost of this exercise was so much higher than the caloric cost of walking for an hour.

Let's look big picture for a minute. Think of your body as a car. Your skeletal system is the car body, your muscles are the pistons, and your cardiorespiratory system is the engine. It's great that you have a fine-looking car, but you need fuel, and that is what the metabolic system is for—converting ingested food into stored energy, then converting this energy into fuel to support body movements. The strongest muscles in the world or the most powerful heart in the world are completely useless without the metabolic system doing its job of fueling the body with the energy needed to perform.

Calories are essential—don't treat them as the enemy. Food is fuel. Fuel your body properly for optimal body composition and performance in any aspect of your life—mental or physical. For most of us, our main energy source during exercise comes in the form of muscle glycogen. Your body has plenty of fuel to perform most exercises—generally about 2 hours of moderate-to-high intensity exercise.

But sometimes we do run out—which is part of the reason you see athletes collapse from time to time. Their bodies have run out of the ability to access and utilize fuel. If you are a runner or were a runner, then I'd be willing to bet that you have experienced a time when you've hit the wall or bonked during a long run. You have the mental fortitude to continue, but the body simply won't run—and the body's systems begin to shut down.

The body is absolutely remarkable at properly operating all of its intricate systems most of the time—from muscles to enzymes to atoms—in complete unison. But it requires good quality fuel. We've already talked about how a calorie isn't a calorie—but you already know this. You wouldn't drink a 6-pack of soda or eat five cupcakes before a morning run to get some calories in your body right? Of course not.

Still, it is understandable that you may be confused with what the right way is. Maybe you ask yourself, What do I eat; How much do I eat; How often do I eat; when you think about taking energy in. And, I bet the same thing goes for your exercise and energy expenditure in order to keep your energy in balance and your weight under control. Do you ever ask What workout should I do, or What about that new workout I read about in that magazine?

So let's cover what we do know about exercise and your metabolism and see if we can clear up some of that confusion.

Exercise increases your caloric expenditure above resting levels or your resting metabolic rate based on how long and how intensely you exercise. But here's an interesting question I get asked: does this increase in metabolism last after I finish exercising? In other words, does this increase in caloric expenditure help you burn more calories throughout the day?

Research has shown that your energy expenditure, in fact, does remain elevated after cessation of exercise. But it is important to note that the amount of elevation in metabolism is dependent primarily on the intensity of the exercise and, to a lesser degree, the duration of your exercise. I'll say that again. The amount of elevation in resting metabolic rate you get depends mostly on the intensity of the exercise, and to a lesser degree, on the duration.

For example, if you walk or jog for 30–60 minutes, you'll likely return to a baseline of energy expenditure within an hour—and probably only burn 30 more calories during that hour than if you didn't exercise. Ultimately this after burn won't play a big additional role on your total daily energy expenditure. But if you do a more highly intensive exercise, it may play a big role in your total daily energy expenditure. What you do during exercise makes a difference in your resting metabolic rate. This is a very important point to understand.

Let's look at an elite marathon runner who works at an extremely high intensity for over 2 hours. Her post-exercise energy expenditure will remain elevated for an extended period of time and could potentially play a large role on your total daily energy expenditure, or calorie expenditure.

Once again whether you'll get a lasting higher RMR after exercise is primarily a factor of intensity and to a lesser extent duration. Pretty much the same concept applies to lifting weights. Plenty of research has shown that vigorous weight training can increase your metabolic rate for hours after exercise. However, the average person who takes long breaks between sets will likely not see a large enough elevation to play a significant role on total daily energy expenditure.

So there is the potential that you could increase your caloric expenditure once you finish exercise, but you would have to work out hard and long enough to reap the really beneficial effects. You may have heard too that exercise increases your resting metabolic rate, or RMR, all day long—literally 24 hours or more.

There has been quite a bit of research showing that the combination of high exercise energy expenditure and high energy intake in endurance-trained people can elevate resting metabolic rate for a short period of time from a few hours all the way up to about 24 hours but not permanently. However, there doesn't seem to be substantial evidence that this elevated resting metabolic rate will occur at all with normal, recreationally-active people, though some research has shown benefits in the elderly.

Now the effect of weight training on RMR is really interesting. Weight training may play a large role in total daily energy expenditure—but there is a caveat that comes with that. It is estimated that 1 lbs of muscle burns between 5–10 Calories at rest per day. So if you are thinking of gaining muscle to increase your total daily energy expenditure, you would have to add quite a bit of muscle in order to have any real effect on total daily energy expenditure.

But think about what we have talked about early in the course about dieting versus dieting and exercise. Although it is less common to see someone recreationally lift weights and gain 10 lbs of muscle, it is not uncommon for someone to diet and lose that amount of muscle mass, especially if exercise is not included in their fat loss plans. In a scenario like this, with a loss of 10 lbs of muscle, yes, muscle mass would play a significant role in total daily energy expenditure. If we take an average of 7 Calories per lbs and say you lost 10 lbs of muscle, this would add up to 700 calories per week. Can you see how easily this would change your energy balance equation?

Ultimately, while exercise of almost any intensity and duration certainly carries many health benefits along with it, the effect of recreational endurance exercise or weight lifting is not likely to play a large role in increasing RMR or post-exercise energy expenditure outside of the exercise time itself. Unfortunately, a lot of the magazine and media claims that it will increase resting metabolic rate, or post-exercise energy expenditure don't hold any water.

So although weight training may play a large role in your total daily energy calorie expenditure—the caveat is that it's not likely to increase your resting metabolic rate dramatically. So what about other forms of exercise—for example, High-Intensity Interval Training, or HIIT? How does High-Intensity Interval Training or HIIT compare to the endurance training we have just talked about—in burning calories and raising your resting metabolic rate? We will talk much more about this later, but let's touch on this here.

For those of you who try to lose weight and improve body composition through exercise, it's likely that you have been told to do aerobic exercise because it's thought to increase both cardiorespiratory fitness and to help lose weight and fat. Most aerobic exercise interventions consist of moderate-intensity steady-state exercise, for about 30 to 40 min for 3 to 4 days per week, over 4–6 months of time. Unfortunately research on these kinds of exercise programs—more often than not—have shown only a minimal fat loss. In contrast, a lot of the research shows that HIIT exercise actually results in significant fat loss.

Now, this may sound counterintuitive because you know that higher intensity exercise burns more carbohydrates—while lower intensity exercise burns more fat—however, the key to body fat manipulation is all about the total amount of calories burned—as we discussed earlier. Luckily, some research has directly compared traditional aerobic exercise to HIIT.

Researchers split young women into two groups. One did three, 20-minute HIIT workouts per week on a bike for 15 weeks. The exercise consisted of an 8-second sprint followed by 12 seconds of low-intensity cycling—this continued for 20 minutes. The other group did aerobic exercise at a moderate pace, 3 times per week working from just 10 minutes up to 40 minutes over the 15-week study. The most interesting part was that the women in the HIIT group lost 2.5 kg, or 5.5 lbs, of subcutaneous fat, the kind directly underneath your skin, whereas no change in fat occurred with steady state aerobic exercise.

What is this telling us? This study shows that HIIT in these young women— lost 2.5 kg, or about 5.5 lbs, of fat over the course of a 15-week exercise plan more than the aerobic group in about half the exercise time. So, what this study is saying is that higher intensity exercise may be much more time efficient for weight loss and improvement in body composition. The caloric cost of this type of exercise will benefit us all. In fact, much of the research regarding HIIT is showing that individuals can exercise for a shorter duration, but still lose more fat, gain more muscle, and thus improve body composition and health to a greater degree than they can with a traditional aerobic program.

But what about caloric expenditure when you're not exercising? What do you do the rest of your day can also make a big difference in your physical activity levels and your body composition. Let's tackle your daily work practices. Do you find yourself sitting for hours on end? Do you ever just stand up and walk around during the day? And what does that have to do with body composition and health?

Now a common misperception is that only physical activity or exercise like running, biking, walking, lifting weights, and so forth is needed to get any sort of health benefit. However, just like snacking on the wrong things throughout the day can make you gain weight, small acts of physical activity throughout the day can make you healthier—and even improve body composition.

Very simple things like taking the stairs rather than taking the escalator or elevator can improve your health over the course of time by adding to the total caloric expenditure of the day. This is not just exercise propaganda either—research shows that this isn't just lip service. Not only does taking the stairs improve leg strength and cardiovascular fitness, but research has shown that the average person will burn just over 1 calorie per stair they climb or about 15 calories for every flight of stairs.

This caloric expenditure is based on a 150- to 160-pound person, so a lighter person will burn fewer calories, and a heavier person will burn more. In addition, research has shown that walking down stairs burns about a third the number of calories as climbing upstairs—so about 5 calories per flight descended making a total of 20 total calories per time you go up and down a flight of stairs.

Now think about how many stairs you could—or maybe do—climb during a day around the house, around the office, or wherever. Let's just say you go up and down 3 flights of stairs per day on average. A total of 20 calories per flight, in a week, and you will burn over 400 calories by simply modifying your daily habits a little bit—and more likely than not you will actually save time taking the stairs. Over the course of a month or a year, these calories add up and can really improve your health and help you improve your body composition—without even working for it. Simple daily habits can consciously be altered to improve your health.

I go to the American College of Sports Medicine National Conference every year to learn about the research being performed all around the world on exercise, nutrition, and health. They have a great tagline or motto that exercise is medicine that is being promoted around the world. That being said, it is truly amazing to me that at every one of these conferences people who are capable, still take the elevator or escalator instead of the stairs the majority of the time. In fact, I just took a group of exercise science students to South Africa to study sports physiology and sports nutrition—and even they took the escalator or elevator every chance they could. The examples go on and on, but I always get a laugh when people are in the gym parking lot circling and circling trying to find a parking spot close to the door.

Now, of course, I'm not saying that you should never take another escalator or park close to a building, but I just want to illustrate how a choice so small still requires a conscious effort if you want to make a change. Just like something as small as brushing your teeth or flossing, make a daily to-do list at work if you develop good habits, then they simply become part of your day.

I've been working on this too. I noticed that at work I was just sitting down way too much. I exercise most days of the week in a confined period of time, but I was pretty sedentary otherwise. So I got on the bandwagon and bought a stand-up desk for my office.

Did you know that in a typical work week, people spend on average of almost 6 hours per day sitting at their desks? It turns out that changing to a standing desk can reduce your risk of obesity, Type II diabetes, cardiovascular disease, cancer, and overall mortality risk. But, does it help to also improve your body composition? I mean, how many calories can you really burn just by standing more? What is the caloric cost of standing?

Your heart rate naturally increases as you change from lying down to sitting to standing and the difference from sitting to standing is approximately 5–10 beats/minute, which equates to 0.35 to 0.7 calories/minute. While this obviously not much, let's think about big picture. This adds up to somewhere between 25–50 calories/hour from a simple change. Given that the average person spends 5 hours and 41 minutes/day sitting at their desk, simply standing instead of sitting could burn almost 285 calories.

Take note that if you stand, you'll probably want to start standing for short periods and work up to standing longer durations. And make sure you keep shifting around while you do stand. What I want you to take away from this is that by simply walking up or down 3 flights of stairs and standing at your desk instead of sitting—both simple, small habitual changes—you can burn almost 350 more calories per day.

Again, this is without taking into consideration any additional physical activity or exercise you do throughout the day including gardening, doing dishes, or walking your dog. Over the course of a week, a month, or a year, the daily marginal gains add up to great health and body composition implications. The fact is that improved health and body composition are not things that happen overnight. Changing habits over the long haul are what really make the difference; and small changes as well as larger ones matter.

Exercise is important to ensure that your body is strong and healthy enough to meet the challenges that you encounter on a daily basis. And eating less will help you lose weight—sure—but as we discussed earlier, weight loss from dieting alone may actually result in losing muscle mass and maybe even rebounding back to a higher weight that you started with.

So, some sort of exercise regimen is vital—and I mean that in every sense of the word—for a healthy expenditure of calories. And exercise needs to be included in any kind of fitness plan in order to improve health and body composition, not simply body weight.

Now, one of the take-home messages from this lecture is that there are many different types of exercise that can help to reach your goals—from small adjustments like taking the stairs at work, walking around more, and perhaps even getting a stand-up desk, if you have a desk job—to full-blown structured exercise plans.

Just like a well-functioning car needs routine care of all is components and parts—the body needs a combination of proper fueling and exercise to optimize its potential. While there may be many ways to alter your body composition—and some are more efficient than others—find a plan that works for you and stick to it.

Often people can get bogged down in the science and the fine details of exercise, nutrition, and health—but it's very simple. If you take calories in, and you do, you must have opportunities to burn them off and keep an energy balance. Plus exercise helps you in so many other ways to improve health. And, at the same time, the quality of your calorie intake is critical to successful body composition change that is permanent.

One of the most important factors in determining whether or not your plan will work—can you guess—adherence and consistency. So keep in mind that as you set your fitness goals the best guarantee that you'll stay consistent with your activity or exercise plan is that you have fun with it and look forward to. If running isn't your thing, try cycling or hiking or tennis or golf or anything. Exercise is a great way to feel good, get outdoors, meet new people, and just enjoy the world you live in.

Make a conscious effort to stay physically active and this will ultimately manifest itself into better nutritional practices and feeling and looking better. Too often people try to make being healthy a very complex idea. It's really not. The fine details may be important to some professional athletes, but just making small adjustments here and there, and committing to being more physically active will ultimately lead you to a healthier lifestyle and body composition.

Try This: Pick a new form of activity and include it at least once per week in your weekly routine.

Exercise for Fat Loss

To lose fat and gain muscle at the same time, you must understand which types of exercise will promote fat loss and which types of exercise will promote muscle gain, and how they can be used in conjunction with each other to achieve the best of both worlds. This lecture will focus on exercise—specifically, aerobic exercise and resistance exercise—to increase fat loss. You will examine these types of exercise and learn the science behind how fat loss works.

Aerobic Exercise versus Resistance Exercise

- There are two major categories of exercise: aerobic exercise (such as walking, running, swimming, or cycling) and resistance exercise (such as lifting weights or doing body-weight strength movements).

- Aerobic exercise is repetitive and relies on the continuous activation of the heart and lungs, often called cardiovascular, or cardiorespiratory, exercise. Most people think that aerobic exercise is the key to fat loss.

- Resistance exercise is less continuous and involves moving or lifting objects with forceful muscle contractions. Resistance exercise is typically related to gains in muscle mass, but plenty of evidence shows that it is actually excellent for fat loss and body composition improvements.

- Most major governing bodies that provide exercise recommendations, such as the American College of Sports Medicine, suggest using both aerobic and resistance exercise. This should provide benefits for both improving health and body composition. A combination of exercise types is also a good idea for fat loss.

Aerobic Exercise: Mode

There are several factors we can manipulate to maximize fat loss when it comes to aerobic exercise.

- The mode, or type, of exercise.
- The duration of the exercise.
- The intensity of the exercise.
- The frequency of exercise, or how often you work out.

In general, keep in mind that something is better than nothing. The more physical work we do, the more calories we burn, and the greater chance for our total calorie deficit to help with fat loss. But there are certain choices we can make to maximize our aerobic exercise, specifically for the greatest fat loss for a given time spent exercising. This includes altering mode, duration, intensity, and frequency of exercise.

Much of the mode of aerobic exercise comes down to your personal preferences.

- What do you enjoy doing?
- What is your accessibility to certain equipment, such as a bike or a pool?
- What time of year is it? Is it snowy or really hot?
- What is your injury history? Certain activities might be less stressful to achy joints or problem areas.

The more movement you do, the better. So, if you run versus just sit on a recumbent bike, for the same amount of time, you will probably have more effective fat loss with running because you are using both your upper and lower body during exercise. With more muscles being worked, more overall energy is usually expended.

Swimming requires both upper- and lower-body muscle groups. But it seems that for a given intensity, swimming will expend fewer calories than either running or cycling. It is thought that the reduced energy expenditure for equally intense swimming exercise might be related to a

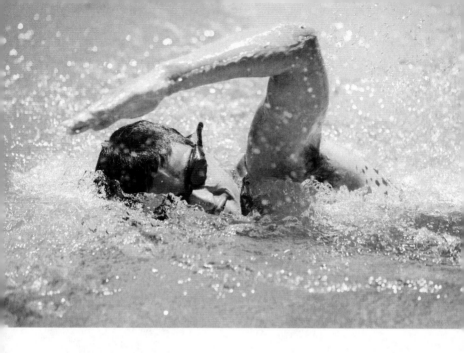

lower heart rate during swimming compared to running or cycling, even when it feels like you are working out at the same effort.

The primary reason for this is your body position during each exercise. In a more upright exercise, such as running or biking, the heart must work to a larger extent against gravity to return blood to the heart. Swimming, however, requires you to lie flat. In this position, blood travels back to the heart quite easily. This requires less work for the heart and a lower heart rate.

Swimming in cool water might also increase your total calorie burn. This is because you not only have to work hard just to swim, but you also have to keep your body temperature within a normal range. This concept also stands for running or cycling outside in the cold.

Aerobic classes, such as step or dance, are not a bad idea, especially if they make exercise more enjoyable for you. However, it is often more difficult to regulate intensity in these types of classes and it also might be a less continuous form of exercise than some other choices, with small breaks given occasionally.

In general, running might actually be the most optimal aerobic exercise type for fat loss specifically. However, if you loathe running or cannot run due to musculoskeletal limitations or injuries, every other form of movement is good and can result in significant improvements in your body composition when paired with solid nutritional choices and lifestyle habits.

Aerobic Exercise: Duration and Intensity

The length of time you exercise and the number of calories you burn are directly and linearly related. The longer you work, the more calories you burn.

If you want the body composition changes that two hours of exercise would give you but you only have 45 minutes to spare in a day, you can burn the same number of calories in 45 minutes that you could over two hours by changing one thing about the way you exercise: the intensity of your exercise.

Intensity is king when it comes to fat loss. Intensity is a measure of how hard you are working. This can be measured by how you feel or quantified by heart rate, exercise speed, or incline.

A major misconception is the idea that low-intensity exercise is better for fat loss. Low-intensity exercise is often called the "fat burn zone." You can actually lose a whole lot of fat by exercising for far less time per day, but you must work out very hard.

This is where high-intensity interval training (HIIT) enters the picture: You simply intermix rest periods with very high-intensity work. So, you might run fast for 1 minute and then "recover" at a slow jog pace for 1 minute and repeat this for 20 minutes.

High-intensity exercise will burn more fuel than low-intensity exercise. When we exercise at higher intensities, we will burn more carbohydrates for energy, and when we exercise at lower intensities, we will burn more fat for energy. However, using fat for fuel during exercise will not result in the greatest overall losses to total body fat over time. So, the fat burn zone might not be named appropriately, and it's misleading.

With a high-intensity workout, you will burn energy during and after the exercise, too. But just how much will you burn is dependent on, most importantly, how hard you exercise and somewhat on how long you exercise.

If your main reason not to exercise is your time, then this technique of going very hard but for a short time eliminates that excuse. Try warming up with a few minutes of walking and things like jumping jacks, lunges, or body-weight squats, and then break your workout session into segments of high-intensity efforts and easy recovery.

You can find access to a number of interval or HIIT workouts online, in training books, or from a coach. Some interval workouts go by minutes, some go by distance, and some just go by how you feel. But the goal is always to work hard during the active, or work, phase and then recover for a period of time before the next active phase.

As you become more fit, you can extend the "hard" work phase and decrease the recovery time. A reasonable place to start could be 30 seconds of very hard work followed by 1 minute of easy recovery.

You might even find interval exercise to be more enjoyable, because it breaks down your workout into segments and makes the time go by more quickly.

Research shows that interval training results in a greater overall adherence to exercise and might be more enjoyable than continuous lower-intensity exercise. Research also shows that interval training combined with resistance training is incredibly effective for reducing

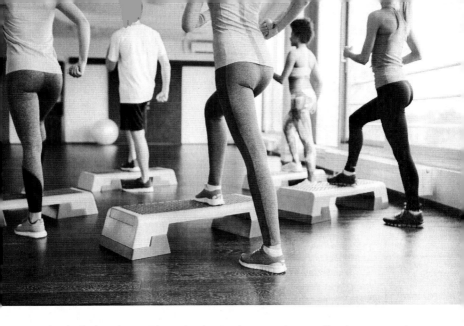

body fat levels. HIIT has also been shown to be as effective, or maybe even more effective, at improving heart health than low-intensity exercise that burned the same number of calories.

- A high level of activity is very difficult, so you really shouldn't do it every day. It is best to mix in days of HIIT and days of slow- to moderate-intensity aerobic exercise. This should help maximize fat loss and keep you from getting hurt.

- And start with an amount of time that you can fit into your schedule. We have shown great results with HIIT for just 20 to 30 minutes! Essentially, you can start with very little exercise and have a great response for improving your body composition.

Aerobic Exercise: Frequency

- Frequency refers to the number of times you exercise per week. For general health, you should exercise three to five days per week, according to the American College of Sports Medicine guidelines.

For fat loss, it's best to incorporate multiple types of exercise, such as aerobic, HIIT, and resistance. But for aerobic endurance exercise, there are a few ways to get the most possible fat loss from your workouts.

- Move lots of muscles.
- Choose higher-intensity exercise through interval training rather than low-intensity exercise, even when the caloric cost is the same.
- Exercise longer rather than shorter when comparing exercises of the same intensity.
- Exercise at least five days per week to see the most improvement.

If you are feeling overwhelmed, don't worry. It is best to only make one change at a time. For example, try to change up your exercise in one small way today that is practical for you. Then, little by little, you can incorporate more of these options to maximize fat loss. It is not a good idea to change everything at once—in fact, that is a sure way to failure.

Resistance Training

A number of research studies have demonstrated that combining HIIT and resistance training is most effective for fat loss and improving body composition. Resistance training is a very powerful tool for changing body composition.

With only aerobic exercise, it is far easier to change your overall size but much more difficult to alter the way it looks physically. You can change from a "big pear" shape to a "small pear" shape, but you need to add resistance exercise if you want to add lean muscle and change the way you look.

Adding lean mass from resistance training is important for fat loss specifically. The addition of resistance training to your activity might kill two or three birds with one stone.

- It will add lean muscle mass, which is metabolically active. This means that it uses a few more calories than other tissues and contributes to your total daily caloric output.
- Resistance training increases lipolysis, or fat mobilization.

Resistance training also increases excess postexercise oxygen consumption (EPOC), just like aerobic exercise, but maybe even more.

Combining the fat-burning effects of aerobic and resistance exercise seems to offer the maximal benefits for fat loss. The combination also looks to be more favorable than aerobic exercise alone in combating certain types of chronic disease, including muscle wasting, osteoporosis, and perhaps even type 2 diabetes.

Try This

Replace one of your longer, slower exercise sessions with short, high-intensity intervals each week.

Questions to Consider

1. What exercise barriers to losing fat do you see in your lifestyle?

2. Where in your week can you fit in aerobic and resistance exercise?

Exercise for Fat Loss

I can't tell you how many times I've worked with people who want to improve their body composition. When I first asked them what they were doing about it, they typically tell me I started to jog, or I started to walk. Of course, this is a great start towards getting in better shape. These slower, aerobic exercises can help to reduce the risk of a number of health issues. They may also reduce body fat and improve your body composition. But improving body composition not only has to do with losing body fat it has a lot to do with either maintaining or increasing muscle mass as well.

So, is it possible to lose fat and gain muscle at the same time? Maybe. To do so, you must understand which types of exercise will promote fat loss, and which types of exercise will promote muscle gain, and how they can be used in conjunction with each other to achieve the best of both worlds.

This lecture will focus specifically on exercise to increase fat loss. In doing so, we'll examine several types of exercise, and discuss the science behind how fat loss actually works.

Fat loss is a process that really takes place in your mitochondria. That's the place where you have all the fat burning machinery inside each cell. It is the place where you use oxygen to break down fat and carbohydrates to create ATP for energy.

So it makes sense that one way to burn more fat is to increase the number of mitochondria that you have in your cells—this is called mitochondrial density. Basically, the more mitochondria you have, the more fat you can burn and the more ATP you can supply to your muscles.

It is well known that aerobic endurance exercise training, something like cycling or jogging at a slow to moderate pace, will increase your mitochondrial density. But are there other ways to do the same thing?

We hear phrases like fat burning, belly busting, trimming, and slimming in the exercise industry all the time. Some of these phrases even suggest that you can spot reduce or lose weight from one specific body area. But is this true? The answer is no. There is no such thing as spot reduction. You cannot work out specifically on your stomach or your arms and expect to lose fat from these areas only. I realize that this goes against many TV and magazine advertisements but trust me, when we lose fat weight, it is not solely coming from the areas that we work out. So you might ask, where does most fat loss occur? And what dictates where this fat loss will come from?

Well, consider your own body. You've probably noticed predictable patterns of where you gain or lose weight. Have you ever said, It all goes to my hips? Or, it all goes to my belly?

Where your body stores excess fat has a lot to do with your genetics and your sex, these factors will determine the pattern and relative concentration of certain receptors within fat tissue that either inhibit or activate fat mobilization from each fat cell and eventually fat burning in the mitochondria of your muscles. Alpha-receptors are the brakes on fat mobilization—they inhibit it. Beta-receptors, are the accelerators of fat mobilization—they activate it.

So it makes sense that the more alpha cells inhibiting fat mobilization that you have in a specific body area, the more trouble you might have losing fat from that area and vice-versa for the beta-receptors. More beta-receptors in an area of your body, the more fat burning or fat mobilization you will have in that area.

A good example is the typical fat distribution patterns among men and women. Men tend to store excess fat in the abdomen or belly, and, as you probably suspect, have a higher concentration of alpha-receptors or inhibitors in that area. Women often store excess fat in their hips and thighs, and also have a greater number of alpha-receptors in these tissues. But, men doing crunches or women doing glute exercises will not necessarily accelerate fat loss more so than any other exercise—either at those specific sites or elsewhere on their bodies.

So, you should think of doing much more than specific body part exercises. Instead, for fat loss, you need to do an assortment of exercises that involve and impact your whole body.

So what are those exercises? Well, first, there are two major categories of exercise. One is aerobic exercise like walking, running, swimming, or cycling, and the second is resistance exercises like lifting weights or doing body weight strength movements

Aerobic exercise is repetitive and relies on the continuous activation of the heart and lungs, often called cardiovascular, or cardiorespiratory, exercise. Most people think that aerobic exercise is the key piece needed for fat loss. Resistance exercise is less continuous and involves moving or lifting objects with forceful muscle contractions. Resistance exercise is typically related to gains in muscle mass. But plenty of evidence shows that it is actually an excellent fat loss tool and way to improve body composition.

Most major governing bodies that provide exercise recommendations, like the American College of Sports Medicine, suggest that using both aerobic and resistance exercise—this should provide benefits for both improving health and body composition. A combination of exercise types is also a good idea for fat loss.

With this in mind, you probably are asking yourself: which types of aerobic exercise and which types of resistance exercise will maximize fat loss specifically?

Let's begin with aerobic exercise. There are several factors we can manipulate when it comes to aerobic exercise. We can change the mode or the kind of exercise, for example, swimming to running to cycling to dancing and back again. We can change the duration of the exercise, 20 or 30 minutes or an hour or more. We can change the intensity of the exercise, how difficult it feels, often based on your heart rate zone or your own subjective feeling. And finally, we can change the frequency of this exercise or how often you work out. Say, over the course of a week or month.

In general, just keep in mind that something is better than nothing. The more physical work we do, the more calories we burn, and the greater chance for our total calorie deficit to help with fat loss. But, there are certain choices we can make to maximize our aerobic exercise specifically for the greatest fat loss for a given time spent exercising. Personally, I still compete in triathlon races of various distances every year. Triathlon involves swimming, biking, and running in that order. So altering mode, duration, intensity, and frequency of exercise is a very common occurrence for me. I'll change all of these factors over the course of training in order to optimize my body composition, performance, and health.

Let's first consider the mode, or the type of aerobic exercise. Much of this comes down to your personal preferences. What do you enjoy doing? What is your accessibility to certain equipment, like a bike or a pool? What time of year is it? Is it snowy or really hot? What is your injury history? Certain activities may be less stressful to achy joints or problem areas.

Now, it might make sense that the more movement you do, the better. So if you run versus just sitting on a recumbent bike, for the same amount of time, you will probably have more effective fat loss because you are actually using both your upper and lower body during exercise. With more muscles being worked, more overall energy is usually expended.

What about swimming? Swimming requires both upper and lower body muscle groups. But, it seems that for a given intensity, swimming will expend fewer calories than either running or cycling. Why? Well, the answer is not as clear as we would like.

It is thought that the reduced energy expenditure for equally intense swimming exercise may be related to a lower heart rate during swimming compared to running or cycling—even when it feels like you are working out at the same effort. The primary reason for this is your body position during exercise. In a more upright exercise like running or biking, the heart must work to a larger extent against gravity to return blood back to the heart. Think of the blood vessels in your body as a column, with the heart resting at the top. In relation to gravity, the larger the distance between the heart and the bottom of the column, the greater distance that must be overcome.

With upright exercise, your heart rate must be increased to overcome this greater vertical distance and assist with getting blood back to your heart. Swimming, however, requires you to lie flat, either supine or prone. In this position, the distance from the heart to the bottom of our column is considerably smaller in terms of gravity so blood travels back to the heart quite easily. This requires less work for the heart and a lower heart rate.

But, if you are an avid swimmer, don't worry. Most times you swim in cool water, which may also increase your total calorie burn. This is because you not only have to work hard just to swim, but you also have to keep your body temperature within a normal range. Similarly, this concept stands for running or cycling outside in the cold. Try to remember this next time you are dreading your cold morning workouts. Maybe this knowledge will help it a little more to make worth it to step outside into the frigid air.

Okay, what if you're not a runner, cyclist, or swimmer? Aerobic classes like step or dance are not a bad idea, especially if they make your exercise more enjoyable for you. However, it is often more difficult to regulate the intensity of these types of classes and also, it may be a less continuous form of exercise than some other choices, with small breaks given occasionally.

In general, running may actually be the most optimal aerobic exercise type for fat loss. However, if you absolutely loathe running, or cannot run due to musculoskeletal limitations or injuries, every other form of movement is good and can result in significant improvements in your body composition when paired with nutritional choices that are good and lifestyle habits.

The next aspect of aerobic exercise that you can manipulate to improve fat loss is the length of time you exercise or exercise duration. It is known that the length of time you exercise and the amount of calories you burn are directly and linearly related. Makes sense—the longer you work, the more calories burned. This is pretty simple. But, how much time out of your day are you willing to give?

Sure, if you run for 2 hours you will burn more calories than if you run for 45 minutes, resulting in more overall fat loss. However, this option may not be feasible or desirable. I even see a lot of people who actually exercise for a long time but never change or improve. This is because the exercise is not intense enough or their eating habits preclude the loss of fat.

Let's say you want the body composition changes that 2 hours of exercise would give you, but you've only got 45 minutes to spare in the day? What if you could burn the same amount of calories in 45 minutes that you could over 2 hours by simply changing one thing about the way you exercise? You can—and that one thing is the intensity of your exercise.

If there is one thing that you take away from this lecture, it is that intensity is king when it comes to fat loss. Intensity is a measure of how hard you are working. As I mentioned before, this can be measured by how you feel, or quantified by heart rate, exercise speed, or incline. A major misconception is that the idea that low-intensity exercise is better for fat loss. We discussed this in the last lecture, but it's a point that bears repeating. Low-intensity exercise is often called the fat burn zone. There is even a button on many exercise machines called The Fat Burning Zone for the low-intensity setting.

But here's a nice fat-loss tip. You can actually use a whole lot of fat by exercising for far less time per day, but there is one caveat. You must work out very hard. This is where High-Intensity Interval Training or HIIT comes into play—you simply intermix rest periods with very high-intensity work. So you might run fast for 1 minute and then recover at a slow jog pace for 1 minute and repeat this for 20 minutes.

First, remember that two major fuel sources are used during exercise: stored fat and stored carbohydrate. The use of each exists along a continuum and is never only stored fat or only stored carbohydrate. However, a greater proportion of fat will be metabolized at rest and during lower intensity exercise, while a greater proportion of carbohydrate will be metabolized at higher intensities. This is where the fat burn at low-intensity myth comes into the picture.

Based on this principle, we, of course, want to work out at low intensities right? The fat burn zone? Well actually, no. It is true that at rest and lower intensities, we will use fat for fuel primarily but, think about this. If the relative proportion of fat used for metabolism dictated actual fat loss, wouldn't the best exercise be sitting on the couch, when relative fat metabolism is at its highest? We know this isn't the case. So how could low-intensity exercise be any different?

Instead, change your thinking. The best way to think of exercise for fat loss is how much fuel you are burning overall, not which fuel type you are using. High-intensity exercise will burn more fuel than low-intensity exercise. Running a mile burns more fuel than walking a mile. When we exercise at higher intensities, we will burn more carbohydrates for energy. And when we exercise at lower intensities, we will burn more fat for energy. But, using fat for fuel during exercise will not result in the greatest overall losses to total body fat over time. So the fat burn zone may not be named appropriately—and it's misleading.

So, how then will higher-intensity exercise result in greater fat loss? The best way to think of this is in terms of oxygen consumption. We all have an oxygen consumption demand at rest in order to maintain normal body processes that we've discussed throughout this course.

When you exercise, the oxygen demand is increased to bring oxygen to your working muscles. Just think about the last time you hustled up a staircase and began breathing hard—this is in part due to a greater need for oxygen to help out your muscles. The greater intensity at which we exercise, the greater our oxygen demand Well, once we come down from our high oxygen consumption after exercise, our resting oxygen consumption will also run a little high in the next several hours for a number of reasons. It is believed that this elevated oxygen consumption is necessary to replenish certain energy systems and help bring down your elevated body temperature. Your body is taking care of itself to restore order, and prepare to do it again if needed.

This time after exercise where you require more oxygen is called excess post-exercise oxygen consumption, or EPOC. Exercise that is really tough results in a greater magnitude of EPOC. Like I just mentioned, this period of heightened oxygen consumption is similar to your car's engine staying warm after you drive. Your body expends more energy after exercise to come back to normal or back to homeostasis. Your body will work on processes like restoring ATP and glycogen that were used during exercise, bringing your body temperature back to normal, and starting to repair damaged muscle tissue.

So, with a high-intensity workout, you will burn energy during and after the exercise too. But just how much will you burn? Well, that is dependent on, most importantly, how hard you exercise and somewhat, on how long you exercise. If your number one reason not to exercise is your time which is the number one excuse that I hear all the time, then this technique of going very hard but for a short time eliminates that excuse.

Well, how do you start? Just go out and sprint? Chances are we won't last very long and, if you're like me, you'll probably injure yourself. Instead, warm-up with a few minutes of walking and things like jumping jacks, lunges or body-weight squats, and then break your workout session into segments of high-intensity efforts and easy recovery.

You can find access to a number of interval or HIIT workouts online, in training books or from a coach. Some interval workouts go by minutes, some go by distance, and some just go by how you feel. But the goal is always to work hard during the active phase and then recover for a period of time before the next active or work phase.

As you become more fit, you can extend the hard work phase and decrease the recovery time. A reasonable place to start could be 30 seconds very hard followed by 1 minute of easy recovery. You could even try mailbox or telephone pole intervals where you simply run hard from mailbox 1 to mailbox 2, then go easy until mailbox 3 and then repeat.

You might even find interval exercise to be more enjoyable, as it breaks your workout down into segments and makes the time go by more quickly. Actually, it does go by more quickly because you can work out for less total time.

Research shows that interval training results in a greater overall adherence to exercise, and may be more enjoyable than continuous lower-intensity exercise. This is just one of many reasons for its effectiveness. In fact, in my own research, we've shown that interval training combined with resistance training is incredibly effective for reducing body fat levels.

HIIT is thought to have this effect in part because it has been shown to increase mitochondrial density and to increase the number and activity of enzymes like citrate synthase, malate dehydrogenase, and others needed to break down carbohydrates and fat to make ATP. In some HIIT research, changes in these enzymes were shown after just 7 weeks of exercising 3 days per week by doing 4 to 10, 30-second maximal sprints on a bike, followed by 4 minutes of recovery. HIIT has also been shown to be as effective or maybe even more effective at improving heart health than low-intensity exercise that burned the same number of calories.

So when it comes to exercise intensity for fat loss, choose higher over lower. And, the best way to do this may be through interval training. Keep in mind though that this level of activity is very hard, so you really shouldn't do it every day. It is best to mix in days of HIIT and days of slow-to-moderate intensity aerobic exercise. This should help to maximize fat loss and keep you from getting hurt.

And start with an amount of time that you can fit into your schedule. We have shown great results with HIIT for just 20–30 minutes. Essentially, you can start with very little exercise and have a great response for improving your body composition.

This brings up the next question. How often should you be exercising? Frequency is the last important aspect of exercise to help with weight and health. This refers to the number of times you exercise per week. For general health, you should exercise 3–5 days per week, according to the American College of Sports Medicine guidelines. But what about for fat loss specifically? These same guidelines suggest aerobic exercise should be completed at least 5 days a week to maintain or increase weight loss.

Think about it: the more often you exercise, the more opportunities throughout the week you have to burn calories both during the actual exercise and after exercise too. It is in your best interest, then, to slowly increase the number of planned workout sessions per week to take advantage of both of these opportunities.

For fat loss, you now know that it's best to incorporate multiple types of exercise—aerobic, HIIT training, and resistance. But for aerobic endurance exercise, here are a few ways to get the most possible fat loss from your workouts. First, move lots of muscle. This is why running may be most effective for fat loss. Second, choose higher intensity exercise through interval training rather than low-intensity exercise, even when the same caloric cost is happening. Third, exercise longer rather than shorter when comparing exercise of the same intensity. And fourth, exercise at least 5 days per week to see the most improvement.

If you are feeling overwhelmed, don't worry. It is best to only make one change at a time. For example, try to change up your exercise in one small way today that is practical for you. Then, little by little try to incorporate more of these options to maximize fat loss. It is not a good idea to change everything all at once—in fact, this is a sure way to failure.

Let me explain. You will not begin your program at 6 days a week or for 60 minutes at a time doing intervals. Instead, you will follow another principle of exercise science, which is progression. Be sure to progress your exercise plan and push yourself within reason.

Why? Because if you incorporate all of these suggestions immediately, chances are you will become overwhelmed and drop the fitness thing altogether. But something is better than nothing and more is better than less in most cases. And as you feel comfortable, you can begin to tailor that something to fat loss. This way you can achieve more than you already do each and every day.

Now that we've talked about aerobic exercise what about resistance training for fat loss? In a number of research studies that I've been working on over the years, we've demonstrated that combining HIIT and resistance training is most effective for fat loss and improving body composition.

It turns out that resistance training is a very powerful tool for changing body composition. You see, with only aerobic exercise, it is far easier to change your overall size but much harder to alter the way that it looks physically. I often say that you can change from a big pear shape to a small pear shape, but you need to add Resistance Exercise if you truly want to add lean muscle and change the way you look.

Adding lean mass from resistance training is important for fat loss specifically. Why and how is this the case? The addition of resistance training to your activity may kill two or three birds with one stone. It will add lean muscle mass, which is metabolically active. This means that it uses a few more calories than other tissues and contributes to your total daily caloric output. In a previous lecture, I described muscle tissue as a very metabolically active tissue or hungry tissue. This means that muscle tissue specifically requires a little bit more energy to be maintained than fat mass. Therefore, the greater amount of muscle mass on your body, the greater energy demands overall, which equals more calories expended each day just for body maintenance.

Resistance training actually increases lipolysis or fat mobilization. In fact, our research group published a few research papers on this in the *Journal of Applied Physiology*. We found that resistance training alone was effective for increased lipolysis from belly fat in healthy young men and in both sedentary lean and obese men. Resistance training also increases EPOC excess post-exercise oxygen consumption just like aerobic exercise, but maybe even more. For example, after 45 minutes of cycling at 70% of maximum, metabolism stayed high for another 14 hours—burning about 190 calories over a control group. Similarly, traditional resistance training with 4 sets of 8 exercises done for 8–12 repetitions has been shown to burn about a 100 extra Calories over the 22 hours following resistance exercise.

However, the authors of this study also found that if the resistance exercise was completed at a much higher intensity, this time using heavy weight to complete exhaustion for 6 repetitions, with only 20 seconds of rest between sets, the calorie burn was 23% greater than the traditional group. The High-Intensity group burned 452 Calories over the same 22 hour period. And, best of all, most of the extra burn was from fat. Now these studies were done in men, but the authors suggested that when body mass is equated, no difference between men and women exists.

So, combining the fat burning effects of aerobic and resistance exercise seems to offer the maximal benefits for fat loss, as described in several recent studies from my lab and others.

The combination also looks to be more favorable than aerobic exercise alone in combating certain types of chronic disease, including muscle wasting, osteoporosis, and perhaps even Type II Diabetes. Exactly which kinds of resistance exercises will increase muscle mass, referred to as hypertrophy, will be covered later. But for now, realize the incredibly important role of resistance exercise for fat loss.

We have discussed the basis for aerobic exercise and resistance exercise for fat loss. How can we determine if we are successful? How quickly or slowly should we expect to lose fat based on these described principles? I will end our discussion with a few more rules of thumb for rating your fat loss success.

It is important to mention first that your rate of fat loss will be different from others depending on your age, your sex, how much fat you have to lose, as well as your unique physiology. In general, fat loss should be gradual. A small amount should be lost every week, which will add up to big gains over time. Again, just like it took a while to put the fat on your body, give it time to come off your body too.

To me the most important factor is how you answer these questions: Are you feeling good? And is your energy level good? These are real world questions, and if they are not a resounding yes, then something in your life has to change. Once you see some results, you may want to work with a professional to continue to make progress in your workouts and nutrition and to continue to meet your body composition goals. Later in the course,

I'll go over some important things to look for if you choose to work with a personal trainer.

So, if you really want to change your body composition the important thing to worry about is how much fat you burn and how many calories you use and the bigger picture; like over a week, a month, or a year. To do this, you probably need to be exercising vigorously at least a few times a week. Recently, the *Journal of the American Medical Association* reported that the more vigorous activity you do, the lower your mortality. Keep in mind, though that you still need to incorporate rest days or days where you simply take a walk and stretch or hike with a friend in order to recover from your hard exercise sessions.

Just remember to tailor your program to target fat loss and your own needs, with fat loss success defined as you feeling the best you ever felt and achieving gradual fat loss over the long-term. Implementing both aerobic endurance exercise and resistance exercise allows for changes that will last a lifetime.

Try This: Replace one of your longer, slower exercise sessions with short, high-intensity intervals each week.

Exercise for Healthy Muscle Mass

T his lecture will tackle one of the most widely discussed, and often misguided, topics of interest in this field: muscle. You will learn why you want to increase muscle mass and how to do it, as well as how to properly maintain it and the health benefits of doing so, especially as you age. You will also learn about the type, volume, frequency, and intensity of exercises that induce muscle growth, and you will explore some of the new schools of training that are becoming increasingly popular.

Resistance Training and Aging

As we age, a phenomenon called sarcopenia occurs, which is the natural, progressive loss of muscle mass as we grow older. Studies have shown that between the ages of 40 and 50, we can lose more than 8 percent of our muscle mass, and that can accelerate to more than 15 percent per decade after the age of 75 if measures are not taken to prevent it. Fortunately, there is a lot we can do to slow down this process.

Most people think that aging alone causes us to lose muscle. But now research is clearly showing that it is more the lack of physical activity that is the major player here. Long-term exercise training can aid in preserving muscle mass. It might also prevent increases in body fat as we age.

Resistance training adds muscle, too—if you specifically plan your program with muscle gain as one of your goals. Data show that as you age, the importance of strength is critical. In fact, just being stronger in your chest and legs is associated with the least risk of premature death.

Resistance training must be included in your exercise program, and there might be some nutritional supplements that can help even more with improving body composition and performance.

Finding a Personal Trainer

What specifically should you do to increase your muscle mass? As with most well-designed exercise training programs, you should have a balance between strength and endurance training (with your ultimate goal the key factor in how much or little of each you do). You know the difference between low-intensity/steady-state aerobic exercise and HIIT training and the benefits of both.

Considering that most of the best athletes hire a coach or trainer, you might want to consider hiring a personal trainer, too. If you are an elite athlete or if you are new to exercise, hiring a personal trainer or coach is a great way to start or work on a new goal or to prepare for a race or competition. This way, you can try new exercises, avoid injury, learn about your exercise and lifting options, and figure out how to lift safely while also working around past injuries.

When choosing a personal trainer, the first step is to figure out if you want to work out in a gym setting or have a personal trainer come to your house. Both are great options, and you just need to find what suits your lifestyle, personality, goals, and budget.

Some trainers offer gentle encouragement, and others are "in your face" to try and motivate you. The last thing you want is someone giving mild-mannered instruction when you know that does nothing to motivate you. And, likewise, you don't want a drill sergeant type if you respond best to gentle but persistent encouragement.

Personal trainers should also be held to some educational and certification standards. Don't be shy about directly asking them about these things. Then, take note—because there are some so-called certifications that you can get with an hour of free time and Internet

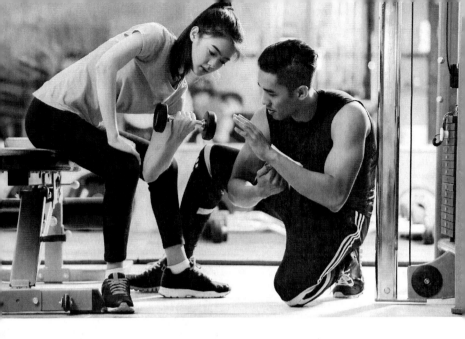

access. Some of the top certifications require a bachelor's degree before you can even sit to take the exams.

Just like any skilled profession, referrals will help you decide, too. Trainers should be able to provide you with some contact information for people they have trained with similar goals.

Also ask about how they measure your success and how they progress clients. Observe them with another client and see how they behave. Does the trainer ignore the client and mindlessly count reps while texting or talking on the phone? Do not hire this type of trainer. Training sessions should be about you, your safety, and your goals.

If you have any special needs (for example, surgeries, sore joints, or known muscle imbalances), be sure to ask if the trainer has credentials and experience with these situations. You also want to ask about the payment structure and make sure that suits your needs. In the end, a good trainer should be extremely transparent so that the client-trainer relationship works for everyone.

It's not as scary as it sounds once you ask the right questions. Realize, too, that you don't need a personal trainer forever. It is a great tool to have, but if you just want some instruction from time to time, personal trainers can assist with that, too.

Developing an Exercise Program

With or without a trainer, you need to develop an exercise program. The most important thing to keep in mind is that every program should be individualized. Everyone's goals are different, and that is extremely important to consider.

A person new to exercise will have a different plan than an elite collegiate athlete or a power lifter. And as research into the science and application of sports science grows, new insights will emerge.

The American College of Sports Medicine (ACSM) guidelines take into account the recommendations of experts across many disciplines, such as exercise science, physiology, athletic training, and medicine. The ACSM recommends lifting weights a minimum of two to three days per week if you use a full-body workout. But if you really enjoy strength training, you can easily spread it out over four or more days per week and change up the order of the muscle groups you exercise each time. Training each major muscle group twice per week is sufficient.

What fits into your schedule now? If it is only exercising one day per week, then doing it one day per week is great. Over time, you can add more days, time, and intensity to your training once you get the hang of it all.

It is recommended to start with 1 to 3 sets of exercises that target each major muscle group. Aim for 8 to 12 repetitions—for example, back, chest, glutes, shoulders, arms, and legs. Often, beginning with machines instead of using free weights is your best bet because they help reinforce proper alignment and form and might be safer until you feel more comfortable with the process.

As you begin to get more comfortable and advanced with your program and your goals become even more specific, your goals can become better defined, and you'll want to develop a specific plan tailored to help you meet those goals.

For example, when designing a plan to build muscle mass or improve muscle quality, there are a few things to think about and include that are unique to these plans.

- Muscular strength is a measure of how much force your muscles can produce in one effort. To improve strength, you want to do 5 to 8 repetitions at a weight that progresses up to about 80 percent of your maximal strength for 1 repetition, or 1 RM. Think higher weight and low to moderate reps for 3 sets.

- Muscular endurance ultimately leads to hypertrophy, or the increase in the muscle fiber size. For muscular endurance/hypertrophy, you would use a lower weight, roughly 65 to 85 percent of your 1 RM— for 8 to 12 repetitions and 1 to 3 sets.

- Muscular power is the amount of work performed per unit of time. This is a quick movement. Aim for a heavy load, typically more than 90 percent of your 1 RM and with only 1 to 4 repetitions.

To increase your muscle mass, you're going to have to put in effort when you're at the gym. If you like to lift and do aerobic exercise, that's great. And don't worry about whether you do cardio or resistance training first when you work out; it's based on personal preference.

Types of Routines

Assuming that you want to lift weights, you might think you should do a total-body routine or split the body segments up and work your legs one day and your upper body on a second day. But many other variations exist, such as lifting your chest and triceps on day one; then back, biceps, and shoulders on day two; and legs on day three. It can be confusing without proper guidance.

To settle this argument, researchers recruited 20 resistance-trained young men and had them perform 2 to 3 sets of 8 to 12 reps for a total of 18 sets per session for 8 weeks. They used either a one-day-per-week split-body routine, where multiple exercises were done for 2 to 3 muscle groups per session; or a three-day-per-week total-body routine, where one exercise was performed per muscle group per session with all muscle groups trained.

The researchers tested the upper- and lower-body strength and muscle size. After 8 weeks, there were no differences (except for greater increases in the size of the forearm flexors) in the total-body routine compared to the split-body routine.

Select a resistance-training program that you like and can stick to—one that you think is fun and keeps you engaged. The chances of you continuing this kind of program are probably far greater than if you follow some plan that you don't think is fun.

Blood Flow Restriction

There are other techniques that are now becoming common that are designed to help optimize muscle protein synthesis and muscle growth. If you're working with a trainer, you can discuss whether any of these would work well for you.

One of these is called blood flow restriction, or occlusion training. Essentially, you perform low-intensity resistance training—only about 20 percent of your one-repetition maximum. You do this while also occluding blood flow with a tourniquet, or tight wrap.

This type of training has many proposed benefits—from improved endurance during aerobic exercise, to increased muscle protein synthesis through one of the main growth-promoting signaling proteins, to the recruitment of more muscle fibers during an exercise. Some research has even shown occlusion training to increase growth hormone, which might result in beneficial physiological outcomes.

Supporters of occlusion training say that it can produce the same responses as if you were lifting heavy weights due to the buildup up of some specific metabolites, such as adenosine monophosphate, inorganic phosphate, and lactate, as well as the depletion of phosphocreatine and a decrease in muscle pH, meaning increased acidity, or muscle "burn."

It's not really any better than traditional training. It can be added as a supplement but shouldn't replace your normal training regimen. You might use it when you are injured and can't lift the same weight as usual. This way, you can still use light weight and get pretty good muscular adaptations.

Try This

See if you can find a great personal trainer and start lifting weights at least one time per week.

Questions to Consider

1. How will you incorporate resistance training into your exercise routine?

2. How can you modify gym-based routines for exercises at home?

Exercise for Healthy Muscle Mass

In this lecture, I want to tackle one of the most widely discussed, and often misguided, topics of interest in this field, muscle. I'll go over why you want to increase muscle mass and how to do it and also how to properly maintain it and the health benefits of doing so, especially as we age. We'll also talk about why lifting weights won't make you bulky, which is one of the most common reasons that clients, especially female clients, tell me they don't lift weights.

In this lecture, we'll cover why this doesn't automatically occur if you lift weights. Now, you may think that lifting weights is only for teenagers, bodybuilders, and athletes, but you're mistaken. Maintaining muscle is not only important for these individuals, but for a person of any age or ability. Research has repeatedly shown that it can help prevent clinical chronic disease like osteoporosis and Type 2 Diabetes. It also is a major factor in allowing you to move around and maintain your independence. You need at least enough muscle mass to walk unassisted, to get out of a chair, and to carry groceries. The best part about lifting weights is that there are no age restrictions.

Now, you may need a modification of an exercise or two but that is where a certified personal trainer can come into play and show you proper form to prevent injury, and make any changes you may need to accommodate any physical limitation. I'll talk about finding a personal trainer a little later in this lecture. Just look up people like Ernestine Shepherd who began to lift weights at age 56 and started competing as a competitive bodybuilder in her 70s. We are also going to talk about the type, the volume, frequency, and intensity of exercise that induce hypertrophy, or muscle growth, and some mechanisms that induce these changes, and we'll explore some of the new schools of training that are becoming increasingly popular. Sound good? All right, let's get into it.

As we age, an interesting phenomenon called Sarcopenia occurs, which is the natural, progressive loss of muscle mass as we grow older. How fast does this happen? Studies have shown that between the ages of 40 and 50 years old, we can lose more than 8% of our muscle mass, and that can accelerate to more than 15% per decade after the age of 75 if measures are not taken to prevent it. Fortunately, there's a lot we can do to slow this process down. Most people think that aging alone causes us to lose muscle. But now, research is clearly showing that it's not simply aging, but more the lack of physical activity that is the major player here.

One study looked at people who were life-long exercisers to determine if chronic exercise could prevent the loss of muscle mass and strength in aging adults. They took 20 men and 20 women between the ages of 40 and 81 years old who exercised at least 4 to 5 times per week and competed as triathletes. These older athletes were put through a series of tests to study their health, their strength, and their body composition using magnetic resonance imaging or MRI technology. MRI gives us an amazing view of the fat and muscle that you have in specific regions of your body. This study used it on the quadriceps muscles of the thigh to look at muscle quality.

As you might expect, the younger people in the study did have a lower body mass index, or BMI, and lower body fat percentage compared to older athletes. But, the fascinating part is that the lean muscle mass and strength were no different between the younger and the older athletes. What's more is that these benefits were similar in both men and women. This highlights the fact that long-term exercise training can aid in preserving muscle mass. It may also prevent increases in body fat as we age. Plus, this study helps to debunk a common myth by showing that aging alone doesn't cause the dramatic drop in muscle mass that we often see—rather, it's the chronic disuse and inactivity that are primarily to blame.

One of the most interesting people to discuss is a man who is a prime example of how exercise, and a healthy diet can improve your muscle mass and quality of life. He's John Nagy. Mr. Nagy is a participant in the Physical Activity Centre of Excellence at McMaster University in Canada. What makes him so unique is that not only does he exercise vigorously, but he is also

97 years old. Yes, you heard me right, 97. A recent interview described his daily routine like this: his warm-up begins with movements in the shower, followed by floor, and ball exercises for his core and his back. He'll then walk to the University—2 miles each way—or make up for it on his treadmill, followed by a 90-minute workout at the University. He also keeps dumbbells, resistance bands, and a Swiss Ball in his apartment next to the treadmill, and a stationary bike. Pretty impressive, right? Mr. Nagy embodies the idea of using regular exercise to maintain his quality of life; to stay able bodied so that he can live to the fullest. Just like Ernestine Shepherd. Maybe we should all take a page, or maybe a few chapters, out of their books.

But, what about adding muscle mass with exercise? Maybe you noticed that you've lost quite a bit of strength or function and want it back, or maybe you just think exercise for muscle mass is the right step for you now. It turns out that resistance training, or lifting weights, adds muscle, too, if you specifically plan your program with muscle gain as one of your goals. In another study, we put 24 men who were familiar with lifting weights in a periodized resistance-training program 3 times per week for 6 weeks. During this training program, the subjects consumed either a placebo or a multi-ingredient performance supplement containing whey protein, casein protein, branched chain amino acids, creatine, beta-alanine, and caffeine. Both groups of participants took their supplement—either the placebo or the multi-ingredient performance supplement—both before and after exercise. Now, you might be asking what periodized resistance training means. This means that the exercise was systematically designed to change the amount of weight lifted and the volume of training. The goal of the exercise was to improve strength and muscle size. Basically, they all lifted 3-days-per-week and every two weeks the subjects lifted more weight for fewer repetitions in order to meet the goals of the training plan.

Subjects in both groups improved body composition, showing us that the training plan worked. But, the subjects who also supplemented with the multi-ingredient supplement increased lean mass more and lost a little bit more fat—although not statistically more—than the group that did resistance training alone that is, those who drank the placebo. Other great news was that by doing resistance exercise, both groups improved their upper and lower body strength and some measures of power. This is extremely important. Data show that as you age, the importance of strength is critical. In fact, just being stronger in your chest and legs is associated with the least risk of premature death. What this shows is that resistance training must be included in your exercise program and that there may be some nutritional supplements that can help even more with improving body composition and performance.

All too often in this area of research, women get excluded from studies. I'd like to shed some light on part of the reasoning for this. It is mainly due to the hormone fluctuations that females go through month-to-month before menopause, which can influence certain variables that are measured. In order to minimize these variations, studies that include women typically track menstrual cycles so that the pre- and post-testing are completed about a month apart and during the same phase of the cycle. This way hormone levels will stay at as consistent a level as possible. With that said, more and more nutrition and exercise research is being done with female subjects.

You can also test postmenopausal women to minimize hormonal fluctuations. For example, in one of our collaborative studies, we explored the extent to which nutrition, resistance training, or the combination could improve body composition in obese postmenopausal women. The results showed that resistance training alone improved strength but not muscle mass, whereas diet alone lost a significant amount of weight, but it was from both fat and muscle mass. However, the diet plus resistance training combo improved most variables, including a loss of body weight from fat mass specifically and they were also able to maintain muscle mass and improve strength—just as a diet and resistance exercise combination did in the study with male subjects. So for those women out there that are afraid of looking too big and muscular, this study should help you realize that it's physiologically impossible to look like you're on steroids unless, well, you're on steroids. So resistance training is needed for both women and men.

Overall, we see time and time again that in order to optimize your health and performance, it's the combination of both nutrition and exercise that creates a synergistic effect to induce the greatest amount of positive change.

This is true particularly if you are overweight. The example I often give is that if you are a large pear-shaped individual, long-slow cardio will likely make you a smaller pear-shaped individual. The reason for this is that while yes, you are likely decreasing body fat, you are also losing a bit of muscle along with it—so your lean mass to fat mass ratio stays relatively the same because they are both lower. However, if you add dynamic weight lifting to your plan, you can actually change your body shape entirely by building lean mass and decreasing fat. Now, this isn't spot reducing; this is actually changing your entire body shape as you work to lose fat and build muscle. I've seen this over and over in our research and while working directly with clients.

Another important factor to note is that even with the training program lasting three months or more, these women did not transform into walking around like the Hulk. In a study that we published last year in the *Journal of Applied Physiology*, we found the 16 weeks of resistance training plus protein intake resulted in maintenance of muscle mass but no increase or decrease. So add resistance training to your routine. It's the addition of weights to your exercise routine that truly transforms your body.

Now, that you know exercise can maintain or improve muscle mass in both the young and the elderly across different training statuses, you are probably wondering what specifically you should do in order to increase your muscle mass? As with most well designed exercise training programs, you should have a balance between strength and endurance training with your ultimate goal the key factor here in how much or how little of each of these that you do. You know the difference between low-intensity steady state aerobic exercise and HIIT training, and the benefits of both.

Considering that most of the very best athletes on earth hire a coach or trainer, you might want to consider hiring a personal trainer too. If you are an elite athlete or a brand new person to exercise, hiring a personal trainer or coach is a great way to start or work on a new goal or to prepare for a race or competition. This way you can try new exercises, avoid injury, and learn about your exercise and lifting options, and figure out how to lift safely while also working around past injuries. But, how do you even begin the process of choosing a personal trainer? The first step is to figure out if you want to work out in a gym setting or have a personal trainer come to your house. Both are great options, and you just need to find what suits your lifestyle, personality, goals, and budget. Some trainers offer gentle encouragement, and others have an in-your-face style and try to motivate you. The last thing you want is someone giving you mild mannered instruction when you know that does nothing to motivate you. And likewise, you don't want a drill sergeant type if you respond best to gentle and persistent encouragement. Personal trainers should also be held to some educational and certification standards.

Some good certifications to look for are from the National Strength and Conditioning Association, or NSCA, and include Certified Strength and Conditioning Specialists and Certified Personal Trainers. Other excellent certifications include those from the American College of Sports Medicine, or ACSM, The National Academy of Sports Medicine, or NASM, the American Council on Exercise, or ACE, and the Aerobics and Fitness Association of America, or AFAA. Just like any skilled profession, referrals help you decide too. Trainers should be able to provide you with some contact information for people they have trained with similar goals. And besides asking about what certifications they have, or if they have advanced education in exercise physiology or a related field, ask about how they measure your success and how they progress clients? Observe them with another client and see how they behave. One of my all-time pet peeves is watching a trainer ignore a client and mindlessly count repetitions while busily texting or talking on the phone. Do not hire this type of trainer. Training sessions should be about you, your safety, and your goals.

If you have any special needs; for example, surgeries, sore joints, or known muscle imbalances, be sure to ask if he or she has credentials and experience with these situations. Of course, you also want to ask about the payment structure and make sure that suits your needs as well. In the end, a good trainer should be extremely transparent so that the client-trainer relationship works for everyone. I promise it's not as scary as it sounds once you ask the right questions. Realize too, that you don't need a personal trainer forever. It's a great tool to have, but if you just want some instruction from time to time, personal trainers can assist with that too. With or without a trainer, you need to develop an exercise program. The most important thing to keep in mind is that every program should be individualized. Everyone's goals are different and that is extremely important to consider. A person new to exercise will have a different plan than an elite collegiate athlete, a weekend warrior, or a power lifter. And, as research into the science and application of sports science grows, new insights will emerge.

So let's start by looking at the American College of Sports Medicine—ACSM—guidelines, which takes into account the recommendations of experts across many disciplines like exercise science, physiology, athletic training, and medicine. ACSM recommends lifting weights a minimum of 2 to 3 days per week if you use a full-body workout. But, if you really enjoy strength training, you can easily spread it out over 4 or more days per week and change up the order of the muscle groups you exercise each time. We'll talk more about this in just a minute, but for now, just know that training each major muscle group twice per week is sufficient. To begin, ask yourself what fits into your schedule now? If it is only one day per week, great, then do it one day per week. Over time, you can add more days, time, and intensity to your training once you get the hang of it all.

It is recommended to start with 1 to 3 sets of exercises that target each major muscle group. Aim for 8 to 12 repetitions and just think about you back, your chest, and your glutes, shoulders, your arms, and legs; for example. Often times, beginning with machines instead of using free-weights is your best bet because they help to reinforce proper alignment and form, and may be safer until you feel more comfortable with the process. As you begin to get more comfortable and advanced with your program, and your goals become even more specific, your goals can get better and more defined, and you'll want to develop a specific plan tailored to help you meet those goals. For example, when designing a plan to build muscle mass or improve muscle quality, there are a few things to think about and include that are unique to these plans.

Muscular strength is a measure of how much force your muscles can produce in one effort. To improve strength, you want to do 5 to 8 repetitions at a weight that progresses up to 80% of your maximal strength for 1 repetition, or 1 RM. Think higher weight, low to moderate reps, for 3 sets. For example, if you can lift 100 lb, or 46 kg, on the bench press then you would start with about 65–70 lb, or 29-31 kg, and work up to using around 80 lb, or 36 kg, for 5 to 8 repetitions. You would repeat this 2 more times before switching exercises.

The second type of muscular training is muscular endurance, which ultimately leads to hypertrophy, or the increase in muscle fiber size. For muscular endurance and hypertrophy, you would use a lower weight, roughly 65–85% of your 1 RM, and 8 to 12 repetitions for 1 to 3 sets. Again, if you can do a 1 RM bench press of 100 lb, or 46 kg, you would use 65 lb, or 29 kg, and do more repetitions—up toward 12 or more—to improve muscular endurance and optimize muscle growth.

The third type of muscular training is called muscular power, which is the amount of work performed per unit of time. This is a quick movement. There are two strategies—the most traditional is to aim for a heavy load, typically over 90% of your 1 RM, and with only 1 to 4 repetitions. Again, using our example of 1 RM bench press of 100 lb, or 46 kg, you would lift 90–95 lb, or 41–43 kg, for just 1 to 2 reps. You would likely take long breaks between sets with this style of lifting. Alternatively, because muscular power is based on how fast the movement can be completed, you can also use a light load—it could even be your body weight—or a load that is somewhere around 50% of 1 RM and then perform the movement fast. Of course, the style you choose is based on your goals, and working with a coach is highly recommended given the technical aspects of doing this safely. The main idea is to move the load as fast as possible.

So you can see that in order to increase your muscle mass, you're going to have to put in the effort when you're at the gym. If you like to lift and to do aerobic exercise, then great, and don't worry too much about whether you do cardio or resistance training first when you work out, it's based on personal preference. Let's assume you want to lift weights. You might think you should do a total body routine or split the body segments up into working your legs one day and your upper body on a second day. But, many other variations exist like chest and triceps on day one, then back, biceps, and shoulders on day two, and legs on day three. It can be confusing without proper guidance. Well, to settle this argument, researchers recruited 20 resistance-trained young men and had them perform 2 to 3 sets of 8 to 12 repetitions for a total of 18 sets per session for 8 weeks. They used either a one-day per week split-body routine where multiple exercises were done for 2 to 3 muscle groups per session, or a 3 day per week total body routine where one exercise was performed per muscle group per session with all muscle groups trained. The researchers tested the upper and lower body strength and muscle size. After 8 weeks, there were absolutely no differences, except for greater increases in the size of the forearm flexors, in the total-body routine compared to the split-body routine. So my suggestion is that you select a resistance-training program that you like, and you can stick to—one that you think is fun and keeps you engaged. The chances of you continuing this sort of program are probably far greater than if you follow some plan that you don't think is fun.

There are also other techniques that are now becoming common that are designed to help optimize muscle protein synthesis and muscle growth. If you're working with a trainer, you can discuss whether any of these would work well for you. One in particular is called blood flow restriction, or occlusion training. So what is it? Essentially, you perform low-intensity resistance training, and by low-intensity I mean really low—only about 20% of your 1 repetition maximum. You do this while also occluding blood flow with a tourniquet or tight wrap. Does this sound more like a torture device than an exercise routine? Well, what's interesting about this type of training is that it does have many proposed benefits. These range from improved endurance training during aerobic exercise such as walking; to increased muscle protein synthesis through one of the main growth promoting signaling proteins called mTOR; to the recruitment of more muscle fibers during exercise. Some research has even shown occlusion training to increase growth hormone, which may influence many beneficial physiological outcomes.

Supporters of occlusion training say it can produce the same responses if you were to lift heavy weights due to the buildup up of some specific metabolites like adenosine monophosphate, inorganic phosphate, and lactate, as well as the depletion of phosphocreatine and a decrease in muscle pH meaning increased acidity or muscle burn. Is it any better than doing traditional training, though? The short answer is not really. It can be added as a supplement, but it shouldn't replace your normal training program. In my opinion, you might use it when you are injured and can't lift the same weight as usual. This way you can still use light weight and get a pretty good muscular adaptation.

So now you know how to maintain and/or increase muscle mass and a few ways to do it for the young and old, and for women and men. There are a ton of exercises and routines that you can perform to achieve an increase in muscle mass. You just have to find what works best for you. It has to be fun, motivating, challenging, and safe. If your exercises are fun, you will be far more likely to stick to the program. Evidence also shows that you'll be more likely to choose healthy eating habits when you enjoy your workout. So now you have all this information about lifting weights, and I hope that you're convinced that you must add this to your workout plan. The key to finding what works best for you is to continue to explore new types of exercise and training styles.

Keep in mind that for real changes to occur you're going to have to sweat and that means pushing yourself and putting in hard work. It also means you're going to have to pay attention to what you eat and how you fuel yourself to feel better, look better, and perform better. What this will do is change your body composition by helping you lose fat mass and increase muscle mass. This is the one-two punch combination that will lead to the most optimal improvements in body composition. Again, we need to shift to a mindset of body composition, not body weight. Try this, see if you can find a great personal trainer and start lifting weights at least one time per week.

Hormones and Body Composition

Your nutrition, exercise, normal physiological processes, and body composition could not occur without the help of hormones, or chemical messengers that act on specific target organs and tissues to cause cellular responses. These responses are essential to help you gain muscle and lose fat. In this lecture, you will learn about hormonal influences on body composition and consider the uncontrollable factors of sex differences and aging changes as well as the controllable factors of diet and exercise.

Insulin

- Insulin is one of the more commonly known hormones. This is because of the huge prevalence of diabetes in the United States and globally. Insulin acts on the liver, fat tissue, and muscles and is one of many hormones required for human growth and development.

- Insulin's main function is to help regulate blood sugar levels. After you eat and your blood sugar begins to rise, the beta cells of your pancreas secrete insulin, which help take glucose out of your blood and put it into cells, where it can be stored or used as energy. At the same time, insulin releases signals to your brain that you are fed, and this can act like a satiety signal, which help you feel full.

- Insulin is a storage hormone. It not only stores sugar, but it also helps you store fat. When insulin is released, it activates an enzyme called lipoprotein lipase, which not only moves fat into fat cells for storage, but also simultaneously inhibits lipolysis (fat breakdown).

- Insulin can also increase your ability to add muscle mass. This is because insulin-stimulated glucose uptake into muscle cells also enhances muscle protein synthesis by increasing the transport of amino acids into your muscles. When insulin is released, you essentially go into "storage" mode rather than "burn" mode and turn off your ability to use fat as a fuel.

Very high-carbohydrate meals tend to raise insulin levels the highest. Also, the glycemic index, or the relative amount that a food raises your blood glucose, can predict your insulin response. The higher the glycemic index of the carbohydrate, the more it will raise insulin.

This acute rise in insulin is normal and really not a problem; your body handles it, and then blood glucose and insulin will return to lower concentrations. However, if you constantly bombard your system with overloads of high-carbohydrate meals, your insulin levels will always be high. This means that you are likely spending more time in fat-storing mode than fat-burning mode.

If this pattern continues for long periods of time, you might become insulin resistant. This is when your cells don't respond to the insulin well, so your blood sugar is not as well controlled and your body is forced to produce more and more insulin to have the same impact on reducing your blood glucose levels.

It is best to avoid massive swings in insulin concentrations. Instead, aim to keep your insulin levels stable by consuming most of your carbohydrates as vegetables and whole grains. These foods tend to have lower glycemic index values—meaning that they don't raise your blood glucose very much when you eat them when compared to sweets, some breads, or juice, which have high glycemic index values.

Protein and fat can also influence insulin, but not to the same extent as carbohydrates. So, it might be beneficial to think about building your typical meal as protein first, good-quality fats and vegetables next, and then other low glycemic index carbohydrates.

Cortisol

Cortisol, commonly known as the stress hormone, is often blamed for weight gain, poor health, and a slew of other headline-friendly half-truths. But the truth is that cortisol is actually very important to our overall health, helping our bodies have a healthy response to physical stressors as well as other life stressors, such as crying children, deadlines, and traffic.

Cortisol is produced and released from the adrenal glands as part of a complex pathway known as the hypothalamic-pituitary-adrenal (HPA) axis.

The cortisol that is released in response to normal daily patterns, or even to stress, is very useful for us metabolically. It helps us use our stored glucose, fat, and protein as energy to deal with the stresses we perceive. Additionally, cortisol can temporarily improve brain and immune function to help you overcome a fear, meet a deadline, or try new exercises.

Cortisol also helps to decrease inflammation, which is why you might have cortisone injections into knees, wrists, and other problematic areas as you age. In fact, certain autoimmune disorders, such as rheumatoid arthritis, have been linked to a suppressed HPA axis and chronically low cortisol levels.

Cortisol acts pretty fast. After roughly 30 minutes, cortisol will begin to degrade, and the HPA axis will stop releasing it. So, the cortisol response to an acute stress like exercise is really not all that long and is quite useful.

Very high levels of cortisol over a long time can lead to fat storage, particularly in your visceral fat, surrounding your organs. Chronically high cortisol is also linked to psychological factors, such as depression, anxiety, and grief, and to physical factors, such as extreme levels of exercise combined with little rest and recovery.

In these situations, not only are changes in your metabolism occurring, but your immune system might also become weak. This is why many people associate high stress or extreme exercise over a long period of time with a greater occurrence of sickness.

Even though exercise and other stressors can temporarily increase cortisol and cortisol in chronically elevated situations is associated with fat storage, any change in body weight or body fat is probably due to the fact that many people deal with these stresses by eating more and making bad food choices.

Normal levels of exercise are not likely to cause chronically high levels of cortisol. In fact, exercising for about an hour per day should help keep cortisol levels within normal ranges.

Catecholamines

In response to stress, exercise, or a frightening situation, many other hormones can be released. Two of these hormones are called the catecholamines, and they are also important contributors to body composition changes.

If you are walking through the woods and a bear walks out in front of you, your body immediately and automatically prepares you to deal with the situation. We refer to this as a "fight-or-flight response."

In this situation, two hormones called epinephrine and norepinephrine are secreted in high amounts into the blood. Together, these hormones are called catecholamines. They immediately provide glucose from breaking down stored glycogen and fat to your muscles so that you can either fight or run away.

These same responses will occur when you begin to ramp up the intensity of exercise. With intense exercise, catecholamines will be released, and you will likely notice that your heart rate and respiratory rate will increase to improve blood flow and deliver oxygen to active organs and tissues so that you can have a better fight-or-flight response.

Catecholamines will also begin to break down stored body fat when they interact with specific receptors called adrenergic receptors, or adrenoceptors, which are receptors that respond specifically to the catecholamines.

Because exercise and catecholamines both lead to lipolysis, or fat breakdown, exercise can be effective at burning fat as a fuel.

One way to begin to change your body composition is to simply exercise regularly. This way, you take advantage of the catecholamine response that occurs and will lead to the breakdown of fat. But nutrition must also be considered here, along with the type and intensity of exercise being done.

A long, slow training session would likely have the lowest catecholamine response, and if you combine this with too much food pre-exercise, during-exercise, or postexercise, then you will likely have little fat loss.

But if you work out intensely with enough fuel to go all out but not too much that you stop lipolysis, you might have a great recipe for burning fat—in part because you have elevated your catecholamines the most with this type of workout.

This is a trial-and-error process, though. You have to experiment with your food and your workouts to see how it makes you feel and if your body composition begins to improve over time. Then, you simply adjust accordingly to continue your path toward your optimal body composition.

Remember, too, that if you exercise at an intense level, you might also be setting yourself up best to burn calories even after your exercise bout is finished. This "after burn" effect can last from just minutes to 24 hours, depending on your exercise intensity.

Thyroid

The thyroid hormones also have a powerful influence on metabolism, body composition, and health. They might be the most misunderstood hormones when it comes to body composition.

Contrary to popular belief, while thyroid problems can certainly contribute to weight gain or even weight loss, the situations where this is the primary reason for weight change are pretty rare, particularly when considering the excellent advances in medications for diagnosed thyroid problems.

The thyroid hormones are produced by the thyroid gland, located in the front of your neck. The two hormones released from the thyroid gland are called thyroxine (T_4) and triiodothyronine (T_3). These unique messengers affect most bodily functions and influence nearly every tissue in your body throughout your entire life.

The thyroid hormones regulate body temperature and are required for efficient metabolism, normal growth and development, and the actions of many other hormones. Without normal levels of thyroid hormones and growth hormone, for example, infants and children experience growth and developmental problems.

Because the thyroid hormones are involved in many metabolic processes, they also play a role in maintaining and increasing your resting metabolic rate and production of body heat—a process called thermogenesis. Heat production is another process that uses energy and can influence your body composition over time.

Many of the bodily functions that thyroid hormones influence expend energy, and we need to replenish that energy by eating. Normally, T_3 will increase energy expenditure after we eat, or "burn more calories," as our food is broken down and transported to various cells within the body. This can help regulate weight when the thyroid hormones are within a normal range.

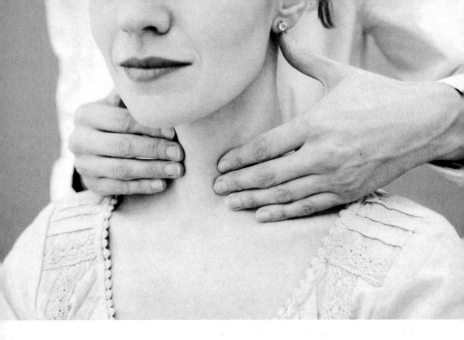

We need to have normal T_3 levels to be healthy in a number of ways. Unfortunately, some people experience chronically low levels of T_3 and T_4, which is called hypothyroidism. In this circumstance, weight gain is likely. If the opposite occurs and T_3 and T_4 are chronically high, this is called hyperthyroidism and would likely result in weight loss.

If you are taking medication for diagnosed hypothyroidism, then your levels are normal because of the thyroid medication that your physician has prescribed.

Your body is capable of maintaining a healthy body composition with smart exercise and quality nutrition, as long as your thyroid levels are regulated.

Hormones, Gender, and Age

Men naturally have more lean muscle compared to women, while women tend to have more total body fat. This is often explained by the location of body fat and the unique reproductive function needs for women. This higher level of fat and lower level of muscle in women typically means that women have metabolic rates that are about 5 to 10 percent lower than men of the same height and weight because muscle mass is more metabolically active. This might explain some of the gender discrepancies in metabolism.

In addition, women are 5 to 8 times more likely to develop hypothyroidism compared to men, which, if not treated, may lead to weight gain. The prevalence of hypothyroidism increases with age, too, affecting about 9 percent of men and women over the age of 60 years old. This might have implications for weight gain in later years, because a decrease in thyroid hormones slows metabolic rate if not treated with medication.

Additionally, decreased muscle mass and strength occurs as we get older, resulting from a gradual loss (about 5 to 10 percent per decade) of skeletal muscle after the age of 30. But these massive changes to body composition only occur if you choose not to exercise or eat properly. In fact, there is other evidence that shows excellent muscle mass quality and function in those who are lifelong exercisers and athletes.

Try This

Limit your intake of added sugars and sugar-sweetened beverages to control your insulin levels, hunger, and body composition.

Questions to Consider

1. What are the primary hormones responsible for dictating body composition?

2. What myths were put to rest in this lecture?

Hormones and Body Composition

When hormones are working properly, life seems to move along, as it should. But, if there are any kinks in the hormonal system, chaos could closely follow—anything from overeating, or under eating, to storing fat, disturbed sleep patterns, or even the inability to feel alert. Hormones control your body and its actions. It all starts in your brain with the hypothalamus and the pituitary glands. These glands are constantly sending out and receiving signals that will adjust how much and what type of hormones the organs like your pancreas, your kidneys, adrenal glands, and thyroid will produce.

These hormones are what keep your body's internal environment stable—what we call homeostasis. For example, if your blood pressure rises, certain hormones send a signal to your brain that will cause a relaxation of your blood vessels, and help bring your blood pressure back to normal. Many times the same thing happens if you have dramatic changes in your body weight—your body resists these changes in order to keep your internal system steady that is, to maintain the body's homeostasis.

You can think about the endocrine system as the thermostat of your body. If your house gets too hot or too cold, the thermostat kicks on and controls the temperature. It's the same way with your body, the endocrine system, and your regulatory hormones. The role of your endocrine system is huge. Have you ever heard people say things like, "My thyroid levels are low that's why I've gained so much weight." Is it true? Are hormones really to blame for all of your perceived body composition issues? In order to answer those questions, let's rewind.

Think about all of the other things your body does for you on a daily basis. Without you even thinking about it blood continues to pump through your veins, and oxygen flows through your lungs, immune cells help to fight off infection, and the kidneys filter out harmful substances from circulation. And what is the common link between your nutrition, your exercise, you're your normal physiological processes, and your body composition? The answer is that these processes could not occur without the help of hormones or chemical messengers that act on specific target organs and tissues to help cause cellular responses. And, as we've discussed, these responses are essential to help you gain muscle and lose fat.

The hormones that initiate these cellular processes are complex and play a critical role in the regulation of metabolism and maintenance of body composition. Your physique and overall health are strongly influenced by certain controllable factors, like diet and physical activity. However, some things beyond your control also contribute to body shape and size, such as genetics, your race or ethnicity, sex, and age. In this lecture I'll talk about hormonal influences on body composition, consider the uncontrollable factors of sex differences, and aging changes, and the controllable factors like diet and exercise. There are many different hormones that we can talk about, but this lecture will focus on insulin, cortisol, catecholamines, and the thyroid hormones.

There are many hormones that can play a role in your ability to store or burn fat, or make you feel hungry or full. Let's start with one I mentioned earlier and that you've probably heard of—insulin. Insulin is one of the more commonly known hormones—this is because of the huge prevalence of diabetes in the United States and globally. Insulin acts on the liver, fat tissue, and muscles, and is one of many hormones required for human growth and development. Insulin's main function is to help regulate blood sugar levels. After you eat and your blood sugar begins to rise; the beta cells of your pancreas secrete insulin, which helps take glucose out of your blood and put it into the cells where it can be stored or used as energy. At the same time, insulin releases signals to your brain that you are fed and this can act like a satiety signal, which will help you feel full. Insulin is a storage hormone. It wants to store everything.

So, not only does it store sugar, but it also helps you store fat. When insulin is released it activates an enzyme called lipoprotein lipase, or LPL, which not only moves fat into fat cells for storage, but it simultaneously inhibits lipolysis, or fat breakdown. This is designed so that you have a storage depot to draw energy from during times when you're not eating. Evolutionarily speaking, human beings could not always just walk into a grocery store and buy food when they were hungry so it really acts as a protection or survival mechanism. Insulin has another role too—it can increase your ability to add muscle mass. This is because insulin-stimulated glucose uptake into muscle cells also enhances muscle protein synthesis by increasing the transport of amino acids into your muscles. So, when insulin is released, you essentially go into storage mode rather than burning mode and turn off your ability to use fat as a fuel.

Now, let's consider this in relation to what you eat. Very high carbohydrate meals tend to raise insulin levels to the highest level. Also, the glycemic index or the relative amount that a food raises your blood glucose level, can predict your insulin response. The higher the glycemic index of the carbohydrate the more it will raise insulin. This acute rise in insulin is normal and really not a problem. Your body handles it, and then blood glucose and insulin will return to lower concentrations. However, if you constantly bombard your system with overloads of high carbohydrate meals, your insulin will always be high. This means that you're likely spending more time in fat storing mode than you are in fat burning mode. If this pattern continues for long periods of time, you may become insulin resistant. This is when your cells don't respond to the insulin well, so your blood sugar is not as well controlled and your body is forced to produce more and more insulin to have the same impact on reducing your blood glucose levels.

So, yes, we need insulin and it is critical to our health and survival. However, it is best to avoid massive swings in insulin concentrations. Instead, aim to keep your insulin levels stable by consuming most of your carbohydrates as vegetables or whole grains. These foods tend to have lower glycemic index values, meaning they don't raise your blood glucose very much when you eat them compared to sweets, some breads, or juice, which all have higher glycemic index values. Protein and fat can also influence insulin, but not to the same extent as carbohydrates. So it may be beneficial to think about building your typical meal as protein first, good quality fats and vegetables next, and then other low glycemic index carbohydrates. This may seem like a lot to think about, but don't let it stress you out because next we'll talk about the stress hormone, cortisol, and the many reasons why it is important to understand.

Cortisol, commonly known as the stress hormone, is often blamed for weight gain, poor health, and a slew of other headline friendly half-truths. But, the truth is that cortisol is actually very important to our overall health, helping our bodies to have a healthy response to physical stressors as well as other life stressors like crying children, deadlines, or even traffic. Cortisol is produced and released from the adrenal glands as part of a complex pathway known as the hypothalamic-pituitary-adrenal axis, or HPA axis.

One interesting thing about cortisol, and many hormones, is that it is released according to your circadian rhythm. This means that it follows a pattern based on the time of day. It is highest in the morning to help with wakefulness and to help provide energy after the overnight fast, and it is lowest at night, allowing for rest and recovery. The cortisol that is released in response to normal daily patterns, or even to stress, is actually very useful for us metabolically. It helps us to use our stored glucose, fat, and protein as energy to deal with the stresses we perceive. Additionally, cortisol can temporarily improve brain and immune function to help you overcome a fear, meet a deadline, or try new exercises.

Cortisol also helps to decrease inflammation, which is why you might have cortisone injections into knees, wrists, or other problematic areas as you age. In fact, certain autoimmune disorders like rheumatoid arthritis have been linked to suppressed HPA axis activity and chronically low cortisol levels. Cortisol has been observed to act pretty fast. After roughly 30 minutes, cortisol will begin to degrade and the HPA axis will stop releasing it. So the cortisol response to an acute stress like exercise is really long and is quite useful. Also, cortisol is going to be produced in your body so even in a theoretical stress free environment you would still produce cortisol according to that circadian rhythm. In fact, if you had chronically low cortisol concentrations, there's a good chance you would feel uncomfortably tired and weak.

So, how would it become chronically elevated and is it making you store fat? In the nutrition and fitness world, the perception is that high cortisol equals high body fat. Well we know that in extreme clinical cases, like those who have Cushing's disease in which cortisol is very high all the time, fat gain is typically seen in the belly, or abdomen, in the face, and neck. In addition, with chronically high cortisol levels muscle can be broken down to provide energy. And over time you see how this would lead to less muscle and more fat. Well, less muscle and more fat is probably not the body composition change that you're going for.

So, yes, very high levels over a long time can lead to fat storage particularly in your visceral fat, the fat surrounding your organs. Chronically high cortisol is also linked to psychological factors like depression, anxiety, and grief, and to physical factors like extreme levels of exercise combined with little rest and recovery. In these situations, not only are changes in your metabolism occurring, but your immune system may also become weak. This is why many people associate high stress or extreme exercise over a long period of time with greater occurrence of sickness.

Even though exercise and other stressors can temporarily increase cortisol, and cortisol in chronically elevated situations is associated with fat storage, any change in body weight or body fat is probably due to the fact that many people deal with these stresses by eating more and making poor food choices. So don't shy away from physical activity. Normal levels of exercise are not likely to cause chronically high levels of cortisol. In fact, exercise for about an hour a day should help keep cortisol levels within normal ranges. The point is that cortisol must be present in your body. It is extremely helpful metabolically, and even if you are completely stress-free, your cortisol values won't drop dramatically. The issues with cortisol happen when cortisol is chronically elevated.

In response to stress, exercise, or a frightening situation, many other hormones can also be released. Two of these hormones are called the catecholamines, and they are important contributors to body composition changes. Let's pretend that you are taking a walk through the woods and a bear jumps out in front of you. In this situation, your body immediately and automatically does something really cool—it prepares you to deal with the situation as best it can. We refer to this as the fight or flight response. In this fight or flight situation, two hormones called epinephrine and norepinephrine will be secreted in high amounts into the blood. These hormones are produced in the adrenal glands, which are positioned on top of each kidney. The adrenal gland is composed of an outer layer called the cortex and an inner layer called the medulla. Epinephrine and norepinephrine produced are from the amino acid tyrosine in the medulla of the adrenal glands. Additionally, norepinephrine can also be produced directly from sympathetic nerve endings throughout your body.

Together, epinephrine and norepinephrine are called the catecholamines. They immediately provide glucose from breaking down stored glycogen and fat to your muscles so that you can either fight or run away. These same responses will occur when you begin to ramp up the intensity of exercise. With intense exercise, catecholamines will be released and you will likely notice that your heart rate and respiratory rate will increase to improve blood flow and deliver oxygen to the organs and tissues, again, so you can have a better fight or flight response.

Catecholamines will also begin to mobilize or breakdown stored body fat when they interact with specific receptors called adrenergic receptors, or adrenoceptors. Adrenergic receptors are receptors that respond specifically to the catecholamines. And because exercise and catecholamines both lead to lipolysis, or fat breakdown, it is easy to see why exercise can be effective at burning fat as a fuel. If you simply exercise regularly, you take advantage of the catecholamine response that occurs and will lead to the breakdown of fat. But, nutrition must also be considered here along with the type and intensity of exercise being done.

For example, a long slow training session would likely have the lowest catecholamine response, but if you work out intensely with enough fuel to go all-out, but not too much that you stop lipolysis, you may have a great recipe for fat burning in part because you have elevated your catecholamines the most with this type of workout. This is a trial and error process, though. You have to experiment with your food and your workouts then you simply adjust accordingly. Remember too that if you exercise at an intense level, you may also be setting yourself up to best burn calories even after an exercise bout is finished. This after burn effect can last from just a few minutes to 24 hours depending on your exercise intensity.

Just like the other hormones we've reviewed so far, the thyroid hormones also have a powerful influence on metabolism, body composition, and health. And they may be the most misunderstood hormones when it comes to body composition. How many of you have blamed your weight gain on a faulty thyroid hormone? I have heard this dozens of times, but the truth is that while thyroid problems can certainly contribute to weight gain, or even weight loss, the situations where this is the primary reason for weight change are pretty rare, particularly when considering the excellent advances in medications for diagnosed thyroid problems.

The thyroid hormones are, as expected, produced by the thyroid gland located in the front of your neck. The two hormones released from the thyroid gland are called thyroxine, or T_4, and triiodothyronine, which is T_3. T_4 is produced in greater amounts, but T_3 is the more biologically active thyroid hormone within the body. In other words, T_3 actually gets the job done. These unique messengers affect most bodily functions and influence nearly every tissue in your body throughout your entire life. Frankly, it would be easier to discuss what they don't do. In short, the thyroid hormones regulate body temperature, and are required for efficient metabolism, normal growth, and development, and for the actions of many other hormones. Without normal levels of thyroid hormones and growth hormone; for example, infants and children experience growth and developmental problems.

Because the thyroid hormones are involved in many metabolic processes, they also play a role in maintaining and increasing your resting metabolic rate and production of body heat in a process called thermogenesis. Heat production is another process that uses energy and can influence your body composition over time. Many of the bodily functions that thyroid hormones influence expend energy and we need to replenish that energy by eating. Normally, T_3 will increase energy expenditure after we eat or burn more calories, as our food is being broken down and transported to various cells within the body. This can help to regulate weight when the thyroid hormones are within a normal range. Now, it's clear that we need to have normal T_3 levels to be healthy in a number of ways.

Take, for example, a study in which obese individuals reportedly had higher concentrations of T_3, increased energy expenditure and metabolic rate. This correlation may sound odd to you. We just said that T_3 increases calories burned. You'd expect people who are obese to have lower concentrations of T_3. But, this increase in T_3 in these obese subjects may be an adaptive response to prevent further weight gain, and T_3 may be increased in an attempt to reduce the amount of energy being stored as fat.

On the other hand, T_3 has been shown to be very low in underweight subjects and during starvation, and this is likely your body's attempt to slow metabolism and conserve energy. These adaptations look like they are in place to reduce fat mass in the obese and preserve or increase fat in the underweight. It is simply a protective mechanism to maintain healthy body weight. Unfortunately, some people do experience chronically low levels of T_3 and T_4, which is called hypothyroidism. In this circumstance, weight gain is likely. If the opposite occurs and T_3 and T_4 are chronically high, this is called hyperthyroidism and would likely result in weight loss.

Now, I want to mention that in otherwise healthy individuals who are taking synthetic thyroid hormones, your doctor has likely brought your blood levels of T_3 and T_4 into normal ranges. So if you are taking medication for diagnosed hypothyroidism—or low thyroid—then you don't have your thyroid problem to blame for weight or fat gain anymore. Your levels are normal because of the thyroid medication that your physician has prescribed. As one endocrinologist that I know stated, "The rate of obesity does not match the rate of thyroid disorder diagnoses." Your body is perfectly capable of maintaining a healthy body composition with smart exercise and quality nutrition so long as your thyroid levels are regulated.

Now, understanding how hormones, sex, and age influence your body composition is also fascinating. We have known for some time that men naturally have more lean muscle compared to women, while women tend to have more total body fat. This is often explained by the location of body fat, and the unique reproductive function needs of women. The higher level of fat and lower level of muscle in women, typically means that women have metabolic rates that are about 5 to 10% lower than men of the same height and weight because muscle mass is more metabolically active. In addition, women are 5 to 8 times more likely to develop hypothyroidism compared to men, which, if not treated, may lead to weight gain.

In an interesting scientific paper on sex differences in body composition and insulin resistance, the authors of this review stated that men who tend to have more fat around their internal organs, were more insulin resistant than women who tend to store their fat around their arms and legs. So the health consequences of excess fat depend not only on the presence of body fat, but where that fat is located. However, as we age, our hormones also change, and this influences our muscle tissue and fat storage.

After menopause; for example, women gain more abdominal fat mass due to the decline in estrogen concentrations. It has also been shown that women burn fat less efficiently after menopause, both at rest, and during exercise. The prevalence of hypothyroidism, or underactive thyroid, increases with age too, affecting about 9% of men and women over 60 years old. This may have implications for weight gain in later years because, as you know, a decrease in thyroid hormones slows metabolic rate if it's not treated with medication. Additionally, decreased muscle mass and strength occurs as we get older, resulting from a gradual loss, about 5 to 10% per decade, of the skeletal muscle after the age of 30. But, it's not all doom and gloom—these massive changes to body composition only occur if you choose not to exercise or eat properly. In fact, there is other evidence that shows excellent muscle mass quality and function in those who are lifelong exercisers and athletes.

We've only scratched the surface of hormones and their influence on body composition and health. However, the hormones we discussed are essential to understand that you have the tools necessary to understand and dispel some common myths about your hormones and their relationship to your body composition. To recap, insulin helps to store glucose and fat. Under stress, cortisol releases stored glucose, and breaks down fat and proteins to provide energy. Catecholamines are released in response to stress and exercise to help us mobilize fuel to fight or run away. Lastly, the thyroid hormones help regulate the amount of energy used by the body. Each of these hormones work with and against each other to try to maintain appropriate amounts of fat mass and muscle tissue, as well as to support the skeletal system.

Another important fact is that you have hormones signaling that you're hungry or that you're full. For example, leptin produced from the fat cells and peptide YY from the intestine makes you feel full and stop eating. But, disruptions in these hormones happen, usually with excess sugar consumption and overall food intake. And sometimes, instead of telling you to stop eating, leptin won't do its job properly, and you will continue to feel hungry. You also have hormones like ghrelin made in the stomach and in the small intestine and neuropeptide Y from the nervous system that make you feel hungry when they are released.

When you consider the entire hormone system, it's clear that we have many different repetitive and redundant ways to regulate our eating, body weight, body composition, and health. And a poor diet, sedentary lifestyle, and chronic stress are all factors that can negatively affect the normal function of your hormones and, as a result, your health, and body composition. Excluding unavoidable health conditions that may alter the function of hormones, a healthy lifestyle can help maintain and prolong normal hormone effectiveness for an extended period of time. Try this limit your intake of added sugars and sugar-sweetened beverages to control your insulin levels, your hunger, and your body composition.

Novel Ways to Change Body Composition

The best method for changing body composition is by increasing the quality of both your exercise and dietary intake. But this can be complicated, leaving some people to search for outside-the-box options—such as using no-calorie sweeteners, using a stand-up desk, wearing ice-cold vests, or simply sleeping more—to help them meet their body composition goals. The rationale behind these methods is generally to either decrease the amount of food you eat or increase your total energy expenditure. This lecture is dedicated to evaluating the efficacy of some of the less-traditional approaches to altering body composition.

Artificial Sweeteners

- There are some tools and tricks that are used to decrease total energy intake to manipulate body composition. To limit calorie intake, many people choose to use low-calorie or no-calorie sweeteners.

- Originally, these artificial sweeteners were for people with diabetes because of their inability to handle large doses of real sugar, but in recent years, they have been incorporated into diets of those looking to lose weight and fat.

- While some research shows that using low-calorie sweeteners instead of full-calorie versions can improve weight loss, there have been some claims that the use of artificial sweeteners can actually increase body weight and might cause negative health effects.

- You might find success using low-calorie sweeteners in moderation to decrease energy intake and help maintain weight loss. Although more research is needed, it seems reasonable to try to choose the artificial

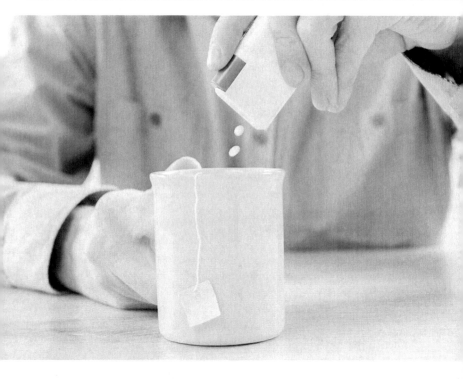

sweeteners that are as natural as you can get. For example, stevia is an herb; you can even grow it in your garden.

But just because they might be more natural does not mean that they are safer. It is probably best to limit added sugars or added artificial sweeteners when possible.

Detox Diets

Another popular dietary method that people use to try to improve body composition and weight loss is the ever-popular detox, or cleanse, diet. Detox regimens normally include pretty serious calorie restriction and focus on the consumption of fruits and vegetables only, many times in the form of juices.

With calorie restriction, you are likely to see weight loss results, but where is this weight loss coming from? The weight loss from detox diets is most likely coming from a loss of stored glucose, also called glycogen.

When you drastically reduce calorie intake, you will deplete glycogen stores from your body in just 24 to 48 hours, which results in even more weight loss, because glycogen is stored with water. So, you end up losing stored glucose and water weight.

Cleanses, or detox diets, only provide short-term fixes for weight loss and do not result in long-term improvements in fat mass. They might even decrease your muscle mass, which is definitely not desirable.

The science does not support the use of detox diets for health or body composition improvements. Until there is consistent research evidence to the contrary, with a healthy liver, you have all the detox power that you need.

Eating Out versus at Home

Probably the easiest way to consume fewer overall calories and create a negative energy balance is to consider how much you eat out at restaurants each week.

Research has shown that eating out at a fast-food or full-service restaurant resulted in an increase in total energy intake, saturated fat, and sodium intake. In fact, eating out results in approximately an extra 200 calories eaten per day.

The typical American adult eats a meal or snack from a restaurant 5.8 times per week. This might cause a long-term positive energy balance, especially if you make poor choices at the restaurant and don't exercise much.

Even with busy schedules, making a conscious effort to prepare more meals at home might make the difference between being stuck in a plateau and reaching the goals you have set for yourself.

It is important to be conscious of portion sizes, regardless of whether you are eating out or cooking at home. Sometimes, you just need to practice eating until you are about 80 percent full. It can take a little while for you to realize that you've had enough to eat—sometimes as long as 15 to 20 minutes.

Sedentary Lifestyle

Americans spend an average of 13 hours per day with no movement. Then, if you add 8 hours of sleep, this makes it a whopping total of 21 hours per day—almost 90 percent of your day.

Studies have found that even if you are doing some physical activity during the day, it can't outdo the harmful effects of sitting during the other time. Sitting for an extended amount of time per day has been related to the development of cancer, diabetes, and cardiovascular disease.

The simple solution is to move more. Research has shown that people who take more breaks from sitting have lower waist circumferences, lower body mass indexes, and better glucose control. And the average length of the breaks was only 4.5 minutes.

No matter how busy you are, you can find a few minutes to get up and move. Try something simple like drinking more water so that you have to get up more to use the bathroom more often. Or instead of calling or sending an email to people in your building for a meeting, walk to their office and meet in person.

Even those who fidget throughout the day might see health benefits. A study from the Mayo Clinic placed sensors on people to measure their daily movement and found that people who commonly paced and fidgeted during the day—including tapping their feet, bouncing their legs, or twiddling their thumbs—were leaner than people who did not fidget as much. Those tiny movements add up over a day.

Another option to cut down on sitting time is to use a standing desk at work, whether this is at the office or at home. You can even add a walking treadmill underneath your desk.

Find a few minutes at lunch to walk, or make a rule to always stand up when you are on the phone. Start small and work up to standing more and more every day.

But just standing isn't the answer, either; it is best to shift around and stand in different positions, such as having one leg up or kneeling. You can find tutorials online about the best positions to stand at your desk.

Cold Exposure

A concept that has taken off in recent years to improve body composition is to use cold thermogenesis as a way to increase energy expenditure. There are cold vests on the market that promise you'll burn up to 500 more calories. Others say to take a cold shower, sit in an ice bath, or simply be exposed to cold environments throughout the day if you want to stay thin and lose fat.

A 2014 study compared the metabolic effects of exercise to the metabolic effects of shivering by covering the study participants with cold water–filled blankets. The energy expenditure was higher with exercise than just being cold, but similar increases in a hormone known as irisin, which is released both during muscle contraction and during shivering, were seen in both conditions.

Although it might increase energy expenditure slightly, there haven't been studies that show that shivering will induce weight loss or fat loss on its own. Some research exists, but the outcomes are scattered, so a more straightforward and practical examination of cold thermogenesis is needed.

Chewing

Research has shown that when you increase the number of times you chew your food, you eat less food and also have a higher thermic effect of food. The thermic effect of food, or diet-induced thermogenesis, means that you increase energy expenditure for digestion, absorption, and storage of food.

Although this technique might seem to have a small impact, think about how quickly you can eat your food when you're really hungry or in a rush. Odds are that you aren't paying attention and taking the time to chew your food very well.

This method certainly isn't going to change your body overnight, but it is something to think about as you eat each meal. When you eat slowly and chew more, you might just increase the thermic effect of that meal and decrease the total number of calories you eat, too.

Sleep

Sleep, or lack of sleep, is more crucial to weight loss and weight gain than most people realize. A 2013 Gallup poll found that 40 percent of adults are getting less than 7 hours of sleep per night, which is below the lowest recommended amount. The national average is only 6.8 hours per night.

In addition, it is estimated that 50 to 70 million Americans have some form of sleep or wakefulness disorder, making it difficult to get a solid 8 hours per night.

It is likely that this ambitious attitude and continuous sleep debt is hurting our health. Sleep can have an effect on metabolic control, insulin sensitivity, food cravings, muscle recovery, body composition, and hormone profile and performance. Sleep debt has also been shown to increase the risk of several chronic diseases.

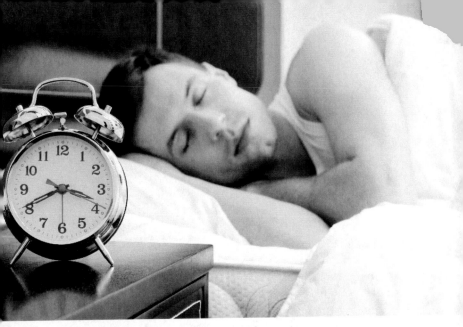

In addition, sleep is a time for your body to heal and recover. Without proper sleep and recovery, it will be more difficult to make the body composition changes you might be looking for. Lack of sleep will cause more fatigue, making your next exercise bout more difficult. Fat loss and muscle gain will suffer.

How can you get more sleep each night?

- Keep a regular sleep schedule by going to bed and waking up at the same times, even on the weekends. This helps your body develop a consistent sleep-wake cycle, making it easier for you to fall asleep at night and feel more rested in the morning.
- Manage stress and try to do something relaxing before crawling into bed each night.
- Turn off your electronics at least 30 minutes before you try to go to sleep.
- When you're restless, try writing down a list of things that are on your mind or wind down by reading a book.
- Take note of what you are eating and drinking in the hours before you doze off. Because bioactive peptides naturally found in milk are

linked to more restful sleep patterns and relaxation, try drinking a small cup of milk before going to bed. It is also important to avoid certain foods and drinks before bed, such as caffeine, nicotine, or spicy foods.

Sufficient sleep is very important, and if you don't get enough, it can seriously affect multiple systems of your body, especially body composition.

Pollutants

There has been a new surge in attention to the influence of environmental pollutants on your body composition.

Obesogens are chemicals in the environment that that could alter metabolism and make you have trouble losing fat. Some examples of obesogens are pesticides, pharmaceuticals, and chemicals in plastics, cans, and personal care products. One of the most common is bisphenol A, which is found in all types of plastic products.

Obesogens are thought to disrupt your endocrine system and affect the number and size of your fat cells and other hormones associated with appetite and satiety. These alterations to the endocrine systems might result in fat gain over time.

We don't know exactly how much exposure will make some of these compounds active in your body, so it is best to avoid exposure. When possible, try filtering water, choosing organic foods, and choosing glassware over plastic when you can.

Exposure to pollutants is not a proven cause of metabolic issues that lead to poor body composition, but they could possibly be a contributing factor.

Try This

As much as possible, aim to get a little more sleep each night.

Questions to Consider

1. What is one nontraditional method of improving your body composition that you will try to incorporate into your routine?

2. Which of the nontraditional methods of improving body composition do you think is the most influential?

Novel Ways to Change Body Composition

U p to this point, the best and most documented method for changing body composition is by increasing the quality of both your exercise and your dietary intake. At first, the simple advice to eat better and exercise more to lose weight and improve your body composition seems like an easy concept, right? But; of course, you also know that it is usually more complicated than that. This is why some people often reach a point where they search for more outside the box options to help them meet their body composition goals.

Maybe you've heard of things like using no-calorie sweeteners, using a stand-up desk, wearing ice cold vests, or simply sleeping more. The theory behind these methods is generally to either one, decrease the amount of food you eat, or two, increase your total energy expenditure. The overarching theme and rationale for these methods is that they help manipulate both energy intake and energy expenditure, which theoretically could result in body composition changes. Does this sound familiar? It makes sense that these less common methods try to create a negative energy balance to increase fat use. This lecture is dedicated to evaluating the efficacy of some of the less traditional approaches to altering body composition.

First, let's talk about tools and tricks that are used to decrease total energy intake in order to manipulate body composition. One very common method comes in a tiny little colorful packet everywhere you go. To limit calorie intake many people choose to use low-calorie or no-calorie sweeteners. Originally, these artificial sweeteners were for people with diabetes because of their inability to handle large doses of real sugar, but in recent years these sweeteners have been incorporated into diets of those looking to lose weight and fat. Sugar consumption in the diet of Americans has increased astronomically too, and not only due to soft drinks, but also from other processed foods like cookies, salad dressing, and condiments.

On average, each American consumes approximately 130 lb—almost 60 kg—of sugar per year. Given that excess of any macronutrient—carbohydrates, fats, or proteins—can be the enemy of ideal body composition, it seems fitting that we look to other options for controlling your sweet tooth. It seems perfect, right? With substitutes like sucralose and aspartame; for example, it is typically thought that we still get the sweet without the negative insulin-stimulating impact of sugar all while lowering caloric intake. There's quite a bit of research to back this up. Even the American Heart Association tells us that replacing sugary foods and drinks with artificial sweeteners is a way to limit calories and achieve or maintain a healthy weight. But there has also been conflicting evidence when it comes to the safety of some of these sweeteners. Let's take a look at both sides of the argument.

In 2014, a meta-analysis tallied the data from over 35 years of research evaluating low-calorie sweeteners and their impact on body weight and body composition. This was actually one of the most comprehensive reviews completed on artificial sweeteners. It was reported that the use of low-calorie sweeteners resulted in a modest, but significant reduction in body weight, body mass index, fat mass, and waist circumference. Based on these results the authors concluded that using low-calorie sweeteners instead of full-calorie versions could improve weight loss. This is a good sign, but conflicting data exist, too. There have been some claims that the use of artificial sweeteners can actually increase body weight, and may cause negative health effects.

For example, one study evaluated the metabolic effects of one sugar substitute called sucralose, which is sold as Splenda. Results showed that one dose of sucralose caused a small increase in blood glucose concentrations, an increase in insulin levels, and a decrease in insulin clearance. Even with no calories, sucralose may still cause an increase in blood glucose, albeit small, which is the exact opposite of the desired effect of artificial sweeteners. Others have looked at sucralose consumption over 12 weeks. This study was in rats, and it also looked at doses of sucralose that were equivalent to what humans would normally eat. Results showed a decrease in the good type of fecal microflora and increased fecal pH. An imbalance of good and bad gastrointestinal microflora, or bacteria in your gut, may be related to weight gain and obesity.

So what is the bottom line here about low-calorie sweeteners? I think you may find success using low-calorie sweeteners in moderation to decrease energy intake, and help maintain weight loss. Although more research is needed, it seems reasonable to try and choose the artificial sweeteners that are as natural as you can get. For example, Stevia is an herb; you can even grow it in your garden. Now, just because they may be more natural, does not mean that they're safer. It is probably best to just limit added sugars or added artificial sweeteners when possible.

Other popular dietary methods that people use to try to improve body composition and weight loss is the ever popular detox or cleanse diet. I'm sure you've known people who have tried these diets, or you have even tried them yourself. Detox regimens normally include pretty serious calorie restriction and focus on the consumption of fruits and vegetables only, many times in the form of juices. Major advocates of these types of diets are celebrities who claim that cleanses provide them with more energy and help them to quickly lose weight. So do the celebrities or the scientists have this figured out?

Well, first it can't be denied that with low-calorie intake you are likely to see weight loss results, but where is this weight coming from? Is it from fat or is it from muscle? Well, the weight loss from detox diets is most likely coming from a loss of stored glucose—also called glycogen. This makes sense because when you drastically reduce calorie intake, you will likely also lower your blood glucose quite a bit. This would make you rely on stored glycogen found in your liver and your muscles to help keep a normal blood glucose concentration. In fact, you will deplete glycogen stores from your body in just 24 to 48 hours, which results in even more weight loss because glycogen is stored with water.

So you end up losing stored glucose and water weight. Cleanses or detox diets only provide short-term fixes for weight loss and do not result in long term improvements in fat mass. They might even decrease your muscle mass, which is definitely not desirable. In my opinion, the science does not support the use of detox diets for health or body composition improvements. Until I see consistent research or evidence to the contrary, with a healthy liver you have all the detox power that you need.

Probably the easiest way to consume fewer calories overall and to create a negative energy balance is to consider how much you eat out at restaurants every week. In 2014, researchers looked at the effects of restaurant food consumption on total calorie intake. Not surprisingly, eating out at a fast food or a full-service restaurant resulted in an increase in total energy intake, saturated fat, and sodium intake. In fact, eating out resulted in approximately an extra 200 calories eaten per day. If you did this every day, that's an extra 73,000 calories per year and possibly up to 20 pounds of fat gain per year. Even if it's not a full 20 pounds, you're still setting yourself up for trouble with your body composition.

The crazy part is that this is not uncommon. The typical adult American eats a meal or snack from a restaurant 5.8 times per week. You can see how this may cause a long-term positive energy balance especially if you make poor choices at the restaurant and don't exercise much. Even with busy schedules, making a conscious effort to prepare more meals at home may make the difference between being stuck in a plateau and reaching the goals you have set for yourself. You'll hear much more about this in an upcoming lecture.

Now let's move away from eating out and think about eating at home. Have you ever heard that it is best to use small plates and bowls to limit how much food you can eat at one sitting? The idea is that if you have bigger plates and bowls you are more likely to increase your portion sizes and overeat compared to if you use smaller versions. Well this may actually be a myth based the science that exists. It turns out that when people are given the option of using a small plate or a large plate, it didn't actually change the number of total calories they ate at that meal. But, it is definitely important to be conscious of portion sizes you are dishing up for yourself when cooking at home or eating out. Sometimes you just need to really try and practice eating until you're about 80% full. It can take a little while for you to realize that you've had enough to eat, sometimes as long as 15 to 20 minutes.

So, what about the energy output side of the energy balance equation? What unusual ways exist to control how many calories you burn in a day? This is a biggie and brings us to the subject of the sedentary nature of our society. Americans spend an average of 13 hours per day with no movement. If you add in 8 hours of sleep this makes a whopping total of 21 hours per day. That's 21 hours—that is almost 90% of your day. And the worst part is, studies have found that even if you're doing some physical activity during the day, it can't outdo the harmful effects of sitting during the other time. So even if you make time for 30 minutes of exercise, all the other sitting is still not good. Sitting for an extended amount of time per day has been related to the development of cancer, diabetes, and cardiovascular disease.

So what should you do? The simple answer is to move more. Here's the research, a 2008 study gave people devices that measured their movement throughout the day. It turns out that people who took more breaks from sitting had lower waist circumferences, lower BMI, and better glucose control. And the best part is the average length of the breaks was only 4 1/2 minutes. No matter how busy you are you can find a few minutes to get up and move. Try something simple like drinking more water so that you have to get up and move to use the bathroom more often. Or instead of calling or sending an e-mail to someone in your building for a meeting, walk to their office, and meet in person.

Even those who fidget throughout the day may see health benefits. A study from the Mayo Clinic placed sensors on people to measure their daily movement and found that people who commonly paced or fidgeted during the day were leaner than people who did not fidget as much. This is called NEAT or non-exercise activity thermogenesis. It includes tapping your feet, bouncing your knees, or even twiddling your thumbs. It seems like nothing, but it looks like those tiny movements add up over a day.

Another option to cut down on sitting time is to use a standing desk at work, whether this is at the office or at home. You can even add a walking treadmill underneath your desk if you get really into it. Find a few minutes at lunch to walk, or make a rule to always stand up when you're on the phone, just start small and work up to standing more and more every day. But just standing isn't the answer either. It's best to shift around and stand in different positions—like one leg up or even kneeling. You can find all sorts of tutorials online about the best positions to stand in at your desk. A concept that has taken off in recent years is to improve body composition with the use of cold thermogenesis as a way to increase energy expenditure. There are cold vests on the market that promise you'll burn up to 500 more calories, and others say to take a cold shower, sit in an ice bath, or simply to be exposed to cold environments throughout the day if you want to stay thin and lose fat. Does this sound a little crazy to you? It might be, but it also might work.

A 2014 study compared the metabolic effects of exercise to the metabolic effects of shivering by covering the study participants with cold water filled blankets. The energy expenditure was higher with the exercise than just being cold, but similar increases in a hormone known as irisin were seen in both conditions. Irisin is a hormone that it is released both during muscle contraction and during shivering. So is cold thermogenesis the answer for weight loss? Although it may increase energy expenditure slightly, there haven't been studies that show shivering will induce weight loss or fat loss on its own. Some research exists, but the outcomes are all over the place. So a more straightforward and practical examination of cold thermogenesis is needed. It could be worth a shot, but it couldn't be counted on to make you have any major changes in body composition.

How about this? When you were a kid, did your mom tell you to chew your food really well? Well not only did she want you to not choke, but perhaps she also was secretly trying to help you improve your body composition. Originally proposed in the early 1900s, Horace Fletcher was the first to tell people to chew each mouthful thoroughly in order to prevent gaining weight. Research has shown that when you increase the amount of times you chew your food, you eat less food, and you also have a higher thermic effect of food. Remember, the thermic effect of food—or diet induced thermogenesis—means that you increase energy expenditure for digestion, absorption, and storage of that food.

Although this technique may seem to have a very small impact, think about how fast you can eat your food when you're really hungry or in a rush. Odds are you aren't paying attention and taking the time to chew your food very well. This method certainly isn't going to change your body overnight, but it is something to think about as you eat each meal. When you eat slowly and chew more, you might just increase the thermic effect of that meal and decrease the total number of calories you eat too. So far, we have talked about outside-the-box methods to limit energy intake and to increase energy expenditure. Now let's change direction and talk about a few odds and ends that may have an impact on your ability to alter body composition. The first very important topic for us to cover is sleep.

Sleep, or lack of sleep, is more crucial to weight loss and weight gain than people realize. A 2013 Gallup poll found that 40% of adults are getting less than 7 hours of sleep per night, which is below the lowest recommended amount. The national average is only 6.8 hours of sleep per night. In addition, it is estimated that 50 to 70 million Americans have some form of sleep or wakefulness disorder making it difficult to get a solid 8 hours of sleep. It is likely that this ambitious attitude and continuous sleep debt is actually hurting our health. Here are just a few of the things that sleep can have an effect on: metabolic control, insulin sensitivity, food cravings, muscle recovery, body composition, hormone profile, and performance.

Not only has sleep debt been shown to increase the risk several chronic diseases, but it is associated with metabolic issues as well. A 2010 study found that adults who got less than 8 hours of sleep per night were hungrier for high carbohydrate foods, putting them at risk for glucose and insulin problems. This is thought to be due to our brains craving the main energy source for it, glucose, when it is in sleep deprivation mode. Another study found that longer sleep duration was associated with lower BMI and better dietary behaviors. And, although more research is needed, it appears that extending or improving your quality of sleep will improve your performance too. Also, sleep is a time for your body to heal and recover; this is a time for your muscles and just about every cell to repair and regenerate.

Without proper sleep and recovery, it will be harder to make the body composition changes you may be looking for. Simply put, lack of sleep will cause more fatigue, making your next exercise bout more difficult. And eventually fat loss and muscle gain will suffer. How can you fix it and catch more sleep each night? The first thing to keep in mind is a regular sleep schedule, and by going to bed and waking up at the same times, even on the weekends. This helps your body to develop a consistent sleep-wake cycle, making it easier for you to fall asleep at night and feel more rested in the morning. I know this is tough in real life, but give it a try.

Second is to manage stress and try to do something relaxing before crawling into bed each night. This does not include spending time on your laptop, iPad, or phone before you go to bed or while lying in bed. Screen time gets your brained revved up and makes it harder for the body to relax and shut down. Turning off your electronics at least 30 minutes before you try to go to sleep is a good idea. Time spent tossing and turning thinking about all of the stuff that needs to get done can prevent you from getting adequate sleep during the night. When you're restless, try writing down a list of things that are on your mind or wind down by reading a book.

Lastly, it's important to take note of what you are eating and drinking in the hours before you doze off. Several studies have found that supplementation with bioactive peptides naturally found in milk were linked to more restful sleep patterns and relaxation. For example, one study in 60 women with sleep difficulties had a 65% improvement in their symptoms when consuming the bioactive peptides from milk proteins before bed. So try drinking a small cup of milk before going to bed. It's also important to avoid certain foods and drinks before bed such as caffeine, nicotine, spicy foods, or anything that you know causes you trouble. Caffeine and nicotine can act as stimulants making it hard to doze off, and spicy foods or eating a large meal may cause uncomfortable heartburn throughout the night. Sufficient sleep is very important, and if you don't get enough it can seriously affect multiple systems of your body, especially body composition.

But, what else can impact multiple systems in your body and make it difficult to improve body composition? This one usually isn't something that you would take notice of right away when looking for ways to alter body composition, but it could be playing a major role. I'm talking about a new surge in attention to the influence of environmental pollutants on your body composition. Obesogens are chemicals in the environment that could alter metabolism and make you have trouble losing fat. Some examples of obesogens are pesticides, pharmaceuticals, and chemicals in plastics, cans, and personal care products, just to name a few. One of the most common is BPA or bisphenol A—this is found in all types of plastic products like storage containers and some water bottles. Others are found in some detergents and certain types of flame retardant materials.

Obesogens are thought to disrupt your endocrine system and affect the number and size of your fat cells, and other hormones associated with appetite and satiety. These alterations to the endocrine system might result in fat gain over time. It makes sense that if you are constantly exposed to these environmental factors early in life, that the negative outcomes may be irreversible and making it harder to manage your weight the rest of your life. We don't know exactly how much exposure will make some of these compounds active in your body so it's best to avoid exposure. When possible, try filtering water, choosing organic foods, and choosing glassware over plastic when you can. Exposure to pollutants is not a proven cause of metabolic issues leading to poor body composition, but they could possibly be a contributing factor.

With a lot of these methods the goal is to make small, obtainable changes in your energy intake or expenditure in order to alter the energy balance equation. In some instances, these efforts could help you cut out a couple hundred calories per day or increase your energy expenditure just a little bit. Will these help produce significant changes in your body? Potentially, but these are best to supplement, not replace your focus on eating quality foods, and using proper exercise techniques to change your body composition. For example, replacing all the sugar in your diet with low-calorie sweeteners may limit your total calorie intake for the day, but I'd rather you focus on a well-rounded diet that is low in refined sugars and just has natural sugars from things like fruit. You'll end up with more nutrient density if you focus on a generally good diet.

What a lot of these methods come down to is, do these work for your body and fit into your lifestyle? Can you stand up more, go for an extra hour of sleep, or add a walk to your lunch break? Don't be quick to dismiss the non-traditional methods used to make body composition changes, but do be wary of things that seem too good to be true. You might just find that something you never thought about helps you reach the results you have been looking for. Try this—as much as possible aim to get a little more sleep each night.

Nutrition and Exercise: Special Needs

E ven though the most common nutrition recommendations might work for many people with many different goals, there are some specific needs for certain populations. In this lecture, you will learn about plant-based eating and nutritional concerns for both young people and older people—some of the most common special dietary categories. In general, total caloric intake, protein content, micronutrient needs, and hydration status are areas to think about as you continue your quest for optimal health.

Vegetarian Eating

- A vegetarian diet is essentially a plant-based diet. There are many reasons for choosing to eat this way, and there are many ways that it's practiced in real life.

- There is a whole continuum of plant-based eating. For example, some plant-based eaters don't eat meat but do eat fish, dairy products, and eggs. Some avoid meat, fish, and eggs but will eat dairy products. Some will just avoid red meat but eat chicken and other poultry and fish. Other plant-based eaters still eat meat, just not much of it.

- The strictest form of plant-based eating is called vegan. Vegans avoid all animal products, and this includes anything that an animal might produce, such as milk, eggs, and even honey.

- Eating more plant foods is a good thing nutritionally. Typically, plants come with a good dose of fiber, vitamins, minerals, and antioxidants— molecules that help maintain your cellular health. If you are eating more plants, you likely will eat less sugar and fat. In addition, there might be fewer incidences of heart disease and cancer from eating more plants.

There are some very important considerations to think about when eating a plant-based diet. There is more that has to be planned and included in a plant-based diet to ensure proper intake of protein, vitamins, minerals, and more.

Combining sources of protein for plant-based eating is necessary to get the essential amino acids required for certain health and growth processes. The key challenge for plant-based eaters is getting the essential amino acids found in animal products into their diet.

Most plant sources of food have incomplete proteins; they lack one or more of the amino acids essential to maintaining and/or building your muscle tissue. But you can combine plant sources of food—such as rice and beans—to create a mixture that is complete in its protein makeup.

Plant-based diets might also be low in other nutrients.

Vitamin B_{12} is only found as a "good" source in animal products. You can get B_{12} in foods like cereals that are fortified with B_{12}, but otherwise, supplementing will be needed.

Iron is also a nutrient that needs some special attention in plant-based diets. Plant-based dieters need almost two times the amount of iron from plant sources to get the same amount of iron as meat eaters.

Vitamin C helps you absorb plant-based iron, but calcium and tannins found in drinks like tea and coffee reduce plant-based iron absorption. Because many plant-based eaters consume a good amount of vitamin C (which is found in foods like peppers, kale, and broccoli), the absorption of iron might not be an issue. But it makes sense to combine iron intake with vitamin C and try to have calcium supplements and tea or coffee an hour or two before you eat iron-rich foods.

Vitamin D is added to dairy foods or drinks during processing. Plant-based eaters who avoid dairy as well as meat might want to supplement with vitamin D.

Omega-3 fats can be found in cold-water fish, but plant-based eaters can consume walnuts, seaweed, hemp, and flax. Because the body uses the plant-based sources for omega-3 fats inefficiently, supplementation with fish oil, krill oil, or an algae-based product is needed.

Calcium and zinc can be consumed in the diet, but absorption for both of these tends to be low compared to nonvegetarians. Plant-based eaters need to take in more calcium and zinc to fulfill the same requirements.

If you are very physically active and trying to train for performance, consuming traditional sports supplements like creatine and beta-alanine might be something to consider.

On a plant-based diet, make sure that you have a combination of plant proteins to meet your goals; have a good variety of nonstarchy vegetables; include good fats; and eat starches, fruit, and starchy vegetables to complete your energy needs.

The Special Nutritional Needs of Children

Both children and adults need carbohydrates, fats, and proteins, but the amount needed changes as we age. The three major nutritional concerns specifically for children are sufficient calories for proper growth, development, and performance; calcium and iron intake; and hydration.

Active children need more calories per kilogram (or per pound) than adults do. They weigh a lot less, so their total intake is lower, but on a relative basis, children need more food per pound of body weight.

Dietary reference intakes (DRIs) exist for children, but they are simply baseline recommendations meant to help children live illness- and disease-free. They were not established for active children looking to perform optimally.

Relative to body weight, children need more protein and a higher percent of essential amino acids than adults because of their extreme rate of growth. The recommendations for boys and girls are identical, with at least 13 grams of protein per day for children ages 1 to 3, 19 grams for ages 4 to 8, and 34 grams for ages 9 to 13.

After age 13, the recommendations differ between girls, who need at least 46 grams of protein, and boys, who need at least 52 grams of protein. This difference is mostly because boys tend to have a larger body size and larger food intake.

A range between about 10 and 30 percent of protein in the diet is considered acceptable. Some resources recommend that children who are athletes (or at least very active) eat about 1.5 grams of protein per kilogram of body weight (or 0.7 grams of protein per pound) per day.

Carbohydrates also come with recommendations. Children need about 130 grams per day; this provides 520 calories from carbohydrates. This might work well for your child, but you have to consider the same factors that you did for total calorie intake—especially their body size, growth rate, and activity level.

These considerations primarily boil down to two basic recommendations: Make sure that children eat enough food, and make sure that they get enough protein to support rapid growth and development.

Of particular concern with children is that, for the most part, they are entirely dependent on adults to purchase, prepare, and pack their food. Depending on the age of the child or adolescent, there are some pretty easy ways to have children get involved with food or cooking. Have them choose a fruit or vegetable at the store or pick a meal they want to help with.

Another resource for children's nutrition are the DRIs of vitamins and minerals. Typically, these are lower at younger ages and progressively increase through the teenage years. Complete lists of DRIs for all age groups can be found online. Calcium and iron intake are of particular concern.

In addition to the calorie and nutrient issues for children, their hydration needs must be considered—particularly if your child is very active. Drinking water or even diluted sports drinks is a good idea, especially during vigorous exercise and outside in warm weather.

Nutrition and Exercise with Age

Your nutrient needs change as you age. While there is no magic drink, potion, or pill for aging, we do know that proper nutrition and exercise are vital for increasing longevity and improving quality of life as you age.

It is not uncommon for exercise to slow down or become nonexistent as we grow older. The World Health Organization recommends at least 150 minutes of activity but says that for real benefits, it's best to exercise roughly 300 minutes per week—about 1 hour per day—for 5 days per week. This should be a mix of moderate and vigorous exercise.

If you don't exercise now, you should start; you can add fitness, muscle, and strength at any age. Research shows that muscle quantity and quality remains excellent if physical activity is consistently part of your daily routine. In addition, it is important to eat properly not only to fuel for a healthy life, but also to help with physical activity, reduce fatigue, and maintain or build muscle mass.

Protein intake for aging people is extremely important. According to the research on protein needs in older people, protein intake should almost be doubled compared to the recommended amount of 0.8 grams of protein per kilogram per day (or 0.36 grams per pound of body weight per day).

This is due to the fact of an age change called anabolic resistance, where we grow resistant to the growth-promoting properties of protein. Anabolic resistance develops as early as roughly age 40.

It is important to also include resistance training or weight lifting in your exercise plan to maintain or improve muscle mass—which is what keeps you moving and healthy. Aiming for about 30 to 40 grams of protein each time you eat might be optimal to improve muscle mass and defend against any age-related decline in muscle mass.

You want to combine this nutrition strategy with resistance training. To fight off sarcopenia, or the age-related decline in muscle mass that affects nearly 50 percent of men and 60 percent of women aged 60 to 69 years old, you have to lift weights and eat enough calories and protein.

Because hunger can decrease with age, it is also important to be aware of your total calorie intake.

Two other nutrient considerations to pay attention to as you age are vitamin D and calcium. To help maintain bone mass and prevent the loss of bone, it is a good idea to eat calcium-containing foods, such as dairy products, green leafy vegetables, and fruit—or you can use a calcium

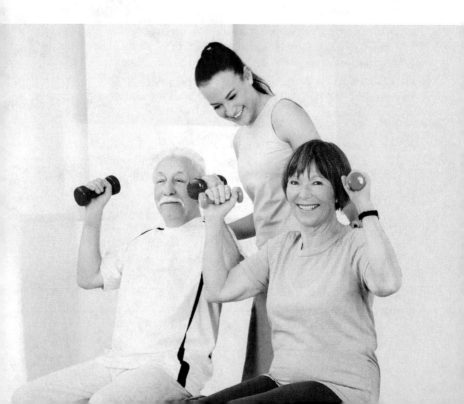

supplement. You should also make an effort to get some sun exposure or supplement with vitamin D to make sure that you are have enough to meet your needs.

Dehydration is also a concern in older individuals. Between the reduced ability to respond to dehydration and a reduction in thirst in older people, they can have major issues with regulating body water content. Even if you don't have the urge to drink fluids, you might need to.

Try This

Get more vegetables into your diet. Aim to eat an additional one to two servings of vegetables per day about three days per week to start.

Questions to Consider

1. What are some nutritional obstacles that people who are new to plant-based eating face?

2. What are some considerations for exercising in the heat if you are an older individual?

Nutrition and Exercise: Special Needs

You might have special needs and considerations when it comes to choosing a particular eating style. In this lecture, I'll discuss some of the most common special needs that I come across. Let's begin with vegetarian- or plant-based eating.

Vegetarian is essentially a plant-based diet. There are all sorts of reasons for choosing to eat this way, and there are many ways that it's practiced in real life. There is actually a whole continuum of plant-based eating. For example, some plant-based eaters don't eat meat but do eat fish, dairy products, and eggs. Some avoid meat, fish, and eggs but will eat dairy products. Some will just avoid red meat, but eat chicken and other poultry, and fish. Other plant-based eaters still eat meat, but just not much of it.

The strictest form of plant-based eating is called vegan. Vegans avoid all animal products, and this includes anything that an animal might produce like, milk, and eggs, and even honey. Eating more plant foods is a good thing nutritionally. Typically plants come along with good doses of fiber, vitamins, minerals, and antioxidants—molecules that help maintain your cellular health. We also know that if you are eating more plants, you likely will eat less sugar and fat. So it's a big benefit to eat more plants—whether you eat meat or not—and there might ultimately be fewer incidences of heart disease and cancer just by eating more plants.

Now, there are some very important considerations to think about when eating a plant-based diet. There is more that has to be planned and included in a plant-based diet to ensure proper intake of proteins, vitamins, minerals and more.

Combining sources of protein for plant-based eating is necessary in order to get the essential amino acids required for certain health and growth processes. Remember that there are 20 amino acids, 9 of which are considered essential—meaning that our bodies don't synthesize them. We have to eat them in our diets.

Here's the key challenge for plant-based eaters—getting the essential amino acids found in animal products like meat, milk, eggs, and the like into your diet. Most plant sources of food have incomplete proteins, meaning they lack one or more of the essential amino acids needed to maintain or build your muscle tissue. The thing to do is to combine plant sources of food in order to create a mixture that is a complete protein. As we've discussed, the most common example of food combined to make a complete protein is rice and beans.

One cup of rice has about 5 g of protein, and a half-cup of black beans has about 9 g of protein. Together you get a complete protein and roughly 15 g of protein. It's easy enough to combine foods. Here's the issue, although—to get this amount of protein, a plant-based dieter must also consider that they are eating roughly 300 or more calories to get that 15 g of protein along with a lot of carbohydrates. However, you certainly can get enough protein and even grow muscle on a plant-based diet—you just need to know what you are doing.

Research has also indicated that we absorb about 95% of animal proteins that we eat, but we only absorb about 85% of plant proteins. So even when you combine plant sources of protein in order to create a complete protein, you would need to eat even over a meat eater to get the protein your body needs for muscle growth and maintenance.

Some other vegetarian options for protein intake can also include eggs or egg whites and milk and dairy products like cottage cheese, Greek yogurt, and whey or casein protein powders. For vegans, those who eat no meat, eggs or dairy products, some protein options include legumes, grains like quinoa and buckwheat, nuts and seeds, and foods like tofu, soy or soy milk, and tempeh.

Now plant-based diets might also be low in other nutrients. It is not uncommon for plant-based eating to lead to low or deficient levels of

Vitamin B12 since B12 is only found as a good source in animal products like meat, fish, eggs, and dairy products. You can get B12 in foods like cereals that are fortified with B12 but otherwise, supplementing might be needed.

Iron is also a nutrient that needs some special attention in plant-based diets. The form of iron that is most readily absorbable comes from animal products—it is called heme iron, and it makes up about 40% of the iron in meat. The less well-absorbed form of iron, found in plants, like nuts, grains, vegetables, and fruit is called nonheme iron. Plant-based dieters need almost 2 times the amount of iron from plant sources to get the same amount of iron as meat eaters.

Another important finding is that Vitamin C helps you to absorb the nonheme, plant-based iron, but calcium and tannins found in drinks like tea and coffee reduce nonheme iron absorption.

Since many plant-based eaters consume a good amount of Vitamin C, found in foods like peppers, kale, and broccoli, the absorption of iron might not be an issue at all. It just makes sense to combine iron intake with vitamin C and try to have calcium supplements or tea and coffee an hour or two before you eat iron-rich foods.

Vitamin D is also a special concern for plant-based eating. Dairy foods are often fortified with vitamin D, meaning that vitamin D is added to the final food or drink during processing. Some plant-based eaters avoid dairy as well as meat. Actually, the best source of Vitamin D is sunlight. So if you're a vegetarian lacking in Vitamin D, and it is winter, or you don't get much sun, then you'll want to supplement with Vitamin D. You'll probably want to talk to your doctor or health care professional about this.

Plant-based eaters should also pay special attention to Omega-3 fats in their diets. Very good sources of Omega-3 fats are cold-water fish, but plant-eaters can go for walnuts, seaweed, hemp, and flax, among choices, to take in something called alpha-linolenic acid or ALA. ALA is then converted to something called docosahexaenoic acid, or DHA, and eicosapentaenoic acid, or EPA—the types of fatty acids that are considered the heavy hitters of the Omega-3-fatty acids. These help with body composition, and also are needed to ward off disease.

The trouble is that the body uses the plant-based sources for omega-3s quite inefficiently. So, once again, supplementation with a DHA or EPA product from fish oil, krill oil, or an algae-based product is needed.

Other needs for plant-based eating include both calcium and zinc. Again, these can be consumed in the diet, but absorption of both tends to be low, compared to non-vegetarians. While Zinc is found in a lot of plant foods like lentils, peanuts, and quinoa, its absorption is lower than it is when you get it from animal products. This just means that plant-based eaters need to take in more zinc to fulfill the same requirements.

If you are very physically active and trying to train for performance, a few other dietary considerations include traditional sports supplements like creatine and beta alanine. Creatine is made naturally in your body, but you also get some from your diet—if you eat meat and fish, that is. Those who only eat plants will have lower levels of stored creatine. Since creatine is used for short, explosive movements and has shown to have some benefits for cognition, neurological disorders, and muscle mass—supplementing with creatine might be something to consider.

It turns out that vegetarians have about 50% less carnosine in their muscle tissues. Due to the link between carnosine concentrations and overall health as well as evidence for exercise performance advantages emerging in the scientific literature, it is likely a good idea to also consider supplementing with beta alanine for the production of carnosine.

On a plant-based diet, make sure that you have a combination of plant proteins to meet your goals, a good variety of non-starchy vegetables, like greens, spinach, arugula, broccoli, and squash, include good fats, like nuts, seeds and healthy oils, and eat starches, like bread, whole grains, and potatoes; fruit, and starchy vegetables like corn and peas, to complete your energy needs.

The health benefits that come from a plant-based diet can be achieved by simply eating more plants. Changing gears, let's talk about some of the special nutrition needs of children. I often get the question from parents about what to feed their kids, and if a kid's diet is really different from the way adults should eat?

Well, yes and no. Both children and adults need carbohydrates, fats, and proteins. But the amount needed changes as we age. So the general recommendations are quite similar, but the details can vary.

The three major nutritional concerns specifically for children are sufficient calories for proper growth, development, and performance, calcium and iron intake, and hydration. Active kids actually need more calories per kg or more calories per lbs than adults do. They weigh a lot less, so their total intake is lower, but on a relative basis, kids need more food per lbs of body weight. Dietary Reference Intakes exist for children, but remember they are simply baseline recommendations meant to help children live illness and disease-free. They were not established for active kids looking to perform optimally, which is what I'd like to focus on.

Relative to body weight, children need more protein and a higher percent of essential amino acids than adults because of their extreme growth rate. The recommendations for boys and girls are identical, with at least 13 g per of protein day for kids ages 1–3, 19 g for ages 4–8, and 34 g for kids aged 9–13. After 13, the recommendations differ between girls. And girls need at least 46 g of protein, and boys need at least 52 g of protein. This difference is mostly since boys tend to have a larger body size and larger food intake. One thing to consider although is that a range between about 10 and 30% of protein in the diet is considered acceptable. So if your 9-year old girl eats 1800 calories per day, she might eat anywhere from 45-135 g of protein.

Some resources recommend that children who are athletes, or at least very active eat about 1.5 g of protein per kg of body weight, or 0.7 g per lbs per day. To make it easy, I would simply use whole numbers and aim for slightly less than 1 gram of protein per lbs of body weight. If your active child weighs 75 lbs, then, aim for just less than 75 g of protein.

Carbohydrates also come with recommendations. Kids need about 130 g per day—this would provide 520 calories from carbohydrates. This might work well for your child, but you have to consider the same factors that you did for total calorie intake—especially their body size, growth rate, and activity level.

These considerations primarily boil down to two basic recommendations: First, make sure that children eat enough food, and second, make sure they get enough protein to support rapid growth and development. Of particular concern with children is that, for the most part, they are entirely dependent on adults to purchase, prepare, and pack their food. So, many times I'll end up giving seminars to both parents and children. It really helps to have the whole family on board for the lifestyle that is created in a household.

Depending on the age of the child or adolescent, there are some pretty easy ways to have children get involved with food and cooking. Have them choose a fruit or vegetable at the store or pick a meal they want to help with.

Another resource for children's nutrition are the Dietary Reference Intakes, or DRIs, of vitamins and minerals. Typically, DRIs are lower at younger ages and progressively increase through the teenage years. Complete lists of DRIs for all age groups can be found online. But calcium and iron intake are of particular concern, so I'll talk about those.

Calcium is required for proper bone growth and strength. The total intake along with calcium and exercise lay the foundation for bone strength into adulthood. In fact, geriatric conditions are caused by lack of physical activity, lack of calcium, and lack of vitamin D as a child and as a young adult; and these include osteopenia, which is low bone mineral density; and osteoporosis, which is very low bone density or highly porous and brittle bones. Both osteopenia and osteoporosis are often considered pediatric diseases with geriatric consequences. This means that how you treat your bones as a child will have an impact on your health when you become older. Check out the current DRI's for specific recommendations. Dairy foods provide about 75% of the calcium in North America, but foods like fortified orange juice and cereals and spinach all contain calcium too. Supplements can also be used if calcium-containing foods can't be added to the diet.

The other major micronutrient to consider for children is iron. Iron is actually one of the most common nutrient deficiencies worldwide. Iron helps transport both oxygen and carbon dioxide throughout the body. When children and adolescents do not get enough iron in their diets, iron-deficiency is likely, and something called iron-deficiency anemia might occur where there is a low level of red blood cell production. Low levels of iron, in general, can lead to fatigue, brittle hair and nails, pale skin, and poor growth.

I think you'll be amazed to learn that an early study from the Department of Pediatrics at Baystate Medical Center found that about 45% of female teenage endurance athletes and about 15% of male teenage endurance athletes were iron deficient following an 11-week competitive season. For active people, the lack of ability to transport oxygen in the blood is not healthy and will reduce performance. These findings are specific to this study, but other studies agree.

During the teenage years, girls need 15 to 18 mg, and boys need 11mg of iron per day. Teen girls need more because of the loss of iron that occurs with menses. But spinach, most beans, steak and fortified cereals all can easily provide enough iron. One caveat is that iron toxicity can occur anywhere around 20 mg per kg of body weight and beyond. While this is isn't likely to occur from eating whole foods, it could happen if a child swallowed about 15-20 iron tablets in supplement form. This sounds odd but for some children, iron supplements or multivitamins might look like candy. So always be cautious with what is available to your children.

Outside of these calorie and nutrient issues for children, their hydration needs must also be considered—particularly if your child is very active. Young children end up with a higher core temperature and they sweat less than adolescents do, despite having more sweat glands per unit skin area than either adolescents or adults.

One thing that is both a disadvantage and advantage for children is their large surface area per unit of body mass compared to adults. This body surface to mass ratio causes them to heat up more quickly from the environment. However, because of their high body surface to mass ratio, children also cool at a faster rate than adults.

The research is actually mixed as to whether or not children are at a disadvantage in terms of regulating their body temperature—a process called thermoregulation. One landmark study had five prepubertal girls and five college-aged women exercise at a slow pace on a treadmill for 50 minutes in three different environmental temperatures. As the temperature increased for each trial, the young girls could not tolerate exercise for quite as long as the college-aged women.

In fact, at all environmental temperatures the girls had higher heart rates and higher temperatures than the women. This likely had to do again with the body surface area to weight ratio that I discussed. Drinking water or even diluted sports drinks is a good idea—especially during vigorous exercise, and outside in warm weather.

On the other end of the spectrum are nutrition and exercise changes that occur as we age. In general, there is a lack of understanding by people that their nutritional needs change as they age. You might be surprised to learn that the United States Department of Agriculture, USDA has found an overall decline in the diet quality of Americans over age 65. The World Health Organization, WHO, also reports alarming rates of obesity worldwide for all of us including those over 65 years old. This correlates with the American data.

While there is no magic drink, potion or pill for aging, we do know that proper nutrition and exercise are vital for increasing longevity and improving quality of life as you age. It is not uncommon for exercise to slow down or become non-existent, as we grow older. In fact, the U.S. Center for Disease Control, or CDC, has reported that only about 28–34% of adults ages 65–74 are physically active. The WHO recommends at least 150 minutes of activity but says that for real benefits, it's best to exercise roughly 300 minutes per week—that comes out to 1 hour per day—for 5 days a week. This should be a mix of moderate and vigorous exercise. If you don't exercise now, that shouldn't stop you. Start. You can add fitness, muscle, and strength at any age.

Keep in mind that there are plenty of examples of older individuals who are not only active but are athletes. For example, at age 84, Lew Hollander completed an Ironman distance triathlon—which is 2.2 miles of swimming, 112 miles of biking, and 26.2 miles of running.

There is also research evidence to show that muscle quality and quantity remains excellent if physical activity is consistently part of your daily routine. In addition, it's important to eat properly to not only fuel for a healthy life but to help with physical activity, to reduce fatigue, and to maintain or build muscle mass. As you'll recall, protein intake for aging people is extremely important. According to the research on protein needs in older people, protein intake should almost be doubled compared to the recommended amount of 0.8 g of protein per kg per day, or 0.36 g per lbs of body weight per day. This is due to the fact of an age change called Anabolic Resistance—where we grow resistant to the growth promoting properties of protein. Anabolic Resistance develops as early as roughly age 40, give or take a few years.

It is important to also include resistance training or weight lifting in your exercise plan in order to maintain or improve muscle mass—the very thing that keeps you moving and healthy. So aiming for about 30–40 g of protein each time you eat might be optimal to improve muscle mass and defend against any age-related decline in muscle mass. It should equal out over an entire day to just less than 1 gram of protein per lbs of body weight.

So if you weight 160 lbs, you would aim for a protein intake of somewhere between 115 and 160 g—which you can get from lean meat, dairy products, protein powders, or proper combinations of plant foods. You want to combine this nutrition strategy with resistance training. Research that looked at 3 months of resistance training and protein intake in over 100 people between 50 and 80 years old, concluded that higher protein intake led to the best improvements in muscle mass.

To fight off sarcopenia, or the age-related decline in muscle mass that affects nearly 50% of men and 60% of women aged 60–69 years old, you have to lift weights and eat enough calories and protein. Since hunger can decrease with age, it is also important to just be aware of your total calorie intake.

Two other nutrient considerations to pay attention to as you age are Vitamin D and Calcium. To help maintain bone mass, and prevent the loss of bone, where something called bone resorption exceeds bone formation, it is a good idea to eat calcium-containing foods like dairy products, green leafy vegetables, and fruit, or you can simply use a calcium supplement.

The average intake of calcium in older populations is between 650 and 800 mg/day, but it should be 1000–1200 mg/day. Omnivores can get the recommended amount by combining multiple food sources throughout the day. For example, 1 cup of milk, 1 packet of oatmeal, 1 cup of yogurt, and a 6 oz portion of salmon would be good. For plant-eaters, you might try a glass of orange juice fortified with calcium, and other foods like an ounce of almonds, 4 ounces of tofu, 1/2 a cup of soybeans, and a slice of calcium-fortified bread. It is pretty easy, but you can also use a calcium supplement. Calcium supplements are available in two forms. These are calcium carbonate and calcium citrate. Calcium carbonate is designed for people with ample stomach acid—typically younger individuals. But as we age, the production of stomach acid can also decline. So, for older people, using a calcium citrate—which is naturally a little acidic—will help with the absorption of calcium.

About 90% of men and women over age 51 do not meet the recommended Vitamin D intake of 600–800 IU. You should make an effort to get some sun exposure or supplement with Vitamin D to make sure you have enough to meet your needs.

Lastly, dehydration is also a concern in older individuals. Usually, your kidneys respond to changes in blood volume and salt concentration by producing a hormone called antidiuretic hormone or ADH. This hormone does what it sounds like, it stops or slows diuresis, or the production of urine, to conserve water. In older people, even though ADH is produced, it turns out that there are fewer nephrons or active components of the kidney, for the ADH to act on, and the nephrons are just less responsive in general.

Dehydration can also be an issue since older individuals have a decrease in thirst sensation. So even when dehydrated, older people just do not respond with the same level of thirst as a younger person.

You can easily see that a lower perceived level of thirst would probably lead to less fluid intake and just exacerbate dehydration. Between the reduced ability to respond to dehydration and a reduction in thirst, older people can have major issues with regulating body water content. A key message is that in older people, even if you don't have the urge to drink fluids, you might need to. Experts have often said thirst cannot be used as a reliable indicator of the fluid requirements of older individuals.

Now you can see that even although the most common nutrition recommendations might work for a lot of people with many different goals; there certainly are some very specific needs for certain populations. In this lecture, we discussed plant-based eating and nutritional concerns for both young people and older people. But there are definitely more special considerations, especially when you begin to incorporate specific diseased populations. In general, total caloric intake, protein content, micronutrient needs, and hydration status are areas to think about as you continue your quest for optimal health.

Try this: Just get more vegetables into your diet. Aim to eat an additional 1–2 servings of vegetables per day, 3 days per week to start.

Set-Point Theory and the Last Five Pounds

A t some point, you've probably wanted to lose "those last 5 pounds" before some upcoming event. Those last 5 pounds are often stubborn. Even with some changes that can be made to fine-tune the last 5 pounds, you'll end up fighting your physiology at some point. The set-point theory describes how and why your body is typically within just a few pounds of your "usual" body weight—the body weight that you just don't seem to budge from. In this lecture, you'll learn about ideal body weight, the set-point theory, and some common habits that make losing those last 5 pounds pretty difficult, but not impossible.

Ideal Body Weight

- Just like many topics in this field, your ideal body composition is different from that of your spouse or your best friend. Simply stop comparing and some of your stress will immediately decrease. But, of course, this is difficult to do.

- For ideal body weight, first think about what weight you were able to sustain, as an adult, where you felt the best you've ever felt. Chances are that this is more reasonable as a target then some former version of yourself with totally different life circumstances, stresses, and priorities.

- Your ideal body weight and body composition is when you feel your best, perform your best, and look your best. This ideal weight might change over time and is dependent on your goals.

- Calculating your ideal body weight is a good first step—although this will involve some trial and error.

First, you'll need to get your body composition measured. This can be done by any of the various measurement techniques, such as a skinfold test, bioelectrical impedance analysis, or DXA scan. Your best bet is to look up exercise science labs at local universities or colleges or speak with some professional staff at your health club. Just be sure to use the same method for measuring each time.

Once you have your body composition measured, take your weight of muscle mass and divide it by (1 − your goal body fat percent). This value is your ideal body weight at your selected percent body fat. This is your new goal weight.

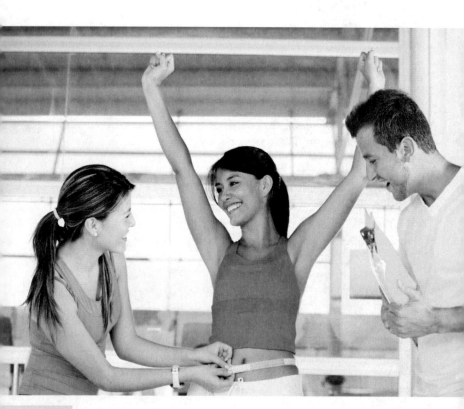

Then, subtract your goal weight from your current weight to determine how many pounds (or kilograms) of fat you need to weigh your goal weight and have your goal body fat percent.

This might be simple to calculate, but making it a reality is the difficult part. Despite implementing the right steps for diet and exercise, sometimes a plateau still hits you unexpectedly.

Set-Point Theory

The concept of set point also goes by names like "lipostat" or "homeostatic control mechanism." The set-point theory states that you have a "set" weight where your body is most comfortable. By this definition, if you were to either gain or lose weight, your body would do all it could to pull you back to the original starting weight.

For example, if you start to diet and exercise properly, it is common to lose weight rapidly at first before this rate of weight loss slows down significantly. In other words, you hit a plateau.

While you might have great intentions and a great start to a new lifestyle, in the end, despite great efforts and initial changes, body fat and weight tend to creep back up, and there is no improved body composition or health.

Often, if you restrict your food intake enough, it just dramatically increases your hunger levels—similar in some cases to starvation. This response is called hyperphagia, or increased hunger.

The truth about most diets is that you eventually return to the ways you used to eat. Typically, this is because you change so many things all at once that you can't keep it up. Other times, the diets are just absurd, and you can't live a real life.

When you do eat again after a severe diet, your fat mass comes back quickly compared to the slower development of lean muscle. You might feel hungry until your muscle mass has fully recovered. You also slow your metabolic rate, in part due to the loss of lean mass.

If you put together reduced energy expenditure with increased hunger, you could end up with more fat mass and body weight after dieting.

It seems that we are just ingrained with a body weight that our bodies work hard to defend. This is the set-point theory.

Essentially, you have a well-regulated internal control mechanism in the hypothalamus that tightly maintains your preset level of body fat and body weight. Your hypothalamus responds to signals from your fat cells, your gastrointestinal tract, and your pancreas to alter your metabolism, hunger, body fat levels, and weight.

Not only do these changes occur but you also have some hormones like ghrelin, leptin, and serotonin that control your hunger and appetite.

And, just as you might expect, if you lose weight, there is a good chance you'll end up hungry, and if you gain weight, you may end up losing your appetite.

With weight loss, your metabolic rate will decrease, so you require fewer calories than you used before you started losing weight. Eventually, the initial decrease in food you eat becomes the "normal" amount of food you require to sustain your new size.

Your body no longer sees that you are eating less, so there is no energy deficit. So, now, at the lower weight, you have to adjust, lowering energy intake again—that is, reducing your calories even more—to spark more weight loss.

The opposite is true, too: If you are trying to gain weight by eating a lot more food, you will increase your metabolic rate in an unconscious effort to bring your weight back to a set point, where it is comfortable hanging out.

Research repeatedly shows that when overfeeding or underfeeding stops, body weight returns to its starting point. So, despite your best efforts, it is really difficult to lose fat and keep it off. But can you change your set point?

If you can reestablish normal hormone functioning and a normal energy balance at the lower or higher target weight—by eating high-quality foods and exercising in a smart way—then your new body weight can be maintained.

If you make the right choices to fuel yourself well with nutrient-dense, high-quality foods and live an active and healthy lifestyle, your body simply regulates your body composition for you. Maybe you just need to consistently choose foods that work with your body composition goals rather than against them.

Breaking through a Plateau

Despite the challenge of losing fat and keeping it off, plenty of success stories exist. So, how do you reset your set point? One theory is that if you need to focus on quality foods, then you have a chance to fix the hormones that were not serving you well and begin to automatically regain control.

Two hormones that have to do with this are insulin and leptin. Insulin is the blood glucose–lowering and fat-storing hormone, and leptin is thought of as the "stop eating" hormone. The problem with these is that people can become resistant to both of them.

With obesity, you have a greater risk for these hormones (among others) to not work properly, and you can become resistant to their actions. This means that even with more insulin or leptin, the normal physiological responses of clearing blood glucose and stopping your hunger do not happen easily.

Research suggests that both eating more nourishing, high-quality foods and exercising can restore normal functioning of hormones like insulin and leptin as well as improve metabolic functioning and overall health.

There are some more ways to break through a plateau. First, consider why you are doing this. You work hard all day long; you have a lot going on in your life. Why even focus on your body composition?

This is very personal, but you must find a real reason for why you care about feeling your best, looking your best, and performing your best. Maybe you set a small bet with a friend. This challenge keeps you accountable and motivated.

You need to set some behavioral goals. You'll feel a sense of accomplishment by checking off the goal of working out 3 times per week instead of just focusing on the long-term goal of improving your muscle mass by 5 pounds or losing 10 pounds of fat.

By simply focusing on the things you can control—such as what you eat, how much and how often you eat, and your workouts—you immediately have achievable goals. This is much better than going after some lofty weight loss goal or body composition change. Like most things, half the battle can just be getting started.

None of us have time to work out, eat well, plan ahead, or make this a priority. But all of us can make time.

Next, consider whether you are getting sloppy—with your exercise, your sleep habits, or your nutrition. Maybe you work out with a little less intensity or for a shorter duration of time than you meant to. Maybe you dropped from a solid 8 hours per night of sleep to only 5 or 6. If you follow the same plan every day, it gets pretty easy to become a bit sloppy with your usual habits.

If breaking a plateau is important to you, you will need to rededicate yourself to exercise basics. Make sure that you are working out for the full amount of time that you promised yourself, instead of taking a bunch of breaks and counting them as exercise.

- You need to lift weights. This is what transforms your body, adds the most muscle mass, and helps ramp up your metabolism little by little. In addition to slowing muscle loss, lifting weights might help you get past that plateau.

- If you've hit a plateau, it's probably a good time to revisit what you do for your overall exercise plan as well and get back in the right mindset to work out.

- Make sure that your workout is fun, entertaining, and rewarding. Recent research determined that exercise adherence and weight loss success were largely determined by your attitude toward the workout session.

- Focus, from time to time, on the bigger reason for needing to change. Is it to be healthy enough to play with your children and grandchildren? Is it to live well rather than just to live long? These larger goals can help, although it's usually the fun of the activity and the smaller, more immediate goals that will drive your day-to-day commitment.

- Finally, consider whether you are getting lazy with your eating habits. This could be a great time to briefly track your calories, even if you think you're eating right. Recheck your "take for granted" habits, such as your usual serving sizes. Are you putting more on your plate than usual?

- Try to pay attention to your hunger. Pay attention to how you feel. You don't need a huge post-workout meal every day. You might consider different food choices and sizes based on how hard you actually push yourself that day.

- Think about your activity level and your food quality; these should be your guiding principles. Once you can get your focus back for your eating habits and exercise plan, you'll probably find that you can continue to move toward your goals.

Make small changes, instead of massively overhauling everything at once. Don't try to start exercising every day, eat completely new foods, drink more water, eat more vegetables and fruits, and skip every happy hour all at once. Find one very easy thing to do, such as drink more water, and begin there.

Try This

Write down three things that you feel you've become a little sloppy with in your daily routine. You'll most likely identify some great places to focus on to reset your set point.

Questions to Consider

1. What nutrition and eating habits do you take for granted that can be tightened up?

2. What are the first two small changes you can make to improve your body composition?

Set-Point Theory and the Last Five Pounds

Chances are that you may be at a healthy weight and perfectly happy with your body composition, and really just want to learn more about the amazing field of exercise and nutrition physiology. Despite your excellent health, though, I would bet that at some point you've said, I'd like to lose these 5 lbs before some upcoming event. And as you probably know, the last 5 lbs are often the one's that people dread losing the most. They just seem to be stubborn—not budging much despite your best efforts.

It could be that you've already come a long way—maybe you've improved your body composition a ton over the past year, for example. So, after all, that time and being so close to your goal, it is no wonder that that last little bit seems like it is so hard to conquer. It is sort of like a long road trip in the car. It's the last hour that always seems like the longest part of the drive.

Most times I can quickly identify easy-to-fix behaviors that can be manipulated to get results. These are basic things that my clients know but have just forgotten over time because they've been at this for so long. For example, it is very easy to go to the gym for 60 minutes, but that is not the same thing as exercising with a specific goal in mind and a specific plan for 60 minutes.

Other times, much more sophisticated nutritional changes can be implemented to help in your final push to optimize body composition. Sometimes I'll employ these changes for athletes before a single race or event, but they are not something I would say is sustainable over the long term. Even with some changes that can be made to fine-tune the last 5 lbs, you'll end up fighting your physiology at some point.

You may have heard of something called the set-point theory which is a theory that describes how and why your body is typically within just a few lbs of your usual body weight. In other words, this is the body weight that you just don't seem to budge from. In this lecture, you'll learn about ideal body weight, the set-point theory and some very common habits I see all the time that make losing those last 5 lbs pretty difficult, but not impossible.

Let's start with a simple question: What is your ideal body composition? Just like many topics in this field, your ideal body composition is different from that of your spouse or your best friend. Simply stop comparing and some of your stress will immediately decrease. But, I know this is tough to do. For ideal body weight, first, think about what weight you were able to sustain, as an adult, where you felt the best you've ever felt. Chances are that this is more reasonable as a target then some former version of yourself with totally different life circumstances, stresses, and priorities.

Many doctors and experts have stated publically that there is no such thing as an ideal body weight. I disagree. To me, your ideal body weight and body composition is when you feel your best, perform your best, and look your best. Now this ideal weight may change over time, and it is dependent on your goals. If your goal is to run a marathon, then clearly a lower body fat levels and body weight will be advantageous to make you feel and perform better well while running. On the other hand, maybe you don't have much muscle mass right now, and this makes doing some basic things like picking up kids or grandkids or being as active as you want to be difficult. Then for you, adding muscle mass and body weight may be ideal for you in order to feel, perform, and look your best.

Calculating your ideal body weight is a good first step—although this will involve some trial and error, of course. Here's what you do: First, you'll need to get your body composition measured. This can be done by any of the measurement techniques that we have discussed. It could be a skinfoldtest, bioelectrical impedance analysis, or a DXA Scan. Your best bet is to look up exercise science labs at local universities or colleges or speak with some professional staff at your health club. Just be sure to use the same method for measuring each time. Once you have your body composition measured, take your weight of muscle mass and divide it by one minus your goal body fat percent. This value is your ideal body weight at your selected percent body fat.

For example, let's say you weigh 195 lbs, or 89 kg, have 137 lbs, or 62 kg, of muscle mass, and 30% body fat. The goal you've set for yourself is to lose 5% body fat. Now, take the weight of your muscle mass or 137 lbs and divide it by 1 minus 0.25, which is your goal percent body fat. So this becomes 137 divided by 0.75. This equals 183 lbs, or 83 kg. This is your new goal weight. Then, just subtract your goal weight of 183 from your current weight of 195 and you'll see that you need to lose 12 lbs, or 5 1/2 kg of fat, to weigh 183 lbs and have 25% body fat.

Well, it may be simple to calculate, but making it a reality is obviously the tough part. Despite implementing the right steps for diet and exercise, sometimes, a plateau still hits you unexpectedly.

Here's where we need to talk about the set-point theory. Set-point also goes by names like your lipostat or your homeostatic control mechanism. The set-point theory states that you have a set weight where your body is most comfortable. By this definition, if you were to either gain or lose weight, your body would do all it could to pull you back to the original, starting weight. For example, if you start to diet and exercise properly, it is common to lose weight rapidly at first before this rate of weight loss slows down—a lot. In other words, you hit a plateau.

Too many times, I've seen great intentions and a great start to a new lifestyle, but in the end, despite great efforts and initial changes, body fat and weight tend to creep back up, and there is no improvement in body composition or health. Often times, if you restrict your food intake enough, it just dramatically increases your hunger levels, some in cases of starvation. This response is called hyperphagia or increased hunger.

Here is the truth about most diets—eventually you simply return to the ways you used to eat. Typically this is because you change so many things all at once that you can't keep it up. Other times, the diets are just absurd, and you can't live a real life. In fact, roughly 78% of people who lose about 5% of their body weight initially, eventually gain it back over 5 years

When you do eat again after a severe diet restriction, here is what happens: Your fat mass comes back quickly compared to the slower development of lean muscle. You actually feel hungry until your muscle mass has fully recovered. You also slow your metabolic rate, in part due to the loss of lean mass. Does that sound good? Very hungry, rapidly putting on fat, and slowly putting on muscle after your attempt to become healthier. This doesn't sound great to me. If you put together reduced energy expenditure with increased hunger—you can see that you could end up with more fat mass and body weight after dieting.

So, this brings us back to the set point. Could it be that we are just ingrained with a body weight that our bodies work hard to defend? Actually, yes, this does seem to be true. Think about your friends who can eat whatever they want without gaining any weight. You probably would say that this type of person has a fast metabolism, right? Well, you can also say they have a low set-point. The same thing goes the other way too. Maybe you are someone who seems to put on weight quickly. You'd probably say this person has a slow metabolism or a high set point.

So, how does the set point work? Essentially, you have a well-regulated internal control mechanism in the hypothalamus that tightly maintains your preset level of body fat and body weight. Your hypothalamus responds to signals from your fat cells, your gastrointestinal tract, and your pancreas to alter your metabolism, hunger, body fat levels, and weight.

Not only do these changes occur but you also have some hormones like ghrelin, leptin, and serotonin that control your hunger and appetite. And, just as you might expect, if you lose weight, there is a good chance you'll end up hungry, and if you gain weight, you may end up losing your appetite.

It's important to know that with weight loss, your metabolic rate will decrease, so you require fewer calories than you used before you started losing weight. Eventually, the initial decrease in food you eat becomes the normal amount of food you require to sustain your new size. What happens here is that your body no longer sees that you are eating less; so there is no energy deficit.

So, now, at your lower weight, you have to adjust, lowering energy intake again, that is reducing your calories even more, to spark more weight loss. For example, in one study, after 10 weeks on a weight loss diet, men and women did lose weight. The trouble is that some of their hormones like leptin, ghrelin, cholecystokinin and others also changed in a way that made them hungrier and lowered their metabolic rates—and these changes persisted for months after the study ended.

The opposite is true too—if you are trying to gain weight by eating a lot more food, you will increase your metabolic rate in an unconscious effort to bring your weight back to a set-point where it's comfortable hanging out. Even in overeating research studies, where people were fed a lot of extra food, the participants ended up gaining far less weight than the researchers predicted. And when the participants went back to eating normally, they went right back to their initial body weights.

Time and time again, research shows that when overfeeding or underfeeding stops, body weight returns to its starting point. Does it make sense now why, despite your best efforts, it is really hard to lose fat and keep it off? So, how then can you change your body composition for good if you are always fighting to stay at your set-point weight?

Can you change your so-called set-point? Yes. And I'll tell you why. The studies we just talked about gave some pretty drastic calorie changes and then, at the end of the study, just stopped. Most of them also don't include a major quality portion to the diets, just quantity of food. Most don't include smart exercise either. It makes sense that if you can re-establish normal hormone functioning and a normal energy balance at the lower or higher target weight—by eating high-quality foods and exercising in a smart way— then your new body weight can be maintained. This is really a great thing.

If you make the right choices to fuel yourself well with nutrient-dense, high-quality foods and live an active and healthy lifestyle, your body simply regulates your body composition for you. Maybe you just need to consistently choose foods that work with your body composition rather than against them. Is this all it takes to burst through a plateau or prevent weight-regain?

It might just be that easy. Despite the challenge of losing fat and keeping it off, plenty of success stories exist—I'm sure you know some of the people who have found one method that just works for them. So how do you re-set your set-point? One theory is that if you need to focus on quality foods, then you have a chance to fix the hormones that were not serving you well and begin to automatically regain control. Two hormones that have to do with this are insulin and leptin. Insulin is the blood glucose lowering and fat storing hormone and leptin is thought of as the stop eating hormone. The trouble with these is that people can become resistant to both of them. With obesity, you have a greater risk for these hormones among others to not work properly, and you can become resistant to their actions. So this means that even with more insulin or more leptin, the normal physiological responses of clearing blood glucose and stopping your hunger, do not happen easily.

Studies in animals have shown that the quality of the food they eat has a major influence on body weight and body composition—and the hormone changes that occur. The research evidence suggests that both eating more nourishing, high-quality foods and exercising can restore normal functioning of hormones like insulin and leptin, improve metabolic functioning, and overall health.

Here are some more ways to break through a plateau. Let's go back to the basics again. The first question you should ask yourself is why am I doing this? You work hard all day long; you have a lot going on in your life. So why even focus on your body composition? Well, this is a very personal thing, but each of you must find a real reason for why you even care about feeling your best, looking your best, and performing your best. Maybe you set a small bet with a friend to start the ball rolling. For example, challenge your neighbor over taking their garbage cans out or washing their car. This challenge keeps you accountable and motivated

Without a doubt, you need to set some behavioral goals, too. You'll feel a sense of accomplishment by checking off the goal of working out 3 times per week instead of just focusing on the long term goals of improving your muscle mass by 5 lbs or losing 10 lbs of fat.

By simply focusing on the things you can control—like what you eat, how much and how often you eat, and your workouts, you can immediately have achievable goals. This is way better than going after some lofty weight loss goal or body composition change. Like most things, half the battle can just be getting started.

When it comes to having time to exercise, I'll let you know a little secret. None of us have time to workout, eat well, plan ahead, or make this a priority. But, all of us can make time. Maybe not every day, but there is no way that you can't get dressed a little faster, check a few less emails, or turn off the TV. That alone might get you the 30 minutes you didn't have time before.

The second question you should ask yourself is, Am I getting sloppy? Sloppy with your exercise, sloppy with your sleep habits or sloppy with your nutrition. Maybe you work out with a little less intensity or for a shorter duration of time that you meant to. Maybe you dropped from a solid 8 hour per night of sleep to only 5 or 6 hours? If you follow the same plan day in and day out, it gets pretty easy to become a bit sloppy with your usual habits. You might be amazed at how something seemingly unimportant like sleep can influence so much. Well, don't underestimate it. Poor sleep is linked to an incredible 55% increased risk of obesity in adults and 89% increased risk in children. If breaking a plateau is important to you, you will need to re-dedicate yourself to the exercise basics that we discussed earlier in the course.

Just think about the last trip you had to the gym. Are you working out for that full hour that you promised yourself, or are you changing for 10 minutes, talking to a friend for a few minutes, warming up for a few minutes, and only really exercising for a few minutes before having to hurry back to work or some other event? Without a doubt, you need to lift weights. This is what transforms your body, adds the most muscle mass, and helps to ramp up your metabolism little by little. In addition to slowing muscle loss, lifting weights will help you past that plateau.

If you've hit a plateau, it's probably a good time to revisit what you do for your overall exercise plan as well as get back in the right mindset to workout. Make sure your workout is fun, entertaining, and rewarding in its own right. This is not a shocker, but recent research determined that exercise adherence and weight loss success was largely determined by the attitude you have towards working out. An interesting study found that calling a 1.4-mile walk a Scenic Stroll resulted in subjects eating far fewer calories when tempted with post-walking snacks than subjects who were told the short walk was simply exercise.

Reshaping how you think about exercise and finding a way to enjoy it can do wonders. Imagine if you actually want to go workout, break a sweat, and make yourself healthy. Doesn't that just sound so much better than having to go or worse, dreading to go work out?

It does to me. Find a way to make your workouts more enjoyable and connected to your true reason for doing all of this in the first place. Maybe you need to make a change to add something fun. Maybe arrange to workout with a friend, join a group fitness class that focuses on strength exercises, create a fitness challenge at work, or simply incorporate exercises or sports that you enjoy to your usual routine.

Focus, from time to time, on the bigger reason for needing to change. Is it to be healthy enough to play with your kids and grandkids? Is it to live well rather than just to live long into old age? Or is it simply to know that you are taking advantage of the body that you were given. These larger goals can help, although it's usually the fun of the activity and the smaller, more immediate goals that will drive your day-to-day commitment.

The third question to ask is, Am I getting a little lazy with my eating habits? This could be a great time to briefly track your calories again. Try a spot-check every now and then for your calorie intake—it can do wonders—even if you think you're doing it all perfectly. Recheck your take for granted habits like your usual serving sizes. Are you putting more on your plate than usual? One I see a lot is people who clean up dinner and decide to finish off the rest of what's on your kid's plate. Those calories count, too.

It is really easy to just eat things out of habit, even if you know that you can make better choices. Try to pay attention to your hunger. Pay attention to how you feel. And realize that you don't need huge post-workout meal every day. You might consider different food choices and sizes based on how hard you actually push yourself that day. For example, on days when you really push yourself and get after it at the gym or on the road or in the pool, then you probably would do best by eating a little more food that day. But on your recovery days and your rest days, you probably don't need as many calories. Again, think about your activity level and your food quality—these should be your guiding principles.

Make sure you are focusing on quality foods again. These foods have an added bonus of being nutrient-dense and filling all at the same time. You've already seen that this strategy also has the ability to rescue some problems that come about with your hormones too. This strategy is likely a key to resetting your set-point.

Once you can get your focus back for your eating habits and exercise plan, you'll probably find that you can continue to move towards your goals. But another thing that I practice and that I have all of my clients practice is to make sure to make small changes, instead of massively overhauling everything all at once. Time and time again, I have seen people try to start exercising every day, eat completely new foods, drink more water, eat more vegetables and fruits, and skip every happy-hour all at once. This does not work.

Dr. John Berardi, a leader in nutrition coaching, has always recommended doing one small thing every day. In his plan, he recommends to make your changes a little too easy. The change you make should not be difficult. Find one very easy thing to do, like drink more water, and begin there. You'll have to fight the urge to change it all and have immediate results. But, at least the results will allow you to move your set-point rather than constantly yo-yo-ing with your weight and body composition.

That's the entire point. Too many people lose and gain weight for decades. We have a wonderful physiological system that tries to take care of us by defending our appropriate and healthy body weight. But we develop unhealthy diet and exercise habits that throw that system off and reestablish new baselines. This is why it is really difficult to make long-lasting changes to body composition.

You may even be the person who has tried every diet out there but with no luck. But, even though our bodies defend our usual body weight—the good news is that we can adjust this. You just need to decide that your transformation begins now and start something today.

Try This: Write down three things that you feel you've become a little sloppy with in your daily routine. I'm sure you'll identify some great places to focus in order to re-set your set-point.

Choosing Your Nutrition Plan

T he fad diet popularity might stem from the belief that maybe there is an easy and quick way to improve body composition. It also stems from the thought that there might be one diet that is best for everyone. But this just isn't the case. Your personal preferences and physiology have a lot to do with your success of changing your body composition through diet and exercise. This lecture will highlight some interesting key points and new research for traditional diets and popular fad diets.

MyPlate

For many years, the conventional approach to eating in the United States was to follow the Food Guide Pyramid. In fact, many countries have some pyramid design to indicate their eating recommendations. The original design had a wide base of grains, indicating that you should build a diet primarily from carbohydrates, leading up to a peak of fat and oils to use sparingly.

In 2011, the traditional pyramid was replaced with something called MyPlate, which is an image of a plate with the food groups on it. The new plate graphic has been both praised and criticized, but it does, at least, seem to make sense to show food on a plate rather than a pyramid. It was designed to remind Americans to eat healthfully, but not necessarily to change consumer behavior.

This guide assumes that most Americans know how to eat healthfully and that "healthfully" has a definition that is the same for everyone. In addition, just by looking at the MyPlate image, it is difficult to interpret which foods should be a priority.

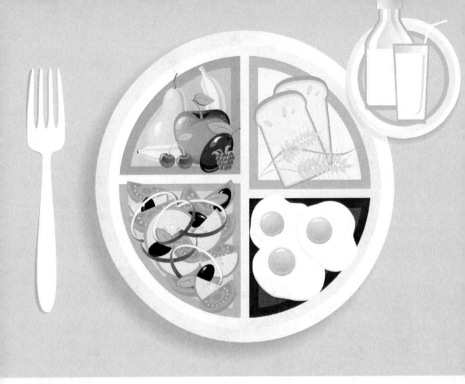

The MyPlate recommendations encourage variety in what we eat, and they provide some visual cues for the proportion of vegetables, fruit, grains, and protein that should be on your plate. It also encourages whole grain consumption rather than simply more grain consumption.

MyPlate recommendations, however, are very general. The MyPlate diet—traditionally thought of as a high-carbohydrate, low-fat diet—suggests that a plate 75 percent full of grains, vegetables, and fruit, which are all sources of carbohydrates, is best for everyone, regardless of how active your lifestyle is.

For very active people, and especially people who like to work out at high intensities, a higher-carbohydrate diet has been supported in the research more times than not. This, though, is usually based on improving exercise or sports performance, but not everyone is concerned with performance. You might be much more interested in body weight or body composition.

- The overall calorie and carbohydrate needs of someone who is physically active will be different from someone of the same size and gender who is sitting still all day at a desk.

- In addition, constantly high blood sugar levels—which you might get following a very high-carbohydrate diet without enough exercise—are at least related to many different kinds of ailments, including type 2 diabetes.

- Carbohydrates are not inherently a problem, but the overconsumption of them combined with a lack of physical activity tends to get people into body composition trouble.

- The MyPlate recommendations suggest that real fruit and 100 percent fruit juice as well as real vegetables and 100 percent vegetable juices are the same. However, the ways we digest and absorb solid food compared to liquids are different in many ways, including how quickly the nutrients get into your body. In addition, many juices are loaded with added sugars that real fruit does not contain.

- Healthy fats—such as olive oil, avocado, and fish or fish oil—are not included, even though healthy fats have a major place in our diets and have some wonderful health benefits.

- Another drawback is that there is not really a distinction between "better" choices and "worse" choices of proteins or carbohydrates.

- Most of the epidemiological scientific literature regarding health and weight loss in overweight individuals recommends consuming more healthy fats and reducing intake of refined carbohydrates. There are both positives and negatives with a high-carbohydrate, low-fat diet, and it is entirely dependent on how you feel, look, and perform when eating this way.

High-Fat, Low-Carb Diets

Over much of the same time that we have been told that a higher-carb, low-fat diet is best for all of us, primarily from the MyPlate recommendations, obesity and diabetes rates have skyrocketed. So, naturally, people have been drawn to drastically different eating styles to see if they can improve their health and body composition.

Thus, the high-fat, low-carb diet was born. This kind of eating goes by many names, such as Atkins, Paleo, and ketogenic diets. While these are different diets, some major similarities exist. Advocates of the high-fat, low-carb diets point to research that shows more fat oxidation (fat burning) with this kind of diet—and rapid weight loss.

Eating a high-fat diet means that fat would make up about 60 to 75 percent of your total caloric intake. The assumption with high-fat diets is that if carbohydrate feeding lowers your ability to burn fat, then a high-fat diet would increase your ability to burn fat as a fuel.

Overall, there is actually a lot of evidence to show improvements in health, body composition, and other physiological functions with a higher-fat, low-carb approach. For example, with this diet, there is higher fat oxidation during exercise, increased availability of free fatty acids, and increased activity of fat oxidation enzymes. Additionally, there is a reduction in enzymes involved with glycolysis—which is the breakdown of sugar to provide energy—along with reduced muscle glycogen and liver glycogen storage.

If you can better control blood sugar with a high-fat, low-carb diet, this could be highly useful for controlling body fat and ultimately your overall body composition. Also, fat and protein tend to keep you feeling full for a longer period of time than carbohydrates alone.

So, you can use a high-fat, low-carb approach to improve some health outcomes and maybe even body composition, but the problem is that this diet is often carried out incorrectly. While on a high-fat diet, people are usually just eating more fast food, fried food, and processed meats—a high fat intake, with no concern of the type of fat, along with a normal amount of carbohydrate intake. Ultimately, with a plan like this, health does not seem to improve.

Additionally, there are some questions as to the feasibility of a high-fat, low-carb diet when you bring exercise into the equation. Some studies show no difference in exercise performance after you eat a high-fat or high-carb diet; however, these studies usually involve exercise that is done at low to moderate intensities. If you exercise at high intensities, then exercise performance might decline on a high-fat diet.

Eat Better, Not Less

There are some general guidelines for changing your body composition in a healthy, effective way.

1. Aim for minimally processed foods.
2. Try for fewer refined starches and sugars.
3. Eat protein with each meal or snack.
4. Eat more fruits and vegetables.
5. Eat more good fats, such as nuts, eggs, avocado, and fish.

The Ketogenic Diet

Traditional high-fat, low-carb diets are 60 percent fat, 20 percent carbohydrate, and 20 percent protein. But there are two very popular diets that manipulate these percentages: the ketogenic diet and the Paleo diet.

The ketogenic diet is a more extreme version of a typical high-fat, low-carb diet. While traditional high-fat diets allow for quite a few carbohydrates in the diet, the ketogenic diet tends to restrict carbohydrate intake to around 50 grams—2 slices of whole wheat bread—of carbohydrate per day. This diet is about 5 to 10 percent carbohydrate, 80 percent fat, and the rest protein.

The ketogenic diet attempts to put a person into nutritional ketosis, where you burn a lot of fat. Almost all of the energy you use is from fat. When you do this, ketones are produced as natural byproducts. Your organs and cells use ketones when you are in ketosis instead of glucose. This typically would happen during periods of fasting or, as in this case, extreme carbohydrate restriction.

The ketogenic diet is being studied for possible use as a treatment for conditions like epilepsy and even brain cancer, as well as body composition and health improvements.

Eating like this, with so little carbohydrate, might be difficult for the first few weeks. Reports of irritability, hunger, and lethargy are common. But experts say that it becomes easier over time, and you can still exercise, perform, think, and concentrate on this kind of diet. But this is definitely not for everyone.

The Paleo Diet

The Paleo diet is a dietary approach based on eating like we imagine our ancestors did to stay healthy, lean, and fit. The idea is that we evolved to eat certain foods but not others.

The Paleo diet emphasizes animal products, nuts and seeds, fruits, and vegetables. Notably, strict followers of the Paleo diet do not eat grains, legumes (such as beans and peas), or dairy products. This is because the designers of the diet say that these foods did not exist 10,000 years ago, and our ancestors did not eat them. It's a sort of radical back-to-nature approach.

Many excellent books and websites dig into the evolution of these Paleo theories, and most do not hold up to scientific scrutiny from evolutionary biologists and archaeologists (because we don't know exactly what foods our ancestors ate 10,000 years ago). Nevertheless, the Paleo diet, overall, is an approach worth considering, but likely not for the reasons that Paleo followers promote.

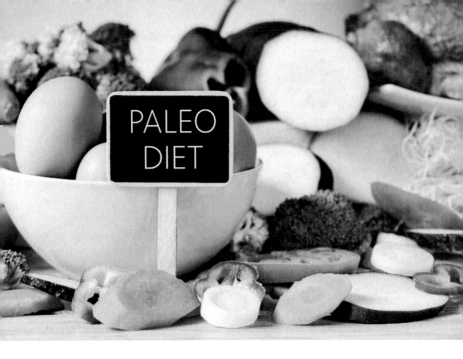

In general, Paleo promotes good-quality foods. Research has also shown that the Paleo diet improves many markers of health and metabolism. This diet promotes quality protein intake and lots of vegetables. Whole foods are also emphasized, so this diet is superior to a typical fast-food diet.

The exclusion of milk, legumes, and grains isn't a one-size-fits-all approach. Those with allergies or sensitivities might fair well, but for everyone else, it doesn't make much sense to eliminate all of these great foods. There are many lean, energetic, and active healthy people who choose to include milk, legumes, and dairy in their diets.

The original Paleo diet has been revised and has changed to a much more reasonable approach that is now mainstream. Things like grass-fed dairy and some starches and wine are allowed.

Intermittent Fasting

- Intermittent fasting is simply a diet plan where you go for extended periods of time without eating. There are many types of intermittent fasting schedules. Some popular ones include alternate-day fasting, where you only eat every other day; eat, stop, eat, where you have a 24-hour fast about 1 to 2 times per week; and the 16:8 diet, where you fast for 16 hours and then have 8 hours where eating is allowed.

- Intermittent fasting is not a new concept. Most people fast for about 8 to 10 hours every night. There are religious observances, such as Ramadan, where Muslims fast from sunrise to sunset for an entire month.

- Research is now accumulating to show some benefits to following an intermittent fasting diet. Health benefits—such as improved blood lipids and blood glucose, reduced inflammation in the body, and improved appetite control—have been shown.

- Theoretically, intermittent fasting could make a difference in body composition. The problem is that there are so many different styles of fasting, so clear-cut answers are difficult to come by.

- For some people, intermittent fasting fits well into their lifestyle. If you don't like breakfast and can't be bothered to take a lunch break, it might work for you. But for others, this style of eating can promote some binge eating at night and less control over what is eaten when you finally get home, feeling starved.

- If you are exercise training while fasted, and you do this regularly, data shows elevated markers of muscle damage and overall stress. And almost all data shows a performance advantage from eating food prior to exercise and a performance decrease if you are fasted.

- The benefits reported with intermittent fasting have also been shown with exercise and a restriction-free diet. So, only choose intermittent fasting if you know it fits your lifestyle and you know you can stick to it.

Try This

Rather than a fad diet, choose a healthy eating habit that you've learned and start by fitting it into your schedule just two times per week.

Questions to Consider

1. What are the positive and negative aspects of a diet that you have tried? Was the diet successful?

2. What would be the first easy-to-change habit that you would focus on?

Choosing Your Nutrition Plan

J ust about everyone I meet has an opinion, mantra, or theory about the best food to eat or diet to try. Nutrition, probably more than most topics, just inherently has some people thinking that their way is the only way. So, some interesting styles of eating have emerged. My friends and family have tried it all: low-fat, high-fat, low-carb, high-carb, vegan, raw, vegetarian, juice cleanses, ketogenic, MyPlate, Mediterranean, If It Fits Your Macros, paleo, intermittent fasting, and everything in-between. The interesting part is that the way you respond to a particular diet may be entirely different than the way your best friend does. The way we digest, absorb and use our food is very personal.

I had one client who was following, to the T, the gluten-free diet that her husband followed. She was surprised when I asked her if she liked to eat this way—her response was no, not particularly. Then I asked her if she had an allergy to gluten? Again, her answer was no. She was also feeling tired all the time. It was obvious to me that the diet simply didn't meet her specific needs.

The fad diet popularity may stem from the belief that maybe there is an easy way, a quick way to improve body composition. It also stems from the thought that there may be one diet that is best for everyone. But this just isn't the case. Your personal preferences and physiology have a lot to do with your success in changing body composition through diet and exercise. However, I know that media attention and the science behind some diets is interesting and appealing, but also, downright confusing.

In this lecture, I will highlight some interesting key points and new research for traditional diets and popular fad diets. Then, I'll wrap it all up with my personal thoughts on choosing your own nutritional path.

For many years, the conventional approach to eating in the US was to follow the Food Guide Pyramid. No doubt you've heard of this pyramid before, in fact, many countries have some pyramid design to indicate their eating recommendations. The original design had a wide base of grains, indicating you should build a diet primarily from carbohydrates, leading up to a peak of fat and oils, to use sparingly. In 2011, the traditional pyramid was replaced with something called MyPlate, which is an image of a plate with the food groups on it.

The new plate graphic has been both praised and criticized, but it does, at least, seem like it makes sense to show food on a plate rather than a pyramid. It was designed to remind Americans to eat healthfully, but not necessarily to change consumer behavior. So this guide is designed to remind us to eat healthfully, but this assumes that most Americans know how to eat healthfully and that healthfully actually has a definition that is the same for everyone.

If you take a glance at The MyPlate recommendations, you'll see that it is a bit hard to interpret which foods should be a priority or which foods are recommended. This may not be the best thing for people who are less informed about food types and quality. The MyPlate recommendations do encourage variety in what we eat, and they provide some visual cues for the proportion of vegetables, fruit, grains, and protein that should be on your plate. It also encourages whole grain consumption rather than simply more grain consumption. These are all good things, right?

MyPlate recommendations, however, are very general. The MyPlate diet traditionally is thought of as a high carbohydrate, low-fat diet, and it suggests that a plate 75% full of grains, vegetables, and fruit—which are all sources of carbohydrates—is the best for everyone—regardless of how active your lifestyle is.

For very active people, and especially people who like to work out at high intensities, a higher carbohydrate diet has been supported in the research more times than not. This, though, is usually based on improving exercise or sport performance, but not everyone is concerned with performance. You may be much more interested in body weight or body composition. You have to keep in mind that the overall calorie and carbohydrate needs of someone who is physically active will be different from someone of the same size and sex who is sitting still all day long typing on a computer, for example.

It's also important to remember that constantly high blood sugar levels—which you might get following a very high carbohydrate diet without enough exercise—are at least related to many different sorts of ailments including the well-known type 2 diabetes. Don't get me wrong; I don't believe that carbohydrates are not inherently a problem. But, it is the over-consumption of them combined with a lack of physical activity that tends to get us into some body composition trouble.

If you review the MyPlate recommendations more closely, they also suggest that real fruit and 100% fruit juice and real vegetables and 100% vegetable juices are the same. However, the ways we digest and absorb solid food compared to liquids are different in many ways, including how fast the nutrients get into your body. In addition, many juices are loaded with added sugars that real fruit does not contain. But, I do like the overall emphasis on eating more fruit and vegetables.

Lastly, it is important to note that healthy fats don't have a place—olive oil, avocado, and fish or fish oil are not included at all. And you may recall that healthy fats have a major place in our diets and have some wonderful health benefits.

Another drawback is that there is not really a distinction between better choices and worse choices of proteins or carbohydrates.

If you check out most of the epidemiological scientific literature, the overall theme is quite consistent for health and weight loss in overweight individuals: you should consume more healthy fats and reduce your intake of refined carbohydrates. There are both pluses and minuses with a high carbohydrate, low-fat diet, and it is entirely dependent on how you feel, look, and perform when eating this way.

Over much of the same time that we have been told that a higher carbohydrate, low-fat diet is best for all of us, primarily from the MyPlate recommendations, our obesity and diabetes rates have skyrocketed. So, naturally people have been drawn to drastically different eating styles to see if they provide their health and body composition improvements. Thus, the high-fat, low-carb diet was born. This sort of eating goes by many names like Atkins, Paleo, and now Keto. While these are actually different diets, some major similarities exist.

So what if we eat fewer carbohydrates and more fat? Advocates of the high-fat, low-carb diets point to research that shows more fat oxidation or fat burning with this sort of diet and rapid weight loss. So what does this really mean? Eating a high-fat diet means that fat would make up about 60–75% of your total caloric intake. The assumption with high-fat diets is that if carbohydrate feeding lowers your ability to burn fat, then a high fat diet would increase your ability to burn fat as a fuel. It sounds like this might improve body composition, doesn't it?

Overall, there is actually a lot of evidence to show improvements in health, body composition, and other physiological functions with a higher-fat, low-carbohydrate approach. For example, with the high-fat/low-carbohydrate approach. There is higher fat oxidation during exercise, increased availability of free fatty acids, and increased activity of fat oxidation enzymes. Additionally, there is a reduction in enzymes involved with glycolysis—which is the breakdown of sugar to provide energy—along with reduced muscle glycogen and liver glycogen storage.

This may be a really critical point—if you can better control blood sugar with a high-fat, low carbohydrate diet—this could be highly useful for controlling body fat and ultimately your overall body composition. Also, as you might remember for an earlier lecture, fat and protein tend to keep you feeling full for a longer period of time than carbohydrates alone.

So, if you can use a high-fat, low-carb approach to improve some health outcomes and maybe even body composition, what's wrong with it? Well, first, it is often carried out incorrectly. What I mean is that when I review what people are actually eating while on a high-fat diet, they usually just eating more fast food, fried food, and processed meats. More often than not, I see a high fat intake, with no concern for the type of fat, along with a normal amount of carbohydrate intake. Ultimately, with a plan like this, health does not seem to improve.

Second, there are some questions as to the feasibility of a high-fat, low carbohydrates diet when you bring exercise into the equation. Let me explain. Some studies show no difference in exercise performance after you eat a high-fat or a high-carb diet, however, these studies usually involve exercise that is done at a low to moderate intensities—like 45% of your VO2max or your maximal oxygen consumption—that's likely a slow walk. As you know, this relatively low level of intensity should rely more on fat as a fuel. So it makes sense that exercise performance was no different.

But what happens if you exercise at a high intensity or for prolonged periods of time say 2–3 hours or more at one time? If you exercise at high intensities, above 70–75% of your maximal ability, then exercise performance may decline on a high fat diet. Of course, there are exceptions, but this is likely the outcome. For example, in one study, untrained people were asked to follow either a high-fat diet or a high carb diet for 4 days. When the subjects were asked to exercise as long as possible at a relatively high intensity of 70-75% VO2max, the subjects on the high-fat diets did not perform as well as those on high-carbohydrate diets.

It is important to note that people who do a lot of aerobic exercise are able to use fat as a fuel at a much higher exercise intensities than the average person. They may be able to use fat above the 75% mark—although this is uncommon unless you really work at it and consistently stay on these high-fat diets.

Additionally, most experts say that it may take far more than 3–4 days of a certain diet for all of the advantages or disadvantages to take shape. So it might just be that these studies were too short to show a difference because the subjects are not fat adapted yet. Traditional high-fat, low-carb diets would shake out like this: 60% fat, 20% carbohydrates, and 20% protein. But, I must briefly mention two very popular diets that manipulate these percentages.

The first is the ketogenic diet. This is really a more extreme version of a typical high-fat, low carbohydrate diet. While these traditional high-fat diets allow for quite a few carbohydrates, the keto diet tends to keep carbohydrate intake to somewhere around 50 g of carbohydrates per day. To put that into perspective, that is 2 slices of whole wheat bread or 1 cup of oatmeal for the entire day. This diet is about 5–10% carbohydrates, 80% fat, and the rest protein.

The ketogenic diet attempts to put a person into nutritional ketosis. Nutritional ketosis is where you burn a lot of fat. Almost all of the energy you use is from fat. When you do this, ketones are produced as natural byproducts. Your organs and cells use ketones when you are in ketosis instead of glucose. This typically would happen during periods of fasting or, in this case, during extreme carbohydrate restriction. If you test your blood, urine or breath for these ketones, you would be considered in ketosis if you had a value above 1.0 mmol/L.

But, don't confuse nutritional ketosis with the dangerous condition of ketoacidosis. They are not the same. Ketoacidosis is dangerous and occurs in severe, uncontrolled diabetes. Ketoacidosis occurs when extremely high levels of ketones make your body very acidic, so much so that your normal metabolic physiology can shut down. Nutritional ketosis, however, does not alter your pH nearly as much. Nutritional ketosis will not harm you.

The ketogenic diet is being studied for possible use as a treatment for conditions like epilepsy and even brain cancer, and, now, for body composition and health improvements. There are entire books written on this type of eating, and they are gaining popularity all the time.

Eating like this, with so little carbohydrate might be difficult for the first few weeks. Reports of irritability, hunger, and lethargy are common. But the experts say that it becomes easier over time, and you can still exercise, perform, think and concentrate on this sort of diet. You simply switch your primary fuel source away from carbohydrates and instead run on ketones.

But, this is definitely not for everyone. In fact, in my opinion, cutting out entire food groups isn't necessary. Most of the elimination diets—meaning ones that eliminate an entire macronutrient—help with controlling calorie intake. Let's face it, by not eating an entire nutrient category, you're likely to eat less food overall, particularly in the short-term. So while this diet may work for some people, there are certainly alternatives that provide more options, variety, and pleasure in eating.

The second very popular diet to mention is called the Paleo diet. This is a dietary approach based on eating like we imagine our ancestors did in order to stay healthy, lean and fit. The idea is that we evolved to eat certain foods but not others.

The Paleo diet emphasizes animal products, nuts and seeds, fruits, and vegetables. Notably, strict followers of the Paleo diet do not eat grains, legumes like beans and peas, or dairy foods. This is because the designers of the diet say that these foods did not exist 10,000 years ago, and our ancestors did not eat them. It's a sort of radical back-to-nature approach. Many excellent books and websites dig into the evolution of these Paleo theories, and most do not actually hold up to scientific scrutiny from evolutionary biologists and archaeologists because we don't really know exactly what foods our ancestors ate 10,000 years ago. Nevertheless, the Paleo diet—overall—is an approach worth considering, but likely not for the reasons that Paleo followers promote.

In general, Paleo promotes good quality foods. Research has also shown that the Paleo diet improves many markers of health and metabolism. This diet promotes quality protein intake and lots of vegetables—that must be a good thing. Whole foods are also emphasized—so any way you cut it, this diet is superior to a typical fast-food diet.

The exclusion of milk, legumes, and grains isn't a one-size fit all approach. Those with allergies or sensitivities might fair well, but for everyone else, I'm not sure why you'd eliminate all these great foods. Honestly, I know many very lean, energetic and active healthy people who choose to include milk, legumes, and dairy in their diets.

While the arguments about the evolution of our ancestors and farming and eating practices that the Paleo diet suggest don't hold up, I do think that there are some really great parts to this diet, as well as the other diets that I've talked about in this lecture.

As I mentioned earlier, I have analyzed a number of dietary plans of Keto and Paleo followers. What I see more than anything is increases in dietary fat overall—not specifically good fat like avocados, nuts and seeds. I have also seen extremely high blood triglyceride levels and total body inflammation with this approach. It just seems like there is a lot of confusion about how to implement this dietary approach, particularly for highly active people. Interestingly, the original Paleo diet has been revised and has changed to a much more reasonable approach that is now mainstream. Things like grass-fed dairy and some starches and wine are now allowed.

Another diet called intermittent fasting has also gained a lot of attention recently. Intermittent fasting is simply a diet plan where you go for extended periods of time without eating. There are many types of intermittent fasting schedules. Some popular one's include alternate day fasting—where you only eat every other day; another one called eat, stop, eat—where you have a 24-hour fast about 1–2 times per week, and the 16–8 Diet—where you fast for 16 hours and then have an 8 hours window where you're allowed to eat.

This may sound odd, but it intermittent fasting is not really a new concept. Most people fast for about 8–10 hours every night. There are religious observances like Ramadan where, for an entire month, Muslims fast from sunrise to sunset. That sounds pretty close to the 16–8 diet, doesn't it?

Research is now accumulating to show some benefits to following an intermittent fasting diet. Health benefits like improved lipids and blood glucose, reduced inflammation in the body, and improved appetite control have all been shown. It seems like common sense too that if you eat fewer times in a day, you simply have less time to eat. Some research has shown reductions in body weight and body fat while maintaining muscle mass when one meal per day was compared to eating 3 meals per day in healthy men and women who were between the ages of 40 and 50. Also, animal studies have demonstrated increased lifespan following intermittent fasting diets.

So, theoretically, intermittent fasting could make a difference in body composition. The trouble is that there are so many different styles of fasting. So clear-cut answers are tough to come by.

For some people, intermittent fasting fits well into their lifestyle. If you don't like breakfast, and can't be bothered to take a lunch break, it might work for you. I have one client who has maintained a 16 hour fast, and 8-hour feeding window for over 5 years now. But, for others, this style of eating can promote some binge eating at night and less control over what is eaten when you finally get home feeling starved.

It is important to note that if you are exercise training while fasted, and you do this regularly, data shows elevated markers of damage and overall stress. And, almost all data shows a performance advantage from eating food prior to exercise and a performance decrease if you are fasted. For example, research on athletes that are fasted indicates a reduction in speed, agility, endurance, and a decrease in mood and alertness. Occasionally using a fasted workout is fine as part of a larger plan for a specific goal, but I wouldn't recommend it for every single workout.

The bottom line is that the benefits reported with intermittent fasting have also been shown with exercise and a restriction-free diet. So, I would only choose intermittent fasting if you know it fits your lifestyle and you know you can stick to it.

As you might be able to tell by now, people are serious about supporting or bashing either the high-carbohydrates, low-fat approach or the low-carbohydrates, high-fat approach. For some reason, this riles people up as much as an argument about politics. You may even feel this way about the various fad diets that you've tried.

But let's be smart about this. I think there are certain good points to most of the diets that exist. These include controlling calorie intake, attempting to have more people eat more high-quality foods and limiting highly processed and sugar-filled foods as well as trying to make it easy to follow. You'll see these commonalities regardless of the diet plan.

So, how do we get it right? Which diet do we choose? Well, the bookstore probably won't help too much—you'll see thousands of dietary books on the shelves. This, more than almost anything, shows that we don't have it right yet and that we are still searching for the optimal way to eat. In a book called *Faster, Higher, Stronger*, author Mark McClusky says that it is the execution of what you know to be true that's most helpful, and not getting lost chasing some magic bullet. I agree. It's all about taking care of the most basics first. For example, maybe just eat more vegetables for 3 weeks until it becomes part of your daily routine. Then, and only then, try a new habit like eating more lean protein for a few weeks.

Handle your basic nutrition needs and see how you respond to the foods you eat. What makes you feel good, energetic and healthy? These questions are often lost in the sea of concerns about body weight. The best approach is to pick just one or two attainable goals and master them—avoid all the other stuff you hear about. For example, McClusky described this recommendation for athletes: Eat one g of protein daily for every lbs of body weight to support muscular growth and eat at least eight fist-sized servings of vegetables per day. The mantra has become to eat better to change your body composition, not less.

Here are a few strategies that I use personally: Aim for minimally processed foods. Try for fewer refined starches and sugars. Eat protein with each meal or snack. Eat more fruits and vegetables, and eat more good fats like nuts, eggs, avocado, and fish

The goals of any of these strategies are simple—emphasize quality in your diet and understand that one positive habit you adopt, no matter how simple, so long as you can adhere to it, can make a great long term impact on your body composition and health. Try this: Rather than a fad diet, choose a healthy eating habit that I outlined and start by fitting it into your schedule just two times per week.

Motivation to Change Your Body Composition

The goal of this course has been to provide you with tools to implement change as you see fit. What you now have is a knowledge base and a tool set. Together, they offer a way to achieve more and live life as a fit and healthy person. You have the science behind the basics of nutrition and exercise and how they work to alter your body composition, improve your performance, and optimize your health. But how do you best implement these changes? This lecture discusses major motivational concepts and ideas for how to change your daily behaviors to reach your optimal body composition, health, and performance.

Successfully Changing Your Body Composition

- Changing your exercise habits alone is probably not enough to drastically change your body composition. To significantly change body composition, both smart exercise and a healthy diet are necessary.

- In addition, the type of exercise you do makes a difference. For example, research has shown that simply eating a higher-protein diet and doing both resistance training and HIIT training leads to more body fat and belly fat loss compared to eating a more traditional lower-protein diet and simply walking or jogging most days of the week.

- If your goal is to improve body composition, simplify both your diet and exercise routine, and do not change everything at once. Creating a complex meal plan and exercise schedule does you no good if you can't stick to it. It might just set you up for failure and disappointment.

No change is too small. And the more confident you are with your goal, the more likely you are to be successful.

Another strategy is to simply be aware and fully present when you make nutrition and exercise choices. This is more difficult than it seems.

How many times do you try to eat a meal, finish a few emails, take a call, watch television, and talk to your spouse all at the same time? If you're too busy and distracted to pay attention to what you're eating and drinking throughout the day, it is easy to overeat or overdrink.

Researchers have shown that distracted eating leads to eating more food at that meal and in subsequent meals. In addition, simply being mindful—or paying attention—leads to eating less later in the day.

The type of distraction that leads to more food consumption is probably individualized. But there are many different types of mindless acts that can sabotage everything you have worked so hard for during your workouts.

The simple act of paying attention and being physically and mentally present when you eat can make a real difference in the number of calories you consume. It's much easier to eat until you are about 80 percent full if you pay attention. There is no clear way for how to only eat until you are 80 percent full, so you will have to experiment with this.

Research has shown that people who know about and practice being fully present when they eat—called mindful eating—take in fewer calories throughout the day and lose significantly more weight than people who do not.

To start, slow down. Simply eating slowly might give your brain a chance to process your hunger cues and help you figure out when to stop eating. It takes a little time to feel full. If you don't give yourself that time and just keep shoveling your food in, it's pretty easy to get a few hundred extra calories down in just a few minutes.

- Also, try to eliminate distractions. Just like when you drive, if you can stop all the distractions—such as television, tablets, cell phones, and any number of gadgets—when you eat, you'll have a better chance of making it to your destination.

- You can also practice being fully present and engaged during your workouts. If you're outside, try to look around a bit (safely, of course) and notice the landscape and trees and smell the fresh air. If you always jog or run with music, then from time to time, try unplugging and listening to your breathing and heartbeat as you exercise.

- Think about what muscles are working and what these exercises are doing for you. Think about how much stronger you are becoming both physically and mentally from each successful workout.

- Some people call this the mind-body connection. You think about your progress, the blood flowing through your body and nourishing your cells, and the fuel you ate to power your workout and make you strong and energetic.

- This ability to focus and connect with your workout could be the one thing that turns the corner for you and makes you truly love being physically active.

- Also, find activities that you enjoy doing. They might be traditional things, such as walking, running, or swimming, or other options, such as yoga, hiking, group exercise, or sports. There are endless options for getting in your recommended amount of exercise, and it doesn't have to be something you dread.

- To improve health, you need to exercise. Doing a wide variety of exercises, including resistance training and high-intensity intervals, can be pretty simple to include and can also be fun, especially if you are in the right mindset for change.

Adherence to your diet and exercise plans are going to make or break your efforts. No matter the diet or exercise regimen, a participant's adherence to the program is most strongly associated with their weight loss. Simply making changes that you can stick to is the key to success with body composition change.

Grocery Shopping Tips

One way to improve adherence is to understand how to set up your home for success, and it starts with knowing some grocery shopping tips. This is one of the most fundamental concepts that sets the stage for making successful dietary changes. If your grocery shopping is organized, it makes it so much easier for you to make better and healthier choices at home.

Make a list before you go to the store. You arrive prepared, and you save time. Just get what you need. If it isn't on the list, don't buy it. This doesn't mean to exclude any items that you consider treats—but only buy small amounts, because if it's in your house, you'll probably eat it.

Making a list also helps you think about your meals for the week, rather than just one meal or one day's meals. You have a broader perspective on your dietary choices. Making a list helps you prepare for meals in advance so that you're more likely to have a go-to option that fuels you right.

If you don't use a list, especially if you are new to eating well, you are more likely to buy the food you've always bought, and that might be the problem. Use a list to remind you of the healthier choices you want to start making.

Don't get confused by labels like "natural," "gluten-free," and "low-fat." The food industry bombards you with thousands of options, which leads to confusion and often poor choices. The health halo effect occurs when you see a label on the front of a package that says "good source of vitamin C" and believe that it is automatically better for you or lower in calories.

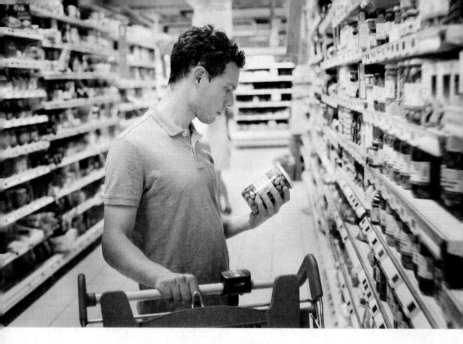

These claims can actually mean very little, but we often believe that they are better for us. Your best bet is to investigate the product for yourself by looking at the Nutrition Facts label that can be found on each item. Or, better yet, aim for minimally processed foods with as few ingredients as possible.

It isn't practical to think that you can avoid processed foods altogether. Almost everything we buy to eat is processed in some way. But aim for products that require the least amount of processing to get onto your plate.

When you get home, you might even immediately wash and cut fruits and vegetables and store them in a visible place or keep a bowl of fruit out on the counter for an easy grab-and-go option. Keep things like nuts, seeds, and vegetables accessible for snacks.

Simple changes to your grocery habits and kitchen setup will enable you to make better choices and help you meet your goals. Several facets of your lifestyle play a role in your ability to successfully make behavior changes, so take note of these and slowly address them over time.

What Progress Looks Like

- As you implement one change at a time, you might wonder what sort of results you can anticipate. Patience is key. If it took 20 years to put on, give it more than 20 days to come off.

- Losing massive amounts of weight quickly might not be the best approach. If you lose 5 pounds (2.3 kilograms) in a week, it is most likely due to changes in water weight or even from muscle loss with extreme calorie restriction. Neither of these will result in the positive body composition changes you are looking for.

- Some research supports the idea that slower weight loss might be best for actual and permanent changes in body composition, particularly with your muscle mass.

- What kind of changes in numbers should you see if you make a solid effort to improve your body composition? It's difficult to say because it is so individualized, but some experts suggest that average fat loss changes are around 0.5 percent body fat loss every 4 weeks and average muscle gain is around 1 pound (0.45 kilograms) of lean mass every 4 weeks (if those are your specific goals).

- Before focusing on numbers and goals, you should consider how these changes make you feel. Is this working for your lifestyle? And then listen to your body. But if you aren't making any progress, then it is important to reevaluate and make a change that you can stick to, and begin the process again.

- Being aware of what your progress should look like and being prepared to encounter barriers and relapses are both very important to your overall success.

Try This

Write down your shopping list and take it with you to the store to stock your house with foods that support your goals.

Questions to Consider

1. What is one behavior change that you will make to overcome a barrier?

2. What is one goal that you will set yourself to achieve?

Motivation to Change your Body Composition

From the onset of this course, the idea has been to provide you tools to implement change as you see fit. What you now have is a knowledge base and a tool set. Together, they offer a way to achieve more and live life as a fit and healthy person. You have the science behind the basics of nutrition and exercise and how they work to alter your body composition, improve your performance, and optimize your health.

But, how do you best implement these changes? Well, that is the purpose of this lecture. But is no secret because I've been hinting at it throughout all of the lectures in this course. The key is to make small changes in your daily behaviors and habits. Sounds easy enough, right? Well, that's the entire point—to make this journey towards your optimal body composition as easy as humanly possible.

Did you know that about 40% of the actions that we do in a day are habits? This means almost 10 hours of our day is spent doing things we don't consciously think about. That is a significant amount of time. If poor eating and no exercise have developed into habits over time, it makes it much harder to change because they are so ingrained in your daily routine. That's why it always seems crazy to me that people think they can change everything overnight or lose the fat in one week that it took them 20 years to put on. But change is definitely possible if the right approach is taken.

The key is to set small, reachable goals and alter small, daily habits that fit into your lifestyle. Maybe you were expecting me to give you an overall plan that had you eating only chicken breasts and broccoli, drinking herbal teas and practicing yoga for hours on end—but that'll never work.

The changes you make need to work for you. Trying to lift as much as your personal trainer or eat just like her may not work for you. That works for her—and was probably developed over many years.

But only you know what works best for you, and your schedule, and your family, and your goals. Focus on changes you know you can make with the greatest success. Also, keep in mind that the ability to successfully change a behavior is closely related to your confidence. If you set a goal that you are not confident in, then you're likely to make it. Why not make it easier on yourself and choose goals that you are sure to meet. For example, what seems more realistic? Exercising for one hour three days per week or losing 30 lbs of fat? Doesn't it seem much easier to work on the habits that you can control rather than on results that you really can't control? It's far easier to say I'll exercise three days per week, or I'll eat 4 servings of vegetables today.

This lecture discusses major motivational concepts, and ideas for how to change your daily behaviors in order to reach your optimal body composition, health, and performance.

You need to know that changing your exercise habits alone is probably not enough to drastically change your body composition. Of course, there are success stories here and there, but to a large extent exercise alone won't push the dial too far. To significantly change body composition both smart exercise and a healthy diet as we have discussed it are absolutely necessary.

Researchers have looked at the effect of diet alone, exercise alone or the combination on weight and body composition changes in overweight to obese women. The women were randomized into 1 of 4 groups for an entire year—the diet-only group followed a calorie-reduced, low-fat diet; the exercise-only group completed an aerobic exercise program working up to about 45 minutes of exercise, 5 days per week; and the combined group obviously did both of these. They also had a 4th control group had no lifestyle change at all. After a year of this, the diet-only group decreased body fat by 4.2%—which is not bad. The exercise-only group didn't fare nearly as well and only lowered body fat by 1.6%; it was the combined diet and exercise group that did the best and lost 5.9% body fat. Other studies seem to line up most of the time to confirm these results: that diet and exercise must be combined to see significant changes.

The research I've been involved in has also shown that the type of exercise you do makes a difference. For example, simply eating a higher protein diet and doing both resistance training and HIIT training led to more body fat and belly fat loss compared to eating a more traditional lower-protein diet and simply walking or jogging most days of the week. So, what else can you do to better your chances of success?

If your goal is to improve body composition, I recommend you simplify both your diet and exercise routine and do not change everything at once. Creating a complex meal plan and exercise schedule does you no good if you can't stick to it. It may just set you up for failure and disappointment. Honestly, no change is too small. For example, Dr. John Berardi, a leading physique transformation expert, recommends asking yourself how confident you feel on a scale of 1–10 that you could complete a new behavior task, something like eating at least 3 servings of vegetables, 5 days per week. Then, only start this new habit if you answered a 9 or a 10 on the scale. Anything lower and this doesn't seem to stick very well—it's likely too much to expect of yourself—or anyone else. The more confident you are with your goal, the more likely you are to be successful.

Another strategy is to simply be aware and fully present when you make nutrition and exercise choices. This is harder than it seems. How many times do you try to eat a meal, finish a few emails, take a call, watch TV, and talk to your wife all at the same time? I have to work at this all the time too, but if you're too busy and distracted to really pay attention to what you're eating and drinking throughout the day, it is really easy to overeat and overdrink. Researchers from the University of Birmingham in the United Kingdom published an article in 2013 in the *American Journal of Clinical Nutrition* that analyzed all related research for how attention and memory influenced how much food was eaten.

Each study of the 24 studies analyzed had groups that were either distracted or not while eating—such as watching TV or not watching TV. The authors found that distracted eating lead to eating more food at that meal and in subsequent meals. They also reported that simply being mindful—or paying attention—lead to eating less later in the day.

Another study had 60 women eat a cereal bar while watching TV, walking, or talking and measured their desire to eat and total food intake. While the desire to eat was not influenced, the women consumed more calories in the day specifically 5 times more chocolate if the cereal bar was eaten while walking. The authors simply noted that this served as a form of distraction that lead them to overeat.

The type of distraction that would lead to more food consumption is probably quite individualized. In this study walking was a bigger distraction than TV. But there are many different types of mindless acts that can completely sabotage everything you have worked so hard for during your workouts.

The simple act of paying attention and being physically and mentally present when you eat can make a real difference in the number of calories you consume. It's far easier to eat until you about 80% full if you pay attention. There is no clear way for how to only eat until you are 80% full—so you will have to experiment with this. You probably know, though, that feeling of very hungry and also being way too full. So practice stopping at a point when you feel like you are not overly full—perhaps it is that point when you say to yourself—I should probably stop now, but one more serving would be so good. Give it a try—I think you'll find out how to stop when you are about 80% full if you practice enough and make this a real goal.

Along the same line, one study decided to see how this approach, often called mindful eating, worked in middle-aged women who ate out at restaurants at least 3 times per week. They had one group attend small group sessions to learn about behavior change and mindful eating strategies, while the other group had no help at all. As you might expect, the people who knew about and practiced being fully present when they ate, took in fewer calories throughout the day and lost significantly more weight. So, here's how to start—slow down.

Simply eating slowly might just give your brain a chance to process your hunger cues and help you figure out when to stop eating. It is pretty well understood that it takes a little bit time to feel full. If you don't give yourself that time, and just keep shoveling your food in, it's pretty easy to get a few hundred extra calories down in just a few minutes. Also, try to eliminate distractions. Just like when you drive, if you can stop all the distractions when you eat, you'll have a better chance of making it to your destination. TV, tablets, cell phones and any number of gadgets will distract you.

You can also practice being fully present and engaged during your workouts. I can't tell you how many times I'll walk into my gym and notice the same person, day after day, year after year, mindlessly go through the motions. If you're outside, try to look around a bit safely, of course, and notice the landscape, the trees, smell the fresh air. If you always jog or run with music, then from time to time, try unplugging and listening to your breathing and heartbeat as you exercise. Think about what muscles are working, and what these exercises are doing for you. Think about how much stronger you are becoming both physically and mentally from each successful workout.

Some people call this the mind-body connection. You think about your progress, you think about the blood flowing through your body and it nourishing your cells, you think about the fuel you ate to power your workout and make you strong and energetic. Your body is an amazing thing and deserves some attention. This ability to focus and connect with your workout could be the one thing that turns the corner for you, and makes you truly love being physically active.

Also, find activities that you enjoy to do. They may be traditional things like walking, running, swimming or other options like yoga, hiking, group exercise, golf, basketball, or any other sport. There are endless options for getting in your recommended amount of exercise, and it doesn't have to be something you dread.

Without a doubt, to improve health, you need to exercise. If I told you that there was a medication that provided the same benefits as exercise, it would be prescribed to everyone in the world. To truly optimize your body composition, simply walking probably won't cut it. It will improve health and maybe even body weight, but it probably won't change your body composition dramatically. But, doing a wide variety of exercises, including resistance training and high-intensity interval training can be pretty simple to include and can also be fun, especially if you are in the right mindset for change.

The last point to emphasize is that adherence to your diet and exercise plans are going to make or break you. Recently, a short review came out that analyzed studies that evaluated popular diets. No matter what diet was tried, they all consistently had one thing in common. No matter the diet or exercise regimen, the participant's adherence to the prog was most strongly associated with their weight loss. So simply making changes that you can stick to is the key to success with body composition change.

One way to improve adherence is to understand how to set-up your home for success. And it starts with knowing some grocery shopping tips. This is really one of the most fundamental concepts that set the stage for making successful dietary changes. If your grocery shopping list is organized, it makes it so much easier for you to make better and healthier choices at home.

Where do you go first? Make a list before you go to the store. This way you arrive prepared, and you save you time. Just get what you need and get out of there. If it isn't on the list, don't buy it. This doesn't mean to exclude any items that you consider treats—but only buy small amounts. Because if you are like me, if it's in your house, you'll probably eat it.

Making a list also helps you think about your meals for the week, rather than just one meal or one day's meals. You have a broader perspective on your dietary choices this way, and making a list helps you prepare for meals in advance, so you're more likely to have a go-to option that fuels you right. If you don't use a list, especially if you are new to eating well, you are more likely to buy food you've always bought, and that may be the problem. Use a list to remind you of the healthier choices you want to start making. Keep in mind that grocery stores are scientifically set up to encourage you to spend more money and buy more things.

You'll often hear experts tell you to stay on the perimeter of the store because that's where you find fresh fruits and vegetables and foods like lean meats, and dairy products. But, you'll need to dive into the middle of the store as well for some staples like olive oil, tea, nuts, seeds, some legumes, and some whole grain options too.

But, don't get confused by labels like natural, gluten-free, and low-fat. The food industry bombards you with thousands of options, which leads to confusion and often poor choices. There is something called the health halo effect—this happens when you see a label on the front of a package that says good source of vitamin C and believe that it is automatically better for you or lower in calories.

These claims can actually mean very little, but we often believe these foods are better for us. For example, the label natural is not regulated by the Food and Drug Administration. But, the United States Department of Agriculture USDA states that Natural is for meat, egg, and poultry products that must be minimally processed with no artificial ingredients. But this has nothing to do with the farming practices—so it could still have antibiotics and growth hormones in the raising process.

Gluten-Free simply means that a particular food has less than 20 parts per million of gluten. It means nothing about the calorie count, nutrient density, or quality of the food. I have had clients tell me they are eating healthy because they are eating gluten-free. But the gluten-free products showed me were not even close to healthy. Unless you have a doctor's order, eating gluten free is no more or less healthy than eating gluten-full.

The same goes for low-fat products. All this means is that the food can have no more than 3 g of fat per serving. Usually, low-fat foods are also stuffed full of added sugars to improve the flavor due to the lower fat content. Your best bet is to investigate the product for yourself by looking at the nutrition facts label that can be found on each item. Or better yet, aim for minimally processed foods with as few ingredients as you can manage.

Notice I didn't say don't eat processed foods. This just isn't very practical. Most everything we buy to eat is processed in some way. Just aim for products that require the least amount of processing to get onto your plate. When you get home, you might even immediately wash and cut fruits and vegetables and store them in a visible place or keep a bowl of fruit out on the counter for an easy grab and go option. And keep things like nuts, seeds, and vegetables accessible for snacks.

Like I said earlier, if it's in your pantry, you'll probably eat it. So try keeping foods you don't want to be tempted by out of your house. I had a client who told me that she only kept those off limit types of foods in the house for her kids and her husband. You see, she had not yet found support from her family for her body composition and health goals. That is an important part of it, and maybe it can be a family decision to get some foods out of the house during the week.

Maybe you can put the money you'd spend on unhealthy snacks into a fund for a special family outing or some other treat. You might even try keeping a list of non-food treats for yourself for when you're tempted to reach out for food to calm down or distract you. Simple changes to your grocery habits and kitchen set up will enable you to make better choices and help meet your goals. Remember that several facets of your lifestyle play a role in your ability to successfully make behavior changes, so take note of these and slowly address them over time.

As you implement one change at a time, you might wonder what sort of results you can anticipate. Well, let me tell you, patience is key. Again, if it took 20 years to put it on, give it more than 20 days to come off. Losing massive amounts of weight quickly may not be the best approach—even though we see this on TV all the time. If you lose 5 lbs, or 2.3 kg, in one week, it is most likely due to changes in water weight or even from muscle loss with extreme calorie restriction. Neither of these will result in the positive body composition changes you are looking for. Some research supports the idea that slower weight loss might be best for actual and permanent changes in body composition, particularly with your muscle mass.

So what kind of changes in numbers should you really see if you're making a really solid effort to improve your body composition? It's tough to tell because it is so individualized, but some experts suggest that average fat loss changes are around 0.5% body fat lost every 4 weeks, and average muscle gain is around 1 lbs or 0.45 kg, of lean mass every 4 weeks if those are your specific goals. And I know you all want numbers and goals, but you should first ask yourself how does this make me feel? Is this working for my lifestyle? And then listen to your body. But if you aren't making any progress then it's important to reevaluate and make a change that you can stick to and begin the process again.

For example, let's say your goal was to pack your lunch for work at least 4 days per week, but you were only able to do it for 2 days. Now identify what didn't work. Perhaps you waited until the morning to pack your lunch and ran out of time. Maybe you didn't buy the right foods at the store. Recheck some items on those grocery store lists. Well, these barriers should become the focus of your change.

For instance, you might leave a note on your bathroom mirror to remind you to pack your lunch before bed. Being aware of what your progress should look like and being prepared to encounter barriers and relapses are both very important to your overall success.

Behavior change is the ultimate combination of everything we've discussed. The fascinating field of body composition, exercise, nutrition, and health is rigorously scientific, and what we know is growing and changes all the time. Ignore the fads. Possessing real knowledge about the science of nutrition and the science of exercise to improve your body composition will help only if you can put it into action.

Unfortunately, there is a huge difference between knowing what to actually do and then actually doing it. As the popular quote states, The difference between who you are and what you want to be is what you do.

And the time to start is now. There is not a right time and tomorrow is probably not any better than today. Choose one small thing to implement and get after it.

Surround yourself with positive and supportive people too. They say you are the average of the 5 people you associate with most. So be sure some of those people lead you towards good behaviors. This alone could spark some change in you that you never knew existed and allow you to discover your optimal body composition.

I absolutely love this field. I love being in the trenches of the research world and being able to share the science with the public. It is truly a pleasure to work on projects that really impact people in a positive way. I got started in this field in an attempt to improve my own body composition and performance. But, over the years, that goal has evolved to more altruistic endeavors, and there's nothing better than when the research published from my lab can actually be applied to help you improve your health, performance, and body composition.

You have just dedicated your time to improving your knowledge base in the science and application of nutrition and exercise to improve your body composition. Whether you want to make a change or just learn the information so you can continue to enjoy health and vigor, I hope you're excited to know everything that you do now. Let's face it, no matter, if you are an accountant, a salesperson, or a professor—your body composition and health, must be priorities in your life.

Now that you know the nuts and bolts, I suggest that you start simply using the try this recommendations of each lecture in the course to help you make healthy changes. It is never too late to improve the quality of your life.

The science of nutrition and exercise physiology continues to evolve. It is exciting for me to know that what we can measure in the laboratory may provide us insight on better or more efficient ways to achieve more and live life fit. It could be a new superfood or supplement, or just a novel way to use nutrient timing that changes the scope of performance nutrition.

My research team is now answering some questions surrounding these topics. We continue to learn about new ways to optimize body composition, health, and performance. As you continue along your health and body composition journey, make sure to stay open-minded and to seek out the latest evidence.

Try This: Write out your shopping list and take it with you to the store to stock your house with foods that support your goals.

Good luck to you, and stay fit.

Bibliography

Websites/Online Articles

American College of Sports Medicine. "Protein Intake for Optimal Muscle Maintenance." http://www.acsm.org/docs/default-source/brochures/protein-intake-for-optimal-muscle-maintenance.pdf. [Lecture 9]

American Diabetes Association. *Glycemic Index and Diabetes.* http://www.diabetes.org/food-and-fitness/food/what-can-i-eat/understanding-carbohydrates/glycemic-index-and-diabetes.html. [Lecture 6]

American Heart Association. *Monounsaturated Fats.* http://www.heart.org/HEARTORG/GettingHealthy/NutritionCenter/HealthyEating/Monounsaturated-Fats_UCM_301460_Article.jsp#. [Lecture 7]

Ammeson, Jane. "Sleep-Friendly Foods for a Good Night's Rest." *The Times.* http://www.nwitimes.com/niche/get-healthy/healthy-living/sleep-friendly-foods-for-a-good-night-s-rest/article_53cee181-89d6-529c-bcc4-f63a80ad8582.html. [Lecture 20]

Andrews, Ryan. "Body Type Eating: Find Out Whether It's Right for You." *Precision Nutrition* (blog). http://www.precisionnutrition.com/all-about-body-type-eating. [Lecture 2]

———. "Phytates and Phytic Acid: Here's What You Need to Know." *Precision Nutrition* (blog). http://www.precisionnutrition.com/all-about-phytates-phytic-acid. [Lecture 10]

Anello, Robert, Joshua D'Alessandro, and Palmer Johnson. "Dietary Contaminants and Hormonal Disturbances: Is There a Link?" *Mike Ormsbee* (blog). http://mikeormsbee.com/dietary-contaminants-and-hormonal-disturbances-is-there-a-link/. [Lecture 20]

Antonio, Jose. "An Ode to Nutrient Timing." *International Society of Sports Nutrition.* http://www.theissnscoop.com/an-ode-to-nutrient-timing/. [Lecture 12]

Badalaty, Gina. "Obesogens: The Hidden Chemicals That Can Make Your Family Fat." *Mamavation* (blog). http://www.mamavation.com/2015/02/obesogens-hidden-chemicals-can-make-family-fat.html. [Lecture 20]

Berardi, John. "10 Lessons for Your Leanest Summer." *Precision Nutrition* (blog). http://www.precisionnutrition.com/10-lessons-for-2012. [Lecture 22]

———. "Better Version of 'My Plate': Precision Nutrition's Eating Guidelines for Clients." *Precision Nutrition* (blog). http://www.precisionnutrition.com/pn-my-plate. [Lecture 23]

Beyond Vegetarianism. "Comparison of Vitamin Levels in Raw vs. Cooked Foods." http://www.beyondveg.com/tu-j-l/raw-cooked/raw-cooked-2f.shtml. [Lecture 10]

Boston, G. "Why It's So Hard to Lose Those Last 5 Pounds." http://www.washingtonpost.com/lifestyle/wellness/why-its-so-hard-to-lose-those-last-5-pounds/2014/05/20/c15b69f2-dae4-11e3-b745-87d39690c5c0_story.html. [Lecture 22]

Brightcove. "Weight Loss: Where Do Our Calories Go?" Video. http://link.brightcove.com/services/player/bcpid1954212222001?bckey=AQ~~,AAAB xqEDkXE~,hmZyzKR72h2-K9-NOFee3eDD2vff8t15&bctid=3571710062001. [Lecture 3]

Bushak, Lecia. "Obese People Have an Extremely Low Chance of Recovering Normal Body Weight: Study." *Medical Daily.* http://www.medicaldaily.com/obese-people-have-extremely-low-chance-recovering-normal-body-weight-study-343534. [Lecture 22]

Carnell, Susan. "Do You Eat Out of Boredom?" *Psychology Today.* https://www.psychologytoday.com/blog/bad-appetite/201112/do-you-eat-out-boredom. [Lecture 21]

Caroll, Aaron E. "To Lose Weight, Eating Less Is Far More Important Than Exercising More." *The New York Times.* http://www.nytimes.com/2015/06/16/upshot/to-lose-weight-eating-less-is-far-more-important-than-exercising-more.html?_r=1&abt=0002&abg=1. [Lecture 22]

Center for Science in the Public Interest. "Artificial Trans Fat: On the Way Out!" http://www.cspinet.org/transfat/. [Lecture 11]

Centers for Disease Control and Prevention. "Insufficient Sleep Is a Public Health Problem." http://www.cdc.gov/features/dssleep/. [Lecture 20]

————. *Nutrition.* www.cdc.gov/nutrition. [Lecture 7]

Cespedes, Andrea. "Calories Burned Standing vs. Sitting." *LIVESTRONG. COM.* http://www.livestrong.com/article/73916-calories-burned-standing-vs.-sitting/. [Lecture 16]

Dunham, Will. "Weight of the World: 2.1 Billion People Obese or Overweight." *Reuters.* http://www.reuters.com/article/2014/05/28/us-health-obesity-idUSKBN0E82HX20140528. [Lecture 6]

EatingWell (blog). "How to Set Up Your Kitchen for Weight-Loss Success." http://www.eatingwell.com/nutrition_health/weight_loss_diet_plans/how_to_set_up_your_kitchen_for_weight_loss_success?page=2. [Lecture 24]

Ericson, John. "75% of Americans May Suffer from Chronic Dehydration, According to Doctors." http://www.medicaldaily.com/75-americans-may-suffer-chronic-dehydration-according-doctors-247393. [Lecture 10]

Esco, Michael R. "Resistance Training for Health and Fitness." *American college of Sports Medicine.* http://www.acsm.org/docs/brochures/resistance-training.pdf. [Lecture 18]

Fisher, Adjua. "5 Totally Weird Science-Backed Ways to Burn Calories Today (without Exercising)." *Be Well Philly.* http://www.phillymag.com/be-well-philly/2015/03/04/5-science-backed-ways-burn-calories-today-without-exercising/. [Lecture 20]

Ghose, Tia. "Cold-Weather Benefit: Shivering May Count as Exercise." *Live Science.* http://www.livescience.com/43085-shivering-triggers-exercise-response.html. [Lecture 20]

Gorksi, Chris. "What Should Athletes and the Rest of Us Eat at Night?" *Mike Ormsbee* (blog). http://mikeormsbee.com/what-should-athletes-and-the-rest-of-us-eat-at-night/. [Lecture 13]

Greenfield, Ben. "How Much Should You Drink during Exercise?" http://www.quickanddirtytips.com/health-fitness/exercise/how-much-should-you-drink-during-exercise?page=1. [Lecture 10]

Grover, Jenni. "Mindful Eating: 5 Easy Tips to Get Started." *Huffpost Healthy Living.* http://www.huffingtonpost.com/2013/11/12/mindful-eating-tips_n_3941528.html. [Lecture 24]

Harvard Health Publications. *Glycemic Index and Glycemic Load for 100+ Foods.* http://www.health.harvard.edu/newsweek/Glycemic_index_and_glycemic_load_for_100_foods.htm. [Lecture 6]

Helland, L. "35 Lessons from Precision Nutrition's Most Successful Clients." http://www.precisionnutrition.com/35-ways-to-transform-your-body?utm_source=35WaysToTransformBody&utm_medium=Email&utm_campaign=35WaysToTransformBodyEmail. [Lecture 22]

Iowa State University Extension and Outreach. *Fat.* http://www.extension.iastate.edu/humansciences/fat. [Lecture 7]

Ji, Sayer. "Splenda (Sucralose) Found to Have Diabetes-Promoting Effects." *Epoch Times.* http://www.theepochtimes.com/n3/1162919-splenda-sucralose-found-to-have-diabetes-promoting-effects/. [Lecture 20]

Jones, Jeffrey M. "In U.S., 40% Get Less Than Recommended Amount of Sleep." *Gallup*. http://www.gallup.com/poll/166553/less-recommended-amount-sleep.aspx. [Lecture 20]

Keller, Tracy. "The Psychology behind a Grocery Store's Layout." *Notre Dame College Online*. http://online.notredamecollege.edu/psychology/the-psychology-behind-a-grocery-store%E2%80%99s-layout/. [Lecture 24]

Kirkpatrick, Kristin. "5 Strategies to Help You Stop Emotional Eating." *Health Essentials*. http://health.clevelandclinic.org/2015/05/5-strategies-to-help-you-stop-emotional-eating/. [Lecture 24]

Kotulak, R. "Vitamin a Day Just What the Doctor Orders." *Chicago Tribune*. http://articles.chicagotribune.com/2002-06-19/news/0206190305_1_vitamins-rdas-pellagra. [Lecture 10]

Kotz, Deborah. "Are No-Calorie Sweeteners Safe to Eat?" *The Boston Globe*. https://www.bostonglobe.com/lifestyle/health-wellness/2014/01/27/are-calorie-sweeteners-safe/B56kqUuKVJwcEfcWx2PmhO/story.html. [Lecture 20]

Kravitz, Len, and Vivian H. Heyward. "Getting a Grip on Body Composition." http://www.unm.edu/~lkravitz/Article%20folder/underbodycomp.html. [Lecture 2]

Kuzma, Cindy. "The New Math of Calorie Counting." *Men's Health*. http://www.menshealth.com/weight-loss/counting-calories-weight-loss?cm_mmc=DailyDoseNL-_-1755306-_-06302014-_-TheNewMathofCalorieCounting-hed. [Lecture 22]

MacMillan, Amanda. "11 Ways to Stop Overeating after Your Workout." *Time*. http://time.com/3341969/overeating-after-your-workout/. [Lecture 22]

Marie, Joanne. "A List of Leucine-Rich Foods." *LIVESTRONG.COM*. http://www.livestrong.com/article/346375-a-list-of-leucine-rich-foods/ nutritiondata.com. [Lecture 8]

Matilda, Benita. "Increased Chewing Benefits Weight Management." *Science World Report.* http://www.scienceworldreport.com/articles/14587/20140509/increased-chewing-one-of-the-benefiting-weight-management-strategy.htm. [Lecture 20]

May, Kyle P. "What Are METs on a Treadmill?" *LIVESTRONG.COM.* http://www.livestrong.com/article/49231-mets-treadmill/. [Lecture 16]

Mayo Clinic. "Resveratrol in Grapes, Supplements and Other Foods." http://www.mayoclinic.org/diseases-conditions/heart-disease/in-depth/red-wine/art-20048281?pg=2. [Lecture 10]

———. "Sleep Tips: 7 Steps to Better Sleep." http://www.mayoclinic.org/healthy-lifestyle/adult-health/in-depth/sleep/art-20048379?pg=2. [Lecture 20]

Mendez, Elizabeth. "Americans Continue to Adjust Their Ideal Weight Upward." *Gallup.* http://www.gallup.com/poll/158921/americans-continue-adjust-ideal-weight-upward.aspx?utm_source=google&utm_medium=rss&utm_campaign=syndication. [Lecture 2]

Migala, Jessica. "10 Types of Hunger and How to Control Them." *Fox News.* http://www.foxnews.com/health/2014/08/30/10-types-hunger-and-how-to-control-them/. [Lecture 22]

Mosley, Michael. "Calorie Burner: How Much Better Is Standing Up Than Sitting?" *BBC News.* http://www.bbc.com/news/magazine-24532996. [Lecture 16]

Mozaffarian, D. "Dietary Priorities for Preventing Obesity: Are All Calories Created Equal?" https://www.youtube.com/watch?v=GHTsJR0fuIs&feature=youtu.be. [Lecture 23]

MyFoodDiary.com. *Exercise and Avoiding Dehydration.* http://www.myfooddiary.com/resources/ask_the_expert/exercise_avoiding_dehydration.asp. [Lecture 10]

National Heart, Lung, and Blood Institute. *Calculate Your Body Mass Index.* http://www.nhlbi.nih.gov/health/educational/lose_wt/BMI/bmicalc.htm. [Lecture 2]

———. *Portion Distortion: Do You Know How Food Portions Have Changed in 20 Years?* https://www.nhlbi.nih.gov/health/educational/wecan/eat-right/portion-distortion.htm. [Lecture 1]

National Institutes of Health. *Vitamin A.* http://ods.od.nih.gov/factsheets/VitaminA-HealthProfessional/. [Lecture 10]

———. *Vitamin and Mineral Supplement Fact Sheets.* www.cc.nih.gov/ccc/supplements. [Lecture 10]

Nestle, Marion. "FDA's New Food Label: Much Improved!" *Food Politics* (blog). http://www.foodpolitics.com/2014/02/fdasnew-food-label-much-improved/. [Lecture 11]

Newman, Hannah. "Why Not Even Exercise Will Undo the Harm of Sitting All Day—And What You Can Do About It." *Quartz.* http://qz.com/223160/why-not-even-exercise-will-undo-the-harm-of-sitting-all-day-and-what-you-can-do-about-it/. [Lecture 20]

Nierenberg, Cari. "Why Diets Fail: Your Feelings May Dictate Food Choices." *Live Science.* http://www.livescience.com/50803-diets-fail-feelings-food-choices.html. [Lecture 24]

Nutrition.gov. "Questions to Ask before Taking Vitamin and Mineral Supplements." http://www.nutrition.gov/dietary-supplements/questions-ask-taking-vitamin-and-mineral-supplements. [Lecture 10]

Ormsbee, Mike. "Healthy Shopping Tips at the SuperMarket.flv." Video. https://www.youtube.com/watch?v=XA0QCN3YQDI. [Lecture 24]

Orwell, Sol. "Detoxes: An Undefined Scam." *Examine* (blog). http://examine.com/blog/detoxes-an-undefined-scam/?utm_source=Examine.

com+Insiders&utm_campaign=f11d8e46c5-email_Detox1_21_2015&utm_medium=email&utm_term=0_e4d662cb1b-f11d8e46c5-69935085&goal=0_e4d662cb1b-f11d8e46c5-69935085&mc_cid=f11d8e46c5&mc_eid=1ba8bb7558. [Lecture 20]

Pennington Biomedical Research Center. *Single Subject Weight Change Predictor.* http://www.pbrc.edu/research-and-faculty/calculators/sswcp/.

Persistence Market Research. "Sports Nutrition Market Will Reach $37.7 Billion in 2019, Globally." *Globe Newswire.* http://globenewswire.com/news-release/2014/09/23/667761/10099668/en/Sports-Nutrition-Market-Will-Reach-37-7-Billion-in-2019-Globally-Persistence-Market-Research.html. [Lecture 14]

PR Newswire. "New Survey: To Sit or Stand? Almost 70% of Full Time American Workers Hate Sitting, but They do it All Day Every Day." http://www.prnewswire.com/news-releases/new-survey-to-sit-or-stand-almost-70-of-full-time-american-workers-hate-sitting-but-they-do-it-all-day-every-day-215804771.html. [Lecture 20]

Precision Nutrition. "Kitchen Makeover Questionnaire." http://www.precisionnutrition.com/wordpress/wp-content/uploads/2014/11/precision-nutrition-fitpro-starter-kit-assess.pdf. [Lecture 24]

Rosenbrock, Katie. "Give Up These 5 Things to Get Rid of Your Gut for Good." *The Active Times.* http://www.theactivetimes.com/give-these-5-things-get-rid-your-gut-good. [Lecture 22]

Science Clarified. *Lympatic System.* http://www.scienceclarified.com/Io-Ma/Lymphatic-System.html#ixzz3U0bzXGGg. [Lecture 3]

SELFNutritionData. *Nutrition Facts.* http://nutritiondata.self.com/facts/vegetables-and-vegetable-products/2626/2. [Lecture 11]

Smith, Michael A. "Can Lack of Sleep Lead to Carb Cravings?" *Life Extension* (blog). http://blog.lifeextension.com/2011/08/can-lack-of-sleep-lead-to-carb-cravings.html?utm_campaign=normal&utm_source=twitter&utm_medium=social&m=1. [Lecture 20]

St. Pierre, Brian. "Is Nutrient Timing Dead? And Does 'When' You Eat Really Matter?" *Precision Nutrition* (blog). http://www.precisionnutrition.com/nutrient-timing. [Lecture 12]

———. "The Paleo Problem: Examining the Pros and Cons of the Paleo Diet." *Precision Nutrition* (blog). http://www.precisionnutrition.com/paleo-diet. Site visit 8/12/2015. [Lecture 23]

Stone Hearth News. "Eating Out, No Matter Where, Adds 200 Calories a Day." http://www.stonehearthnewsletters.com/eating-matter-adds-200-calories-day/junk-food/#sthash.WbGzT32z. [Lecture 20]

———. "Green, Black, and Oolong Tea Polyphenols May Reduce Visceral Fat, Inflammation." http://www.stonehearthnewsletters.com/green-black-oolong-tea-polyphenols-may-reduce-visceral-fat-inflammation/inflammation/. [Lecture 20]

———. "Not Splendid News for Splenda, Sukrana, SucraPlus, Candys, Cukren and Nevella." http://www.stonehearthnewsletters.com/splendid-news-splenda-sukrana-sucraplus-candys-cukren-nevella/nutrition-food-artificial-sweeteners/. [Lecture 20]

Stromberg, Joseph. "Five Health Benefits of Standing Desks." *Smithsonian*. http://www.smithsonianmag.com/science-nature/five-health-benefits-standing-desks-180950259/?no-ist. [Lecture 16]

Sucralose. "New Research Analyzing 35 Years of Data Confirms Positive Effects of Low-Calorie Sweeteners in Weight Loss." http://sucralose.org/new-research-analyzing-35-years-of-data-confirms-positive-effects-of-low-calorie-sweeteners-in-weight-loss/. [Lecture 20]

SuppVersity (blog). "Can You Become Fat in Only 3 Days? Even with 1,500 Extra Calories, You Can't. All But One Subject Actually Lost Some Body Fat during 3-Day Gluttony on > 50% CHO Diets!" http://suppversity.blogspot.com/2014/09/can-you-get-fat-in-three-days-study.html. [Lecture 22]

———. "Food Is Medicine: Each 10g Fiber Reduce Mortality Risk by up to 34%! Phenols Battle Alzheimer's & Breast Cancer & Two Dozen Dietary GLUT4 Boosters Prevent Diabetes." http://suppversity.blogspot.de/2015/01/food-is-medicine-each-10g-fiber-reduce.html. [Lecture 10]

———. "Prevalent Nutrient Deficiencies in the US: More Than 40% Are Vitamin A, C, D & E, Calcium or Magnesium Deficient and > 90% Don't Get Enough Choline, Fiber & Potassium." http://suppversity.blogspot.com/2015/01/prevalent-nutritient-deficiencies-in-us.html?m=1. [Lecture 10]

Tartar, Jaime. "In Defense of Cortisol." *International Society of Sports.* http://www.theissnscoop.com/in-defense-of-cortisol/. [Lecture 19]

The University of New Mexico Health Sciences Center. "Stairway to Health." http://hsc.unm.edu/wellness/physical/stairs.html. [Lecture 16]

U.S. Food and Drug Administration. *Dietary Supplement Labeling Guide: Chapter IV. Nutrition Labeling.* http://www.fda.gov/Food/GuidanceRegulation/GuidanceDocumentsRegulatoryInformation/DietarySupplements/ucm070597.htm#4-3. [Lecture 14]

———. "Proposed Label/What's Different?" http://www.fda.gov/downloads/Food/GuidanceRegulation/GuidanceDocumentsRegulatoryInformation/LabelingNutrition/UCM387451.pdf. [Lecture 11, Lecture 15]

———. *Proposed Changes to the Nutrition Facts Label.* http://www.fda.gov/Food/GuidanceRegulation/GuidanceDocumentsRegulatoryInformation/LabelingNutrition/ucm385663.htm. [Lecture 11]

Walton, Alice G. "How Much Sugar Are Americans Eating?" *Forbes.* http://www.forbes.com/sites/alicegwalton/2012/08/30/how-much-sugar-are-americans-eating-infographic/. [Lecture 20]

Wood, Sheryl. "Timing of Weight Loss Efforts Matters." *Daily Rx News.* http://www.dailyrx.com/exercise-first-then-diet-prevented-muscle-loss-people-metabolic-syndrome. [Lecture 22]

Zelman, Kathleen M. "Fiber: How Much Do You Need?" *Web MD.* http://www.webmd.com/food-recipes/features/fiber-how-much-do-you-need. [Lecture 6]

Zuckerbrot, Tanya. "5 Ways to Bust a Diet Plateau." *Fox News.* http://www.foxnews.com/health/2014/05/13/5-ways-to-bust-diet-plateau/. [Lecture 22]

Printed Works/Books

Antonio, J., D. Kalman, J. R. Stout, M. Greenwood, D. S. Willoughby, and G. G. Haff. *Essentials of Sports Nutrition and Supplements.* New York: Humana Press, 2008. This is the textbook for the undergraduate course in sports nutrition and sports supplements. [Lecture 5]

Bailor, Jonathan. *The Calorie Myth.* New York: HarperCollins Publishers, 2014. According to this author, by focusing on food and exercise quality rather than calorie quantity, you can burn fat and boost health more easily and enjoyably than you ever thought possible. [Lecture 11, Lecture 22]

Berardi, J., and R. Andrews. *The Essentials of Sport and Exercise Nutrition Certification Manual.* 2nd ed. Toronto, ON: Precision Nutrition, 2010. This is a companion workbook that is meant to accompany a nutritional certification program called Precision Nutrition. [Lecture 1, Lecture 6, Lecture 7, Lecture 8, Lecture 15]

Greenfield, Ben. *Beyond Training: Mastering Endurance, Health & Life.* Riverside, NJ: Victory Belt Publishing, 2014. Offers advice regarding health and lifestyle. [Lecture 5, Lecture 23]

Gropper, S. S., J. L. Smith, and J. L. Groff. *Advanced Nutrition and Human Metabolism.* Edited by P. Adams, A. Lustig, and E. Feldman. Belmont, CA:

Wadsworth/Cengage Learning, 2009. Covers the biochemistry of vitamins, minerals, and energy nutrients. [Lecture 3, Lecture 4, Lecture 19]

Hadley, M. E., and J. E. Levine. *Endocrinology.* 6th ed. Upper Saddle River, NJ: Pearson Prentice Hall, 2007. Offers applications and in-depth coverage of vertebrate hormones. [Lecture 19]

Lieberman, Michael, and Allan D. Marks. *Mark's Basic Medical Biochemistry: A Clinical Approach.* Edited by Susan Rhymer. Baltimore, MD: Lippincott Williams & Wilkins, 2013. Offers a patient-oriented approach that links biochemistry to physiology and pathophysiology.

Mahan, L. K., S. Escott-Stump, and J. L. Raymond. *Krause's Food and the Nutrition Care Process.* St. Louis, MO: Elsevier Saunders, 2012. Provides up-to-date information about nutrition. [Lecture 19]

McArdle, William D., Frank I. Katch, and Victor L. Katch. *Sports and Exercise Nutrition.* 4th ed. Philadelphia, PA: Lippincott Williams & Wilkins, 2012. Offers nutrition and exercise concepts and their practical applications. [Lecture 1, Lecture 5]

McClusky, Mark. *Faster, Higher, Stronger.* New York: Hudson Street Press, 2014. The author explains how today's top athletes are turning to advanced technology and savvy science to improve their performance. [Lecture 23]

Moore, J., and E. Westman. *Keto Clarity: Your Definitive Guide to the Benefits of a Low-Carb, High-Fat Diet.* Riverside, NJ: Victory Belt Publishing, 2014. Explains the powerful therapeutic effects of a ketogenic diet. [Lecture 23]

Straub, R. O. *Health Psychology: A Biopsychosocial Approach.* 3rd ed. New York: Worth Publishers, 2012. With an emphasis on positive health, the new edition examines information from biological, psychological, and social aspects of health. [Lecture 19]

Volek, J., and S. Phinney. *The Art and Science of Low Carbohydrate Performance*. Miami, FL: Beyond Obesity, 2012. Presents more than 130 recipes. [Lecture 22]

Journal Articles

Acheson, K. J., et al. "Protein Choices Targeting Thermogenesis and Metabolism." *American Journal of Clinical Nutrition* 93, no. 3 (2011): 525–534. The objective of this study was to determine the differential effects of three proteins on energy metabolism, satiety, and glucose control. [Lecture 1]

Agarwal, S., et al. "Comparison of Prevalence of Inadequate Nutrient Intake Based on Body Weight Status of Adults in the United States: An Analysis of NHANES 2001–2008." *Journal of the American College of Nutrition* 34, no. 2 (2015): 126–134. The objective of this study was to compare micronutrient intake status of overweight and obese adults with normal-weight adults. [Lecture 10]

Ahmed, T., and N. Haboubi. "Assessment and Management of Nutrition in Older People and Its Importance to Health." *Journal of Clinical Interventions in Aging* 5 (2010): 207–216. Nutrition is an important element of health in the older population and affects the aging process. [Lecture 3]

Alfenas, Rde C., J. Bressan, and A. C. Paiva. "Effects of Protein Quality on Appetite and Energy Metabolism in Normal Weight Subjects." *Arquivos Brasileiros de Endocrinologia & Metabologia* 54, no. 1 (2010): 45–51. The goal of this study was to compare the effects of consumption of different protein sources on food intake and energy expenditure in normal-weight subjects. [Lecture 1]

American College of Sports Medicine, American Dietetic Association, and Dieticians of Canada. "Joint Position Statement: Nutrition and Athletic Performance. American College of Sports Medicine, American Dietetic Association, and Dietitians of Canada." *Medicine & Science in Sports & Exercise* 32, no. 12 (2000): 2130–2145. These three organizations have taken the position that physical activity, athletic performance, and recovery from exercise are enhanced by optimal nutrition. [Lecture 12]

Apolzan, J. W., et al. "Inadequate Dietary Protein Increases Hunger and Desire to Eat in Younger and Older Men." *Journal of Nutrition* 137, no. 6 (2007): 1478–1482. This study was designed to examine the appetitive responses to habitual protein intakes that span the range of adequacy in younger and older men. [Lecture 1]

Aragon, Alan A., and Brad Jon Schoenfeld. "Nutrient Timing Revisited: Is There a Post-Exercise Anabolic Window?" *Journal of International Society of Sports Nutrition* 10, no. 5 (2013): 1–11. The purpose of this paper is to review the existing literature on the effects of nutrient timing with respect to postexercise muscular adaptations and to draw relevant conclusions that allow practical nutritional recommendations to be made for maximizing the anabolic response to exercise. [Lecture 12]

Arazi, Hamid, Arsalan Damirchi, Hassan Faraji, and Rahman Rahimi. "Hormonal Responses to Acute and Chronic Resistance Exercise in Middle-Age versus Young Men." *Sport Sciences for Health* 8, no. 2 (2012): 59–65. In this experiment, researchers examined responses of the endocrine system to moderate-resistance training in younger verses middle-aged men; the men participated in an eight-week moderate-resistance training program three times per week. [Lecture 19]

Arble, D. M., J. Bass, A. D. Laposky, M. H. Vitaterna, and F. W. Turek. "Circadian Timing of Food Intake Contributes to Weight Gain." *Obesity* 17, no. 11 (2009): 2100–2102. This study focuses on the role of the circadian phase of food consumption in weight gain. [Lecture 13]

Arciero, P. J., M. J. Ormsbee, C. L. Gentile, B. C. Nindl, J. R. Brestoff, and M. Ruby. "Increased Protein Intake and Meal Frequency Reduces Abdominal Fat during Energy Balance and Energy Deficit." *Obesity* 21, no. 7 (2013): 1357–1366. The effects of consuming traditional versus higher protein intakes as three or six meals per day on abdominal fat, postprandial thermogenesis, and cardiometabolic biomarkers in overweight individuals during 28 days of energy balance and deficit were compared in this study. [Lecture 9]

Bailey, Regan L., et al. "Dietary Supplement Use in the United States, 2003–2006." *Journal of Nutrition* 141, no. 2 (2011): 261–266. The purpose of this analysis was to estimate dietary supplement use using the NHANES 2003–2006. [Lecture 10]

Bar-Or, Oded. "The Juvenile Obesity Epidemic: Strike Back with Physical Activity." *Gatorade Sports Science Institute* 16, no. 2 (2003): 1–6. Available at http://www.gssiweb.org/Article/sse-89-the-juvenile-obesity-epidemic-strike-back-with-physical-activity. The focus of this article is on combatting juvenile obesity with exercise. [Lecture 1]

Bartlett, J., G. Close, and D. Maclaren. "High-Intensity Interval Running Is Perceived to Be More Enjoyable Than Moderate-Intensity Continuous Exercise: Implications for Exercise Adherence." *Journal of Sports Sciences* 29, no. 6 (2011): 547–553. The aim of this study was to objectively quantify ratings of perceived enjoyment using the Physical Activity Enjoyment Scale following high-intensity interval running versus moderate-intensity continuous running. [Lecture 17]

Bassett, D. R., J. A. Vachon, A. O. Kirkland, E. T. Howley, G. E. Duncan, and K. R. Johnson. "Energy Cost of Stair Climbing and Descending on the College Alumnus Questionnaire." *Medicine and Scence in Sports Exercise* 29, no. 9 (1997): 1250–1254. The goal of this study was to quantify the energy cost of stair climbing and stair descending by measuring oxygen uptake. [Lecture 16]

Bélisle, M., E. Roskies, and J. M. Lévesque. "Improving Adherence to Physical Activity." *Health Psychology* 6, no. 2 (1987): 159–172. This paper consists of two studies that tested the efficacy of Marlatt and Gordon's relapse-prevention approach in increasing attendance during an exercise program and continuation of exercise activities. [Lecture 21]

Berry, E. M. "Are Diets High in Omega-6 Polyunsaturated Fatty Acids Unhealthy?" *European Heart Journal Supplements* 3 (2001): D37–D41. This article reviews the connection between dietary omega-6 fatty acids and atherosclerosis, carcinogenesis, and insulin resistance. [Lecture 4]

Betts, J. A., J. D. Richardson, E. A. Chowdhury, G. D. Holman, K. Tsintzas, and D. Thompson. "The Causal Role of Breakfast in Energy Balance and Health: A Randomized Controlled Trial in Lean Adults." *The American Journal of Clinical Nutrition* 100, no. 2 (2014): 539–547. The aim of this study was to conduct a randomized controlled trial examining causal links between breakfast habits and all components of energy balance in free-living humans. [Lecture 3]

Blackburn, G. "Effect of Degree of Weight Loss on Health Benefits." *Obesity Research* 3 (1995): 211S–216S. This paper reviews the effect of degree of weight loss on specific disease states and risk factors and discusses the impact of ethnic background, fat distribution, age, and mode of weight loss on outcome. [Lecture 1]

Boirie, Y., M. Dangin, P. Gachon, M. P. Vasson, J. L. Maubois, and B. Beaufrère. "Slow and Fast Dietary Proteins Differently Modulate Postprandial Protein Accretion." *Proceedings of the National Academy of Sciences* 94, no. 26 (1997): 14930–14935. The speed of absorption of dietary amino acids by the gut varies according to the type of ingested dietary protein. [Lecture 13]

Børsheim, E., and R. Bahr. "Effect of Exercise Intensity, Duration, and Mode on Post-Exercise Oxygen Consumption." *Sports Medicine* 33, no. 14 (2003): 1037–1060. There are conflicting results regarding the recovery period after exercise and the excess postexercise oxygen consumption. [Lecture 17]

Brose, Andrea, Gianni Parise, and Mark A. Tarnopolsky. "Creatine Supplementation Enhances Isometric Strength and Body Composition Improvements Following Strength Exercise Training in Older Adults." *The Journals of Gerontology Series A: Biological Sciences and Medical Sciences* 58, no. 1 (2003): B11–B19. The goal was to determine whether creatine monohydrate supplementation would enhance the increases in strength and fat-free mass that develop during resistance exercise training in older adults. [Lecture 14]

Brouns, F., and W. Saris. "How Vitamins Affect Performance." *The Journal of Sports Medicine and Physical Fitness* 29, no. 4 (1989): 400–404. This study examined the impact of vitamins on exercise performance. [Lecture 10]

Burd, N. A., S. H. Gorissen, and L. J. C. van Loon. "Anabolic Resistance of Muscle Protein Synthesis with Aging." *Exercise and Sport Sciences Review* 41, no. 3 (2013): 169–173. The level of habitual physical activity might be fundamental to maintain the anabolic responsiveness to protein intake with aging. [Lecture 9]

Calton, Jayson B. "Prevalence of Micronutrient Deficiency in Popular Diet Plans." *Journal of the International Society of Sports Nutrition* 7 (2010): 1–9. Research has shown micronutrient deficiency to be scientifically linked to a higher risk of overweight/obesity and other dangerous and debilitating diseases. [Lecture 10]

Candow, Darren G., et al. "Effect of Whey and Soy Protein Supplementation Combined with Resistance Training in Young Adults." *International Journal of Sport Nutrition and Exercise Metabolism* 16, no. 3 (2006): 233–244. The purpose of this study was to compare changes in lean tissue mass, strength, and myofibrillar protein catabolism resulting from combining whey protein or soy protein with resistance training. [Lecture 12]

Cappuccio, F. P., et al. "Meta-Analysis of Short Sleep Duration and Obesity in Children and Adults." *Sleep* 31, no. 5 (2008): 619–626. This study was conducted to assess whether the evidence supports the presence of a relationship between short sleep duration and obesity at different ages and to obtain an estimate of the risk. [Lecture 22]

Chevion, Shlomit, et al. "Plasma Antioxidant Status and Cell Injury after Severe Physical Exercise." *Proceedings of the National Academy of Sciences* 100, no. 9 (2003): 5119–5123. This is a study of the effects of oxidative stress during strenuous exercise. [Lecture 4]

Clegg, M. E. "Medium-Chain Triglycerides Are Advantageous in Promoting Weight Loss although Not Beneficial to Exercise Performance." *International*

Journal of Food Sciences and Nutrition 61, no. 7 (2010): 653–79. This study reviews medium-chain triglycerdies for use with weight loss and exercise performance. [Lecture 23]

Costa, G. "The Problem: Shiftwork." *Chronobiology International* 14, no. 2 (1997): 89–98. Shift work, such as night work, causes disruption of biological rhythms and perturbation of the social and family life that can negatively affect performance efficiency, health, and social relations. [Lecture 13]

Dashti, Hassan S., et al. "Habitual Sleep Duration Is Associated with BMI and Macronutrient Intake and May Be Modified by CLOCK Genetic Variants." *American Journal of Clinical Nutrition* 10, no. 1 (2015): 135–143. Available at http://ajcn.nutrition.org/content/101/1/135.abstract. The objective of this study was to examine associations between habitual sleep duration, body mass index, and macronutrient intake and to assess whether CLOCK variants modify these associations. [Lecture 20]

Dattilo, M., et al. "Sleep and Muscle Recovery: Endocrinological and Molecular Basis for a New and Promising Hypothesis." *Medical Hypotheses* 77, no. 2 (2011): 220–222. Available at http://www.ncbi.nlm.nih.gov/pubmed/21550729. The authors hypothesized that sleep deprivation decreases the activity of protein synthesis pathways and increases the activity of degradation pathways, favoring the loss of muscle mass. [Lecture 20]

De Castro, J. M. "The Time of Day of Food Intake Influences Overall Intake in Humans." *Journal of Nutrition* 134, no. 1 (2004): 104–111. The hypothesis is that the time of day of food intake would be related to total intake such that intake early in the day would tend to reduce overall intake, whereas intake later in the day would tend to increase intake over the entire day. [Lecture 13]

De Zwaan, M., M. Burgard, and C. Schenck. "Night Time Eating: A Review of the Literature." *European Eating Disorders Review* 11, no. 1 (2003): 7–24. This study reviews the published research on nighttime eating, including the night eating syndrome and the nocturnal eating/drinking syndrome. [Lecture 13]

Dhurandhar, E. J., J. Dawson, A. Alcorn, L. H. Larsen, and E. A. Thomas, et al. "The Effectiveness of Breakfast Recommendations on Weight Loss: A Randomized Controlled Trial." *American Journal of Clinical Nutrition* 100, no. 2 (2014): 507–513. The authors tested the relative effectiveness of a recommendation to eat or skip breakfast on weight loss in adults trying to lose weight in a free-living setting. [Lecture 3]

Diepvens, Kristel, Klaas R. Westerterp, and Margriet S. Westerterp-Plantenga. "Obesity and Thermogenesis Related to the Consumption of Caffeine, Ephedrine, Capsaicin, and Green Tea." *American Journal of Physiology-Regulatory, Integrative and Comparative Physiology* 292, no. 1 (2007): R77–R85. Tools for obesity management—including caffeine, ephedrine, capsaicin, and green tea—have been proposed as strategies for weight loss and weight maintenance. [Lecture 14]

Donnelly, J. E., et al. "American College of Sports Medicine Position Stand. Appropriate Physical Activity Intervention Strategies for Weight Loss and Prevention of Weight Regain for Adults." *Medical Science and Sports Exercise* 41, no. 2 (2009): 459–471. The purpose of this study was to reexamine the evidence from 1999 to determine whether there is a level at which physical activity is effective for prevention of weight gain, weight loss, and prevention of weight regain. [Lecture 1]

Duckworth, A. L., C. Peterson, M. D. Matthews, and D. R. Kelly. "Grit: Perseverance and Passion for Long-Term Goals." *Journal of Personality and Social Psychology* 92, no. 6 (2007): 1087–1101. The authors tested the importance of the noncognitive trait called grit. [Lecture 21]

Duloo, A. G., J. Jacquet, and J. P. Montani. "How Dieting Makes Some Fatter: From a Perspective of Human Body Composition Autoregulation." *Proceedings of the Nutrition Society* 71, no. 3 (2012): 379–389. This paper attempts to address the plausibility and mechanistic basis by which dieting might predispose people to increased fatness. [Lecture 19, Lecture 22]

Fairfield, K., and R. Fletcher. "Vitamins for Chronic Disease Prevention in Adults." *The Journal of the American Medical Association* 287, no. 23

(2002): 3116–3126. Available at http://jama.jamanetwork.com/article.aspx?articleid=195038. This paper reviews the clinically important vitamins with regard to their biological effects, food sources, deficiency syndromes, potential for toxicity, and relationship to chronic disease. [Lecture 10]

Fielding, R. A. "Protein Nutrition Mediates Lean Body Mass Homeostasis in the Aging Warfighter." *Journal of Nutrition* 143, no. 11 (2013): 1857S–1861S. This review highlights selective aspects of protein supplementation in older adults. [Lecture 9]

Figueroa, A., A. Wong, A. Kinsey, R. Kalfon, W. Eddy, and M. J. Ormsbee. "Effects of Milk Proteins and Combined Exercise Training on Aortic Hemodynamics and Arterial Stiffness in Young Obese Women with High Blood Pressure." *American Journal of Hypertension* 27, no. 3 (2014): 338–344. This paper examines the impact of milk proteins and combined exercise training on blood pressure, arterial function, and muscle strength. [Lecture 13]

Figueroa, Arturo, et al. "Effects of Diet and/or Low-Intensity Resistance Exercise Training on Arterial Stiffness, Adiposity, and Lean Mass in Obese Postmenopausal Women." *American Journal of Hypertension* (2013): 1–8. This study evaluates the independent and combined effects of a hypocaloric diet on pulse-wave velocity and body composition as well as low-intensity resistance exercise training with slow movement. [Lecture 18]

Fildes, A., J. Charlton, C. Rudisill, P. Littlejohns, A. T. Prevost, and M. C. Gulliford. "Probability of an Obese Person Attaining Normal Body Weight: Cohort Study Using Electronic Health Records." *American Journal of Public Health* 105, no. 9 (2015): e54–59. This paper examines the probability of an obese person attaining normal body weight. [Lecture 22]

Folch, N., et al. "Metabolic Response to a Large Starch Meal after Rest and Exercise: Comparison between Men and Women." *European Journal of Clinical Nutrition* 57, no. 9 (2003): 1107–1115. The authors hypothesize that net whole-body de novo lipogenesis could be larger in women than men and that glycogen and fat balance could be lower and higher, respectively, following a large pasta meal ingested after rest or exercise. [Lecture 6]

Folch, N., et al. "Metabolic Response to Small and Large 13C-Labelled Pasta Meals Following Rest or Exercise in Man." *British Journal of Nutrition* 85 (2001): 671–680. The metabolic response to a 150- or 400-gram 13C-labeled pasta meal was studied for eight hours following rest or exercise at low or moderate workload. [Lecture 6]

Ford, E. S., C. Li, A. G. Wheaton, D. P. Chapman, G. S. Perry, and J. B. Croft. "Sleep Duration and Body Mass Index and Waist Circumference among U.S. Adults." *Obesity* 22, no. 2 (2014): 598–607. Available at http://www. researchgate.net/publication/247772753_Sleep_Duration_and_Body_ Mass_Index_and_Waist_Circumference_among_US_Adults. This paper aims to examine the form of the relationship between sleep duration and anthropometric measures and possible differences in these relationships by gender and race or ethnicity. [Lecture 13]

Foss, B., L. R. Saeterdal, O. Nordgard, and S. M. Dyrstad. "Exercise Can Alter Cortisol Responses in Obese Subjects." *Journal of Exercise Physiology* 17, no. 1 (2014): 67–77. The aim of this study was to examine the influence of a 22-week lifestyle intervention program on the cortisol response in 35 inactive, obese subjects. [Lecture 19]

Foster-Schubert, K. E., et al. "Effect of Diet and Exercise, Alone or Combined, on Weight and Body Composition in Overweight-to-Obese Post-Menopausal Women." *Obesity* 20, no. 8 (2012): 1628–1638. Available at http://www. ncbi.nlm.nih.gov/pmc/articles/PMC3406229/. The authors conducted a randomized trial among 439 overweight-to-obese postmenopausal sedentary women to determine the effects of a reduced-calorie, low-fat diet, a moderate facility-based aerobic exercise program, or the combination of both interventions, versus a no-lifestyle-change control on change in body weight and composition. [Lecture 24]

Frankenfield, D. C., et al. "Validation of Several Established Equations for Resting Metabolic Rate in Obese and Non-Obese People." *Journal of American Diet Association* 103, no. 9 (2003): 1152–1159. This research evaluates several equations for predicting resting metabolic rate against measured values in obese and nonobese people. [Lecture 15]

Garthe, I., et al. "Effect of Two Different Weight-Loss Rates on Body Composition and Strength and Power-Related Performance in Elite Athletes." *International Journal of Sport Nutrition and Exercise Metabolism* 21, no. 2 (2011): 97–104. Available at http://www.ncbi.nlm.nih.gov/pubmed/21558571. The aim of this study was to compare changes in body composition, strength, and power during a weekly body-weight loss of 0.7 percent slow reduction versus 1.4 percent fast reduction. [Lecture 24]

Gebel, K., et al. "Effect of Moderate to Vigorous Physical Activity on All-Cause Mortality in Middle-Aged and Older Australians." *Journal of the American Medical Association* 175, no. 6 (2015): 970–977. Available at http://archinte.jamanetwork.com/article.aspx?articleid=2212268. This paper examines whether the proportion of total moderate to vigorous physical activity (MVPA) that is achieved through vigorous activity is associated with all-cause mortality independently of the total amount of MVPA. [Lecture 17]

Geer, E. B., and W. Shen. "Gender Differences in Insulin Resistance, Body Composition, and Energy Balance." *Gender Medicine* 6, no. 1 (2009): 60–75. This review summarizes published data on gender differences in insulin resistance, body composition, and energy balance. [Lecture 19]

Gibala, M. "Molecular Responses to High-Intensity Interval Exercise." *Applied Physiology, Nutrition, and Metabolism* 34, no. 3 (2009): 428–432. This paper examines the plausibility that metabolic adaptations to high-interval endurance training could be mediated in part through signaling pathways that are normally associated with endurance training. [Lecture 17]

Goo, R. H., J. G. Moore, E. Greenberg, and N. P. Alazraki. "Circadian Variation in Gastric Emptying of Meals in Humans." *Gastroenterology* 93, no. 3 (1987): 515–518. This paper aims to determine whether gastric emptying could account for circadian changes. [Lecture 13]

Gortmaker, S. L., A. Must, A. M. Sobol, K. Peterson, G. A. Colditz, and W. H. Dietz. "Television Viewing as a Cause of Increasing Obesity among Children in the United States, 1986–1990." *Archives of Pediatrics and Adolescent Medicine* 150, no. 4 (1996): 356–362. This paper examines the relationship between hours of television viewed and the prevalence of overweight children in 1990 and the incidence and remission of overweight children from 1986 to 1990. [Lecture 1]

Greer, B. K., et al. "Branched-Chain Amino Acid Supplementation and Indicators of Muscle Damage after Endurance Exercise." *International Journal of Sports Nutrition and Exercise Metabolism* 17, no. 6 (2007): 595–607. The purpose of this study was to determine whether branched-chain amino acid supplementation attenuates indirect indicators of muscle damage during endurance exercise as compared with an isocaloric carbohydrate beverage or a noncaloric placebo beverage. [Lecture 8]

Groen, B. B. L., P. T. Res, B. Pennings, E. Hertle, J. M. G. Senden, W. H. M. Saris, and L. J. C. van Loon. "Intragastric Protein Administration Stimulates Overnight Muscle Protein Synthesis in Elderly Men." *American Journal of Physiology, Endocrinology, and Metabolism* 302 (2012): E52–60. This study focused on the impact of night feeding of protein on muscle protein synthesis in elderly men. [Lecture 9, Lecture 13]

Grün, Felix, and Bruce Blumberg. "Endocrine Disruptors as Obesogens." *Molecular and Cellular Endocrinology* 304, no. 1–2 (2009): 19–29. This review highlights recent advances in the understanding of the molecular targets and possible mechanisms of action for these compounds as well as areas of future research needed to evaluate the significance of their contribution to obesity. [Lecture 20]

———. "Minireview: The Case for Obesogens." *Molecular Endocrinology* 23, no. 8 (2009): 1127–1134. This review considers the evidence for obesogens, how they might act, and where future research is needed to clarify their relative contribution to the obesity epidemic. [Lecture 20]

Hamilton, M. T., et al. "Role of Low Energy Expenditure and Sitting in Obesity, Metabolic Syndrome, Type 2 Diabetes, and Cardiovascular Disease." *Diabetes* 56, no. 11 (2007): 2655–2667. The purpose was to examine the role of sedentary behaviors, especially sitting, on mortality, cardiovascular disease, type 2 diabetes, metabolic syndrome risk factors, and obesity. [Lecture 1]

Hartman, J. W., J. E. Tang, S. B. Wilkinson, M. A. Tarnopolsky, R. L. Lawrence, A. V. Fullerton, and S. M. Phillips. "Consumption of Fat-Free Fluid Milk after Resistance Exercise Promotes Greater Lean Mass Accretion Than Does Consumption of Soy or Carbohydrate in Young, Novice, Male Weightlifters." *American Journal of Clinical Nutrition* 86 (2007): 373–381. In this study, the effects of milk were compared to those of carbohydrate and soy after resistance exercise in young men. [Lecture 9, Lecture 12]

Haskell, W. L., et al. "Physical Activity and Public Health: Updated Recommendation for Adults from the American College of Sports Medicine and the American Heart Association." *Medicine & Science in Sports & Exercise* 39, no. 8 (2007): 1423–1434. In this article, the American College of Sports Medicine and the American Heart Association make recommendations for adults' physical activity and health. [Lecture 1]

Hoffman, Jay R., et al. "Effect of Protein-Supplement Timing on Strength, Power, and Body-Composition Changes in Resistance-Trained Men." *International Journal of Sport Nutrition* 19, no. 2 (2009): 172–185. The effect of 10 weeks of protein-supplement timing on strength, power, and body composition was examined in 33 resistance-trained men. [Lecture 12]

Hoffman, Jay, et al. "Effect of Creatine and ß-Alanine Supplementation on Performance and Endocrine Responses in Strength/Power Athletes." *International Journal of Sport Nutrition and Exercise Metabolism* 16, no. 4 (2006): 430–446. The effects of creatine and creatine plus beta-alanine on strength, power, body composition, and endocrine changes were examined during a 10-week resistance training program in collegiate football players. [Lecture 14]

Holt, S. H., et al. "An Insulin Index of Foods: The Insulin Demand Generated by 1000-kJ Portions of Common Foods." *American Journal of Clinical Nutrition* 66, no. 5 (1997): 1264–1276. The aim of this study was to systematically compare postprandial insulin responses to isoenergetic 1000-kilojoule (240-kilocalorie) portions of several common foods. [Lecture 6]

Holtcamp, Wendee. "Obesogens: An Environmental Link to Obesity." *Environmental Health Perspectives* 120, no. 2 (2012): a62–a68. Available at http://www.ncbi.nlm.nih.gov/pmc/articles/PMC3279464/. According to this research, obesogens might have a link to obesity. [Lecture 20]

Houston, D. K., B. J. Nicklas, J. Ding, T. B. Harris, and F. A. Tylavsky, et al. "Dietary Protein Intake Is Associated with Lean Mass Change in Older, Community-Dwelling Adults: The Health, Aging, and Body Composition (Health ABC) Study." *American Journal of Clinical Nutrition* 87 (2008): 150–155. The objective of the study was to determine the association between dietary protein and changes in total lean mass and nonboneappendicular lean mass in older, community-dwelling men and women. [Lecture 9]

Isacco, L., P. Duche, D. Thivel, A. Meddahi-Pelle, S. Lemoine-Morel, M. Duclos, and N. Boisseau. "Fat Mass Localization Alters Fuel Oxidation during Exercise in Normal Weight Women." *Medicine & Science in Sports & Exercise* 45, no. 10 (2013): 1887–1896. The purpose of this study was to investigate the effect of low- and high-abdominal to lower-body fat mass ratio on metabolic and hormonal responses during exercise in premenopausal normal-weight women. [Lecture 19]

Ivy, J. L. "Glycogen Resynthesis after Exercise: Effect of Carbohydrate Intake." *International Journal of Sports Medicine*, 19 (1998): S142–S145. This research analyzes how much carbohydrate to ingest after exercise and the effect on glycogen storage. [Lecture 12]

Josse, A. R., S. A. Atkinson, M. A. Tarnopolsky, and S. M. Phillips. "Increased Consumption of Dairy Foods and Protein during Diet- and Exercise-Induced Weight Loss Promotes Fat Mass Loss and Lean Mass Gain in Overweight and Obese Premenopausal Women." *Journal of Nutrition* 141 (2011): 1626–34. The hypothesis of this paper is that participants that consume a high-protein, high-milk-product diet will lose a larger ratio of fat mass to lean body mass than participants consuming an adequate protein diet with moderate or low dairy products during an intervention with energy restriction and an exercise routine. [Lecture 9]

Jówko, Ewa, et al. "Creatine and β-Hydroxy-β-Methylbutyrate (HMB) Additively Increase Lean Body Mass and Muscle Strength during a Weight-Training Program." *Nutrition* 17, no. 7 (2001): 558–566. This paper investigates whether creatine and β-hydroxy-β-methylbutyrate act by similar or different mechanisms to increase lean body mass and strength in humans undergoing progressive resistance exercise training. [Lecture 14]

Kalergis, M., A. Schiffrin, R. Gougeon, P. J. Jones, and J. F. Yale. "Impact of Bedtime Snack Composition on Prevention of Nocturnal Hypoglycemia in Adults with Type 1 Diabetes Undergoing Intensive Insulin Management Using Lispro Insulin before Meals: A Randomized, Placebo-Controlled, Crossover Trial." *Diabetes Care* 26, no. 1 (2003): 9–15. The aim of this paper was to determine the impact of four bedtime snack compositions on nocturnal glycemic control, including frequency of hypoglycemia and morning hyperglycemia, in adults with type 1 diabetes using lispro insulin before meals and NPH insulin at bedtime. [Lecture 13]

Katayose, Y., M. Tasaki, H. Ogata, Y. Nakata, K. Tokuyama, and M. Satoh. "Metabolic Rate and Fuel Utilization during Sleep Assessed by Whole-Body Indirect Calorimetry." *Metabolism* 58, no. 7 (2009): 920–926. sThe purpose of this study was to examine metabolic rate and substrate oxidation during sleep in relation to time of sleep and sleep stage. [Lecture 13]

Katzmarzyk, Peter, et al. "Sitting Time and Mortality from All Causes, Cardiovascular Disease, and Cancer." *Medicine & Science in Sports & Exercise* 41, no. 5 (2009): 998–1005. Researchers examined sitting time and mortality in a representative sample of 17,013 Canadians 18–90 years of age. [Lecture 1]

Keesey, R. E., and M. D. Hirvonen. "Body Weight Set-Points: Determination and Adjustment." *Journal of Nutrition* 127, no. 9 (1997): 1875S–1883S. It appears that hypothalamic mechanisms play a primary role in setting the level at which individuals regulate body weight, and it is likely that the genetic, dietary, and other lifespan influences on body weight are expressed through these mechanisms. [Lecture 22]

Kerksick, Chad, et al. "Journal of the International Society of Sports Nutrition Position Stand: Nutrient Timing." *Journal of the International Society of Sports Nutrition* 5 (2008): 17. The position of the society regarding nutrient timing and the intake of carbohydrates, proteins, and fats in reference to healthy, exercising individuals is summarized by eight points. [Lecture 12]

Kern, Ben D., and Tracey L. Robinson. "Effects of β-Alanine Supplementation on Performance and Body Composition in Collegiate Wrestlers and Football Players." *The Journal of Strength & Conditioning Research* 25, no. 7 (2011): 1804–1815. The purpose of this study was to examine the effectiveness of beta-alanine as an ergogenic aid in tests of anaerobic power output after eight weeks of high-intensity interval, repeated sprint, and resistance training in previously trained collegiate wrestlers and football players. [Lecture 14]

Kinsey, A. W., W. R. Eddy, T. A. Madzima, L. B. Panton, P. J. Arciero, J. S. Kim, and M. J. Ormsbee. "Influence of Night-Time Protein and Carbohydrate Intake on Appetite and Cardiometabolic Risk in Sedentary Overweight and Obese Women." *British Journal of Nutition* 112 (2014): 320–327. This study focused on the acute effect of nighttime feeding in overweight women. [Lecture 9, Lecture 13]

Knab, A. M., et al. "A 45-Minute Vigorous Exercise Bout Increases Metabolic Rate for 14 Hours." *Medicine & Science in Sports & Exercise* 43, no. 9 (2011): 1643–1648. This study investigated the effects of inserting a 45-minute vigorous cycling bout into the daily schedule versus a controlled resting day on 24-hour energy expenditure in a metabolic chamber. [Lecture 17]

Koball, A. M., M. R. Meers, A. Storfer-Isser, S. E. Domoff, and D. R. Musher-Eizenman. "Eating When Bored: Revision of the Emotional Eating Scale with a Focus on Boredom." *Health Psychology* 31, no. 4 (2012): 521–524. This study explored whether eating when bored is a distinct construct from other negative emotions by revising the emotional eating scale to include a separate boredom factor. [Lecture 21]

Koopman, R., L. Verdijk, R. J. F. Manders, A. P. Gijsen, M. Gorselink, E. Pijpers, A. J. M. Wagenmakers, and L. J. C. van Loon. "Co-Ingestion of Protein and Leucine Stimulates Muscle Protein Synthesis Rates to the Same Extent in Young and Elderly Lean Men." *American Journal of Clinical Nutrition* 84, no. 3 (2006): 623–632. This paper investigates the effects on whole-body protein balance and mixed-muscle protein synthesis rates of the ingestion of carbohydrate with or without protein and free leucine after simulated activities of daily living. [Lecture 9]

Kouri, E. M., H. G. Pope Jr., D. L. Katz, and P. Oliva. "Fat-Free Mass Index in Users and Nonusers of Anabolic-Androgenic Steroids." *Clinical Journal of Sport Medicine* 5, no. 4 (1995): 223–228. This paper calculated fat-free mass index in a sample of 157 male athletes, comprising 83 users of anabolic-androgenic steroids and 74 nonusers. [Lecture 2]

Kravitz. L. "Research Sheds New Light on the Exercise 'Afterburn.'" *IDEA Fitness Journal* April (2015): 16–18. Available at http://www.unm.edu/~lkravitz/Article%20folder/ExerciseAfterburn2015.html. Recent research studies help clarify the body's ability to keep burning extra calories long after we stop exercising. [Lecture 17]

Laufs, U., S. Wassmann, T. Czech, T. Münzel, M. Eisenhauer, M. Böhm, and G. Nickenig. "Physical Inactivity Increases Oxidative Stress, Endothelial Dysfunction, and Atherosclerosis." *Arteriosclerosis, Thrombosis, and Vascular Biology* 25, no. 4 (2005): 809–814. Sedentary lifestyle is associated with increased cardiovascular events; the underlying molecular mechanisms are incompletely understood. [Lecture 4]

Lee, T. K., I. J. Clarke, J. St. John, I. R. Young, and B. L. Leury, et al. "High Cortisol Responses Identify Propensity for Obesity That Is Linked to Thermogenesis in Skeletal Muscle." *The FASEB Journal* 28, no. 1 (2014): 35–44. Predisposition to obesity can be predicted by cortisol responsiveness to an adrenocorticotropin challenge, and the response is due to innate differences in muscle thermogenesis. [Lecture 19]

Libotte, E., et al. "The Influence of Plate Size on Meal Composition: Literature Review and Experiment." *Appetite* 82 (2014): 91–96. Available at http://www.sciencedirect.com/science/article/pii/S0195666314003675. This study conducts a literature review and a controlled laboratory experiment to investigate whether plate size influences the composition of a meal and the total meal energy. [Lecture 20]

Madzima, T. A., L. B. Panton, S. K. Fretti, A. W. Kinsey, and M. J. Ormsbee. "Night-Time Consumption of Protein or Carbohydrate Results in Increased Morning Resting Energy Expenditure in Active College-Aged Men." *British Journal of Nutrition* 111 (2014): 71–77. This study focused on the acute effect of nighttime feeding in fit young men. [Lecture 9, Lecture 13]

Mastorakos, G., M. Pavlatou, E. Diamanti-Kandarakis, and G. P. Chrousos. "Exercise and the Stress System." *Hormones* 4, no. 2 (2005): 73–89. There is increasing incidence of exercise-related short-term and long-term consequences on female reproduction. [Lecture 19]

Meredith, C. N., et al. "Dietary Protein Requirements and Body Protein Metabolism in Endurance-Trained Men." *Journal of Applied Physiology* 66, no. 6 (1989): 2850–2856. This study examined endurance runners and nitrogen balance to understand protein needs. [Lecture 8]

Micha, R., and D. Mozzaffarian. "Saturated Fat and Cardiometabolic Risk Factors, Coronary Heart Disease, Stroke, and Diabetes: A Fresh Look at the Evidence." *Lipids* 45, no. 10 (2010): 893–905. Available at http://www.ncbi.nlm.nih.gov/pubmed/20354806. Researchers reviewed the evidence from randomized controlled trials of lipid and non-lipid risk factors, prospective cohort studies of disease endpoints, and disease endpoints for cardiometabolic effects of saturated fatty acid consumption in humans. [Lecture 7]

Michalakis, K., D. G. Goulis, A. Vazaiou, G. Mintziori, A. Polymeris, and A. Abrahamian-Michalakis. "Obesity in the Ageing Man." *Metabolism: Clinical and Experimental* 62, no. 10 (2013): 1341–1349. The aim of this narrative review is to present and discuss the current evidence on the changes in body composition, energy balance, and endocrine environment that occur in the aging man. [Lecture 19]

Miller, M. A., and R. H. Rahe. "Life Changes Scaling for the 1990s." *Journal of Psychosomatic Research* 43, no. 3 (1997): 279–292. In this study, varying influences of gender, age, marital status, and education were explored in more detail. [Lecture 21]

Miller, Paige E., and Vanessa Perez. "Low-Calorie Sweeteners and Body Weight and Composition: A Meta-Analysis of Randomized Controlled Trials and Prospective Cohort Studies." *The American Journal of Clinical Nutrition* 100, no. 3 (2014): 765–777. Available at http://ajcn.nutrition.org/content/early/2014/06/18/ajcn.113.082826.full.pdf+html. The objective of this study was to systematically review and quantitatively evaluate randomized controlled trials and prospective cohort studies, separately, that examined the relation between low-calorie sweeteners and body weight and composition. [Lecture 20]

Misner, B. "Food Alone May Not Provide Sufficient Micronutrients for Preventing Deficiency." *Journal of the International Society of Sports Nutrition* 3, no. 1 (2006): 51–55. The American Dietetic Association has stated that the best nutritional strategy for promoting optimal health and reducing the risk of chronic disease is to wisely choose a wide variety of foods, but this paper aims to show that this is not the only way. [Lecture 10]

Mozaffarian, R. S., et al. "Identifying Whole Grain Foods: A Comparison of Different Approaches for Selecting More Healthful Whole Grain Products." *Public Health Nutrition* 16, no. 12 (2013): 2255–2264. This paper investigates how five recommended whole grain criteria relate to healthfulness and price of grain products. [Lecture 11]

Murphy, C. H., T. A. Churchward-Venne, C. J. Mitchell, N. M. Kolar, and A. Kassis, et al. "Hypoenergetic Diet-Induced Reductions in Myofibrillar Protein Synthesis Are Restored with Resistance Training and Balanced Daily Protein Ingestion in Older Men." *American Journal of Physiology, Endocrinology, and Metabolism* 308, no. 9 (2015): E734–743. This article is about the way dietary protein distribution affects muscle protein syntheis. [Lecture 9]

National Institutes of Health and National Heart, Lung, and Blood Institute. "Clinical Guidelines on the Identification, Evaluation, and Treatment of Overweight and Obesity in Adults." Obesity Education Initiative. Available at http://www.nhlbi.nih.gov/guidelines/obesity/ob_gdlns.pdf. These are guidelines from the National Institutes of Health and the National Heart, Lung, and Blood Institute on how to identify, evaluate, and treat obesity. [Lecture 1]

Nigg, C. R., B. Borrelli, J. Maddock, and R. K. Dishman. "A Theory of Physical Activity Maintenance." *Journal of Applied Psychology* 57 (2008): 544–560. This paper presents the physical activity maintenance theory, which incorporates individual psychosocial variables (goal setting, motivation, and self-efficacy) and contextual variables of the environment and life stress (triggers of relapse). [Lecture 21]

Ormsbee, M. J., A. W. Kinsey, W. R. Eddy, T. A. Madzima, P. J. Arciero, A. Figueroa, and L. B. Panton. "The Influence of Nighttime Feeding of Carbohydrate or Protein Combined with Exercise Training on Appetite and Cardiometabolic Risk in Young Obese Women." *Applied Physiology in Nutrition and Metabolism* 40 (2015): 37–45. This study examined the additive impact of nighttime feeding of whey, casein, or carbohydrate combined with exercise training on appetite, cardiometabolic health, and strength in obese women. [Lecture 9, Lecture 13]

Ormsbee, Michael J., et al. "Fat Metabolism and Acute Resistance Exercise in Trained Men." *Journal of Applied Physiology* 102, no. 5 (2007): 1767–1772. The purpose of this study was to investigate the effect of acute resistance exercise on lipolysis within adipose tissue and subsequent substrate oxidation to better understand how resistance exercise might contribute to improvements in body composition. [Lecture 18]

Ormsbee, Michael J., et al. "Regulation of Fat Metabolism during Resistance Exercise in Sedentary Lean and Obese Men." *Journal of Applied Physiology* 106, no. 5 (2009): 1529–1537. The effect of acute resistance exercise on whole-body energy expenditure and α_2-adrenergic receptor regulation of lipolysis in subcutaneous abdominal adipose tissue was determined in sedentary lean and obese men. [Lecture 18]

Ormsbee, Michael J., et al. "The Effects of Six Weeks of Supplementation with Multi-Ingredient Performance Supplements and Resistance Training on Anabolic Hormones, Body Composition, Strength, and Power in Resistance-Trained Men." *Journal of International Society of Sports Nutrition* 9, no. 1 (2012): 49. The purpose of this study was to investigate the impact of specific pre- and post-workout multi-ingredient performance supplements on anabolic hormones, body composition, muscle strength, and power in resistance-trained men participating in a periodized resistance training program. [Lecture 14, Lecture 18]

Pagoto, Sherry L., and Bradley M. Appelhans. "A Call for an End to the Diet Debates." *The Journal of the American Medical Association* 310 (2013): 687–688. Available at http://jama.jamanetwork.com/article.aspx?articleid=1730520. The results of this study showed that adherence is the key to any dietary intervention. [Lecture 23, Lecture 24]

Paoli, et al. "High-Intensity Interval Resistance Training (HIRT) Influences Resting Energy Expenditure and Respiratory Ratio in Non-Dieting Individuals." *Journal of Translational Medicine* 10 (2012): 237. The authors tested the acute effects of high-intensity interval resistance training versus traditional resistance training on resting energy expenditure and respiratory ratio at 22 hours after exercise. [Lecture 17]

Park, S. K., et al. "The Effect of Combined Aerobic and Resistance Exercise Training on Abdominal Fat in Obese Middle-Aged Women." *Journal of Physiological Anthropology and Applied Human Science* 22, no. 3 (2003): 129–135. This study investigated the effect of both aerobic and resistance exercise on fat loss. [Lecture 1]

Pasiakos, S. M., J. J. Cao, L. M. Margolis, E. R. Sauter, and L. D. Whigham, et al. "Effects of High-Protein Diets on Fat-Free Mass and Muscle Protein Synthesis Following Weight Loss: A Randomized Controlled Trial."

Federation of American Societies for Experimental Biology 27 (2013): 3837–3847. This study measured the effects of high-protein diets on muscle mass after weight loss. [Lecture 1, Lecture 9]

Paul, G. L. "The Rationale for Consuming Protein Blends in Sports Nutrition." *Journal of the American College of Nutrition* 28, no. 4 (2009): 464S–472S. This review focuses on the potential nutritional advantages of combining whey protein, casein, and isolated soy protein. [Lecture 13]

Pelley, Janet. "Plasticizer May Make Boys Less Masculine." *Environmental Science and Technology*. November 12, 2008. This study measured the environmental impact on hormones that influence body composition. [Lecture 20]

Pietiläinen, K. H., S. E. Saarni, J. Kaprio, and A. Rissanen. "Does Dieting Make You Fat? A Twin Study." *International Journal of Obesity* 36, no. 3 (2012): 456–464. The objective of this study is to investigate whether the paradoxical weight gain associated with dieting is better related to genetic propensity to weight gain than to the weight-loss episodes themselves. [Lecture 19, Lecture 22]

Pope, Zachary K., Jeffrey M. Willardson, and Brad J. Schoenfeld. "Exercise and Blood Flow Restriction." *The Journal of Strength & Conditioning Research* 27, no. 10 (2013): 2914–2926. The purpose of this review was to discuss the relevant literature with regard to the type and magnitude of acute responses and chronic adaptations associated with blood flow restriction exercise protocols versus traditional non–blood flow restriction exercise protocols. [Lecture 18]

Prabhakaran, B., et al. "Effect of 14 Weeks of Resistance Training on Lipid Profile and Body Fat Percentage in Premenopausal Women." *British Journal of Sports Medicine* 33, no. 3 (1999): 190–195. The objective of this study was on the effects of a supervised, intensive (85 percent of one-repetition maximum) 14-week resistance training program on lipid profile and body fat percentage in healthy, sedentary, premenopausal women. [Lecture 1]

Raalte, J., W. Brewer, B. Lewis, D. Linder, G. Wildman, and J. Kozimor. "Cork! The Effects of Positive and Negative Self-Talk on Dart Throwing Performance." *Journal of Sport Behavior* 18 (1995): 50–57. The effects of positive and negative self-talk on dart-throwing performance were studied. [Lecture 21]

Reinehr, T. "Obesity and Thyroid Function." *Molecular and Cellular Endocrinology* 316, no. 2 (2010): 165–171. This is a study on thyrotropin and obesity. [Lecture 19]

Ren, R., X. Jiang, X. Zhang, Q. Guan, C. Yu, Y. Li, L. Gao, H. Zhang, and J. Zhao. "Associations between Thyroid Hormones and Body Fat in Euthyroid Subjects." *Clinical Endocrinology* 80, no. 4 (2014): 585–590. The aim of this study was to explore the association between thyroid hormones and body fat in a euthyriod population. [Lecture 19]

Renaud, H. J., J. Y. Cui, H. Lu, and C. D. Klaassen. "Effect of Diet on Expression of Genes Involved in Lipid Metabolism, Oxidative Stress, and Inflammation in Mouse Liver: Insights into Mechanisms of Hepatic Steatosis." *PloS one* 9, no. 2 (2014): e88584. This study examined the molecular changes elicited by nine diets with varying fat, sugar, cholesterol, omega-3 fatty acids, omega-6 fatty acids, and calories in C57BL/6 male mice. [Lecture 4]

Res, P. T., B. Groen, and B. Pennings, et al. "Protein Ingestion before Sleep Improves Postexercise Overnight Recovery." *Medicine & Science in Sports & Exercise* 44, no. 8 (2012): 1560–1569. This paper assessed the effect of protein ingestion immediately before sleep on digestion and absorption kinetics and protein metabolism during overnight recovery from a single bout of resistance-type exercise. [Lecture 13]

Riera-Crichton, D., and N. Tefft. "Macronutrients and Obesity: Revisiting the Calories In, Calories Out Framework." *Economics and Human Biology* 14 (2014): 33–49. Available at http://www.ncbi.nlm.nih.gov/pubmed/?term=Mac ronutrients+and+obesity%3A+Revisiting+the+calories+in%2C+calories+out +framework. The authors conducted dynamic time series and structural vector autoregressions analyses of U.S. data between 1974 and 2006 and a panel analysis of 164 countries between 2001 and 2010. [Lecture 1, Lecture 11]

Roberts, Justin D., et al. "The Effect of a Decaffeinated Green Tea Extract Formula on Fat Oxidation, Body Composition and Exercise Performance." *Journal of the International Society of Sports Nutrition* 12 (2015): 1–9. The aim of this study was to determine whether a decaffeinated green tea extract positively influenced fat oxidation, body composition, and exercise performance in recreationally active participants. [Lecture 14]

Roef, G., B. Lapauw, S. Goemaere, H. G. Zmierczak, K. Toye, and J. M. Kaufman. "Body Composition and Metabolic Parameters Are Associated with Variation in Thyroid Hormone Levels among Euthyroid Young Men." *European Journal of Endocrinology* 167, no. 5 (2012): 719–726. The authors investigated the relationship between thyroid hormone concentrations and body composition with metabolic parameters in a population of healthy euthyroid men. [Lecture 19]

Rognmo, Øivind, et al. "Cardiovascular Risk of High- versus Moderate-Intensity Aerobic Exercise in Coronary Heart Disease Patients." *Circulation* 126, no 12 (2012): 1436–1440. Available at http://www.ncbi.nlm.nih.gov/pubmed/22879367. The authors examined the risk of cardiovascular events during organized high-intensity interval exercise training and moderate-intensity training among 4,846 patients with coronary heart disease in three Norwegian cardiac rehabilitation centers. [Lecture 17]

Romon, M., C. Boulenguez, and P. Frimat. "Circadian Variation of Diet-Induced Thermogenesis." *American Journal of Clinical Nutrition* 57, no. 4 (1993): 476–480. The objective of this study was to assess a circadian variation of diet-induced thermogenesis that could favor weight gain among night workers used to eating a nighttime snack. [Lecture 13]

Santalla, A., C. P. Earnest, J. A. Marroyo, and A. Lucia. "The Tour de France: An Updated Physiological Review." *International Journal of Sports Physiology and Performance* 7 (2012): 200–209. The purpose of this brief review is to summarize what is currently known of the physiological demands of the Tour de France as well as of the main physiological profile of Tour de France competitors. [Lecture 12]

Schoenfeld, Brad Jon, Alan Albert Aragon, and James W. Krieger. "The Effect of Protein Timing on Muscle Strength and Hypertrophy: A Meta-Analysis." *Journal of International Society of Sports Nutrition* 10 (2013): 1–13. The purpose of this paper was to conduct a multilevel meta-regression of randomized controlled trials to determine whether protein timing is a viable strategy for enhancing postexercise muscular adaptations. [Lecture 12]

Schoenfeld, Brad J., et al. "Influence of Resistance Training Frequency on Muscular Adaptations in Well-Trained Men." *Journal of Strength and Conditioning Research* 29, no. 7 (2015): 1821–1829. The purpose of this study was to investigate the effects of training muscle groups one day per week using a split-body routine versus three days per week using a total-body routine on muscular adaptations in well-trained men. [Lecture 18]

Schroeder, E. Todd, et al. "Are Acute Post-Resistance Exercise Increases in Testosterone, Growth Hormone, and IGF-1 Necessary to Stimulate Skeletal Muscle Anabolism and Hypertrophy?" *Medicine & Science in Sports & Exercise* 45, no. 11 (2013): 2044–2051. This paper aims to support that post–resistance exercise increases in certain hormones are "optimal" for maximizing skeletal muscle anabolism and hypertrophy. [Lecture 18]

Schuler, Lou. "Protein: The Manual for Men." *Men's Health.* August 2015. Available at http://www.menshealth.com/meat. This is a guide on meat and health for men. [Lecture 18]

Schutz, Y., U. U. Kyle, and C. Pichard. "Fat-Free Mass Index and Fat Mass Index Percentiles in Caucasians Aged 18–98 Years." *International Journal of Obesity and Related Metabolic Disorders* 26, no. 7 (2002): 953–60. The purpose of this study was to determine reference values for fat-free mass index and fat mass index in a large Caucasian group of apparently healthy subjects, as a function of age and gender and to develop percentile distribution for these two parameters. [Lecture 2]

Simopoulos, A. P. "The Importance of the Ratio of Omega-6/Omega-3 Essential Fatty Acids." *Biomedical and Pharmaceutical* 56, no. 8 (2002):

365–379. Available at http://www.ncbi.nlm.nih.gov/pubmed/12442909. This study analyzed fish oil components and why they are important. [Lecture 7]

Skinner, Tina L., et al. "Factors Influencing Serum Caffeine Concentrations Following Caffeine Ingestion." *Journal of Science and Medicine in Sport* 17, no. 5 (2014): 516–520. The purpose of this paper is to determine whether differences in training status, body composition, and/or habitual caffeine intake influenced serum caffeine concentrations following caffeine ingestion. [Lecture 14]

Skinner, Tina L., et al. "Influence of Carbohydrate on Serum Caffeine Concentrations Following Caffeine Ingestion." *Journal of Science and Medicine in Sport* 16, no. 4 (2013): 343–347. The purpose of this paper is to examine the effect of a high-carbohydrate meal on serum caffeine concentration following caffeine intake. [Lecture 14]

Snijders, T., J. S. Smeets, S. van Vliet, J. van Kranenburg, and K. Maase, et al. "Protein Ingestion before Sleep Increases Muscle Mass and Strength Gains during Prolonged Resistance-Type Exercise Training in Healthy Young Men." *The Journal of Nutrition* (2015). This paper assessed the impact of dietary protein supplementation before sleep on muscle mass and strength gains during resistance-type exercise training. [Lecture 13]

Spear, B. A. "Does Dieting Increase the Risk for Obesity and Eating Disorders?" *Journal of the American Dietetic Association* 106, no. 4 (2006): 523–525. This study examines how dieting might contribute to disordered eating. [Lecture 19]

Stetson, B., A. O. Beacham, S. J. Frommelt, K. N. Boutelle, J. D. Cole, C. H. Ziegler, and S. W. Looney. "Exercise Slips in High-Risk Situations and Activity Patterns in Long-Term Exercisers: An Application of the Relapse Prevention Model." *Annals of Behavioral Medicine* 30, no. 1 (2005): 25–35. The purpose of this study was to examine the relationships among characteristics of exercise high-risk situations, components of the relapse prevention model relevant to exercise slips, and follow-up exercise outcomes in long-term community exercisers. [Lecture 21]

Stunkard, A., R. Berkowitz, T. Wadden, C. Tanrikut, E. Reiss, and L. Young. "Binge Eating Disorder and the Night-Eating Syndrome." *International Journal of Obesity and Related Metabolic Disorders* 20, no. 1 (1996): 1–6. The purpose of this study was to determine in three samples of obese women the prevalence of two eating disorders: binge eating disorder and the night-eating syndrome. [Lecture 13]

Sumithran, P., et al. "Long-Term Persistence of Hormonal Adaptations to Weight Loss." *New England Journal of Medicine* 365, no. 17 (2011): 1597–1604. This paper attempts to figure out the reasons behind the high rate of weight regain after diet-induced weight loss. [Lecture 22]

Symons, T. B., S. E. Schutzler, T. L. Cocke, D. L. Chinkes, R. R. Wolfe, and D. Paddon-Jones. "Aging Does Not Impair the Anabolic Response to a Protein-Rich Meal." *American Journal of Clinical Nutrition* 86, no. 2 (2007): 451–456. Available at http://www.ncbi.nlm.nih.gov/pubmed/17684218. This paper aims to characterize changes in plasma amino acid concentrations and to quantify muscle protein synthesis in healthy young people and elderly people after ingestion of a 113-gram (4-ounce) serving of lean beef. [Lecture 9]

Tang, J. E., D. R. Moore, G. W. Kujbida, M. A. Tarnopolsky, and S. M. Phillips. "Ingestion of Whey Hydrolysate, Casein, or Soy Protein Isolate: Effects on Mixed Muscle Protein Synthesis at Rest and Following Resistance Exercise in Young Men." *Journal of Applied Physiology* 107, no. 3 (2009): 987–992. This study was designed to compare the acute response of mixed muscle protein synthesis to rapidly and slowly digested proteins both at rest and after resistance exercise. [Lecture 9]

Tarnopolsky, M. A., et al. "Evaluation of Protein Requirements for Trained Strength Athletes." *Journal of Applied Physiology* 73, no. 5 (1992): 1986–1995. Leucine kinetic and nitrogen balance methods were used to determine the dietary protein requirements of strength athletes compared with sedentary subjects. [Lecture 8]

Thomas, D. M., et al. "Can a Weight Loss of One Pound a Week Be Achieved with a 3500-Kcal Deficit? Commentary on a Commonly Accepted Rule."

International Journal of Obesity (London) 37, no. 12 (2013): 1611–1613. In this paper, the authors demonstrate the risk of applying the 3,500-kilocalorie rule even as a convenient estimate by comparing predicted against actual weight loss in seven weight-loss experiments conducted in confinement under total supervision or objectively measured energy intake. [Lecture 14]

Thorpe, L. E., et al. "Prevalence and Control of Diabetes and Impaired Fasting Glucose in New York City." *Diabetes Care* 32, no. 1 (2009): 57–62. The purpose of the study was to determine the prevalence of diabetes and impaired fasting glucose and to assess clinical management indicators among adults with diabetes in a representative sample of New York City adults. [Lecture 1]

Thunders, M., S. Mangai, and R. Cooper. "Nutrigenetics, Nutrigenomics, and the Future of Dietary Advice." *Food and Nutrition Sciences* 4, no. 10 (2013): 999–1003. We might need a simpler approach to health care, one that embraces genetic variation yet focuses on the optimum nutritional benefit of dietary components. [Lecture 4]

Tieland, M., K. J. Borgonjen-Van den Berg, L. J. C. van Loon, and L. C. P. G. M. de Groot. "Dietary Protein Intake in Community-Dwelling, Frail, and Institutionalized Elderly People: Scope for Improvement." *European Journal of Nutrition* 51, no. 2 (2012): 173–179. This paper assessed the dietary protein intake, distribution of protein intake throughout the day, and use of protein-containing food sources in community-dwelling, frail, and institutionalized elderly people in the Netherlands. [Lecture 9]

Timmerman, Gayle M., and Adama Brown. "The Effect of a Mindful Restaurant Eating Intervention on Weight Management in Women." *Journal of Nutrition Education and Behavior* 44, no. 1 (2012): 22–28. Available at http://www.jneb.org/article/S1499-4046%2811%2900264-8/abstract. The purpose of this study was to evaluate the effect of a mindful restaurant eating intervention on weight management. [Lecture 24]

Trapp, E. G., D. J. Chisholm, J. Freund, and S. H. Boutcher. "The Effects of High-Intensity Intermittent Training on Fat Loss and Fasting Insulin Levels of

Young Women." *International Journal of Obesity* 32, no. 4 (2008): 684–691. The purpose of this study was to determine the effects of a 15-week high-intensity intermittent exercise program on subcutaneous and trunk fat and insulin resistance of young women. [Lecture 16]

Van Cauter, E., D. Désir, C. Decoster, F. Féry, and E. O. Balasse. "Nocturnal Decrease in Glucose Tolerance during Constant Glucose Infusion." *Journal of Clinical Endocrinology and Metabolism* 69, no. 3 (1989): 604–611. Studies comparing glucose tolerance in the morning versus tolerance in the evening have suggested that the time of day might influence glucose regulation. [Lecture 13]

Veldhuis, J. D. "Changes in Pituitary Function with Ageing and Implications for Patient Care." *Nature Reviews Endocrinology* 9, no. 4 (2013): 205–215. The aim of this article is to critically discuss the mechanisms mediating clinical facets of changes in the hypothalamic-pituitary axis during aging and the extent to which confounding factors operate to obscure aging-related effects. [Lecture 19]

Volek, J. S., et al. "Low-Carbohydrate Diets Promote a More Favorable Body Composition Than Low-Fat Diets." *Strength & Conditioning Journal* 32, no. 1 (2010): 42–47. A low-carbohydrate diet with periodized resistance training promotes greater fat loss while preserving lean body mass and promotes improvements to metabolic health. [Lecture 23]

Wall, Benjamin T., et al. "Chronic Oral Ingestion of L–Carnitine and Carbohydrate Increases Muscle Carnitine Content and Alters Muscle Fuel Metabolism during Exercise in Humans." *The Journal of Physiology* 589, no. 4 (2011): 963–973. The authors determined the effects of chronic l-carnitine and carbohydrate ingestion on muscle total carnitine content and exercise metabolism and performance in humans. [Lecture 14]

Waller, S. M., J. S. Vander Wal, and D. M. Klurfeld, et al. "Evening Ready-to-Eat Cereal Consumption Contributes to Weight Management." *Journal of the American College of Nutrition* 23, no. 4 (2004): 316–321. This study tested the hypothesis that providing a structured snack in the form of a "ready-to-eat" breakfast cereal would help regulate excess energy intake and contribute to weight loss in night snackers. [Lecture 13]

Weigle, D. S. "Appetite Regulation of Body Composition." *Federation of American Societies for Experimental Biology* 8, no. 3 (1994): 302–310. The implications of this adipose tissue–related satiety factor for the pathogenesis of obesity and the possible nature of the factor are discussed within this paper. [Lecture 22]

Werle, C. O. C., B. Wansink, and C. Payne. "Is It Fun or Exercise? The Framing of Physical Activity Biases Subsequent Snacking." *Marking Letters* (2014): 1–12. This paper offers the simple advice to consumers to make certain that they make their physical activity routine fun in order to avoid compensation. [Lecture 22]

Willis, L. H., C. A. Slentz, L. A. Bateman, A. T. Shields, and L. W. Piner, et al. "Effects of Aerobic and/or Resistance Training on Body Mass and Fat Mass in Overweight or Obese Individuals." *Journal of Applied Physiology* 113, no. 12 (2012): 1831–1837. Available at http://www.ncbi.nlm.nih.gov/pubmed/23019316. Researchers compared the effects of similar amounts of aerobic and resistance training on body mass and fat mass in overweight adults. [Lecture 17]

Wilmore, J. H., E. R. Buskirk, EM. DiGirolamo, and T. G. Lohman. "Body Composition: A Round Table." *The Physician and Sports Medicine* 14, no. 3 (1986): 144–162. Four experts assess body fat levels. [Lecture 2]

Wilson, Jacob M., et al. "The Effects of 12 Weeks of Beta-Hydroxy-Beta-Methylbutyrate Free Acid Supplementation on Muscle Mass, Strength, and Power in Resistance-Trained Individuals: A Randomized, Double-Blind, Placebo-Controlled Study." *European Journal of Applied Physiology* 114, no. 6 (2014): 1217–1227. This paper investigated the effects of 12 weeks of beta-hydroxy-beta-methylbutyrate supplementation on skeletal muscle hypertrophy, body composition, strength, and power in trained individuals. [Lecture 14]

Wroblewski, Andrew P., et al. "Chronic Exercise Preserves Lean Muscle Mass in Masters Athletes." *Physician and Sportsmedicine* 39, no. 3 (2011): 172–178. This study evaluated whether high levels of chronic exercise prevents the loss of lean muscle mass and strength experienced in sedentary aging adults. [Lecture 18]

Yang, Quanhe, et al. "Added Sugar Intake and Cardiovascular Diseases Mortality among U.S. Adults." *JAMA Internal Medicine* 174, no. 4 (2014): 516–524. The authors observed a significant relationship between added sugar consumption and increased risk for cardiovascular disease mortality. [Lecture 6]

Yang, Y., L. Breen, N. A. Burd, A. J. Hector, and T. A. Churchward-Venne, et al. "Resistance Exercise Enhances Myofibrillar Protein Synthesis with Graded Intakes of Whey Protein in Older Men." *British Journal of Nutrition* 108, no. 10 (2012): 1780–1788. This study aimed to determine the dose response of myofibrillar protein synthesis with the ingestion of isolated whey protein, with and without prior resistance exercise, in the elderly. [Lecture 9]

Image Credits

NOTES